D1621535

DEALING WITH **HEADACHES**

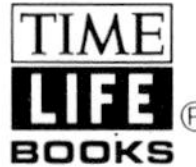

Other Publications:

PLANET EARTH
COLLECTOR'S LIBRARY OF THE CIVIL WAR
CLASSICS OF THE OLD WEST
THE EPIC OF FLIGHT
THE GOOD COOK
THE SEAFARERS
THE ENYCLOPEDIA OF COLLECTIBLES
THE GREAT CITIES
WORLD WAR II
HOME REPAIR AND IMPROVEMENT
THE WORLD'S WILD PLACES
THE TIME-LIFE LIBRARY OF BOATING
HUMAN BEHAVIOR
THE ART OF SEWING
THE OLD WEST
THE EMERGENCE OF MAN
THE AMERICAN WILDERNESS
THE TIME-LIFE ENCYCLOPEDIA OF GARDENING
LIFE LIBRARY OF PHOTOGRAPHY
THIS FABULOUS CENTURY
FOODS OF THE WORLD
TIME-LIFE LIBRARY OF AMERICA
TIME-LIFE LIBRARY OF ART
GREAT AGES OF MAN
LIFE SCIENCE LIBRARY
THE LIFE HISTORY OF THE UNITED STATES
TIME READING PROGRAM
LIFE NATURE LIBRARY
LIFE WORLD LIBRARY

FAMILY LIBRARY:
HOW THINGS WORK IN YOUR HOME
THE TIME-LIFE BOOK OF THE FAMILY CAR
THE TIME-LIFE FAMILY LEGAL GUIDE
THE TIME-LIFE BOOK OF FAMILY FINANCE

This volume is one of a series designed to familiarize readers with the latest advances in medical science as a guide in maintaining their own health and fitness.

DEALING WITH HEADACHES

by Wendy Murphy

AND THE EDITORS OF TIME-LIFE BOOKS

LIBRARY OF HEALTH / TIME-LIFE BOOKS / ALEXANDRIA, VIRGINIA

THE AUTHOR:
Wendy Murphy brings to this work nearly 25 years' experience as a writer and editor in fields as diverse as paleontology and boating, antiques and home repair. Her previous books include *Coping with the Common Cold* in the Library of Health and two volumes of the TIME-LIFE Encyclopedia of Gardening: *Japanese Gardening* and *Indoor Gardening Under Light*.

THE CONSULTANTS:
Dr. Alan M. Rapoport, a neurologist, is Co-Director of The New England Center for Headache, in Cos Cob, Connecticut, a clinic specializing in the diagnosis and treatment of headaches and facial pain. Dr. Rapoport serves as Assistant Clinical Professor of Neurology at Yale University School of Medicine and at New York Medical College, and has written extensively on neurological disorders.

Dr. Fred D. Sheftell, a psychiatrist, is Co-Director of The New England Center for Headache and is Clinical Assistant Professor in the Department of Psychiatry at New York Medical College.

For information about any Time-Life book, please write:
Reader Information, Time-Life Books,
541 North Fairbanks Court, Chicago, Illinois 60611.

First printing. Printed in U.S.A.
Published simultaneously in Canada.
School and library distribution by Silver Burdett Company, Morristown, New Jersey.

TIME-LIFE is a trademark of Time Incorporated U.S.A.

Library of Congress Cataloguing in Publication Data
Murphy, Wendy B., 1935-
Dealing With Headaches
(Library of Health)
Bibliography p.
Includes index.
1. Headache. 2. Headache—Prevention.
I. Time-Life Books. II. Title. III. Series.
RC392.M9 616.8'49 81-21205
ISBN 0-8094-3796-1 AACR2
ISBN 0-8094-3795-3 (lib. bdg.)
ISBN 0-8094-3794-5 (retail ed.)

CONTENTS

CHAPTER 1

"What a head have I!"

Warning: a body out of balance
From a hole in the head to an aspirin pill
Tracking the causes to nerves and arteries
The headaches of everyday life
Aches that can kill
Real pains that are only in the mind

"Lord, how my head aches! what a head have I! It beats as it would fall in twenty pieces."

The anguished words are spoken by the nurse in Shakespeare's *Romeo and Juliet,* and her plaint and painful symptoms are familiar to almost everyone. She is experiencing a headache brought on by stress. Having just returned from a difficult diplomatic mission for her love-stricken mistress, Nurse feels physically and emotionally exhausted. Her head is, in effect, telling her to slow down, relax, remove herself from the fray for a couple of hours. If she heeds these instructions, the painful pulses of blood in her forehead will shortly subside, the taut muscles in her neck will return to their normal, more supple tone, and the splitting headache will end almost as quickly as it began.

Fortunately, headaches usually take this course. Despite their pain, sometimes of frightening and debilitating intensity, and despite their chronic occurrence in some people, most headaches are what physicians call benign—that is, they do not in themselves threaten the survival of the sufferer. Only a small minority—no more than 5 per cent—arise from serious injury or disease, such as brain tumor, cerebral hemorrhage, meningitis, stroke, the aftermath of an internal head injury, or some other life-threatening condition. The other 95 per cent constitute what one pioneer student of headaches, Dr. Harold G. Wolff of New York Hospital, described as biologic reprimands.

These reprimands can strike persons of all ages, and they vary widely in the severity of their pain and in its duration, location and frequency. But they share a similar purpose: They inform the sufferer that something in the body is off balance, forcing the system to make unconscious adjustments in an attempt to regain its equilibrium. These subtle adjustments consist principally of tightened muscles and expanded blood vessels in the head and neck; in turn, the muscles and vessels press upon, or otherwise irritate, various neighboring tissues to produce the painful sensations known collectively as headache.

The events, or triggers, that can throw an individual's system off balance are legion and often unpredictable. They tend to be highly peculiar to the individual—one man's meat may literally be another man's poison when it comes to initiating headaches. An ordinary frankfurter, for example, is a potent headache trigger for some people; others—the vast majority—can eat as many hot dogs as they please, up to the point of indigestion. To make matters even trickier, a factor that triggers a headache in an individual on one day will not necessarily bring one on the following week, because some secondary contributing factor—in effect, one component of a combination of triggers—is absent.

Some triggers are signs of excess—too much physical exertion, too much alcohol, too much of some chemical constituent in food that is eaten or air that is breathed, even too much squinting because of a glaring light or too much slouching because of a badly designed chair. But a trigger may just as well be a form of insufficiency: hunger, thin air at high altitudes or abnormally low barometric pressure. Even

The agony of a headache is imaginatively depicted in this 19th Century colored etching by English artist George Cruikshank. As the sufferer limply clutches a medicine bottle, grotesque demons—contemporary symbols of pain—threaten him with a hot poker, drill holes in his head, hammer in a wedge and assail him with trumpet blasts and raucous singing.

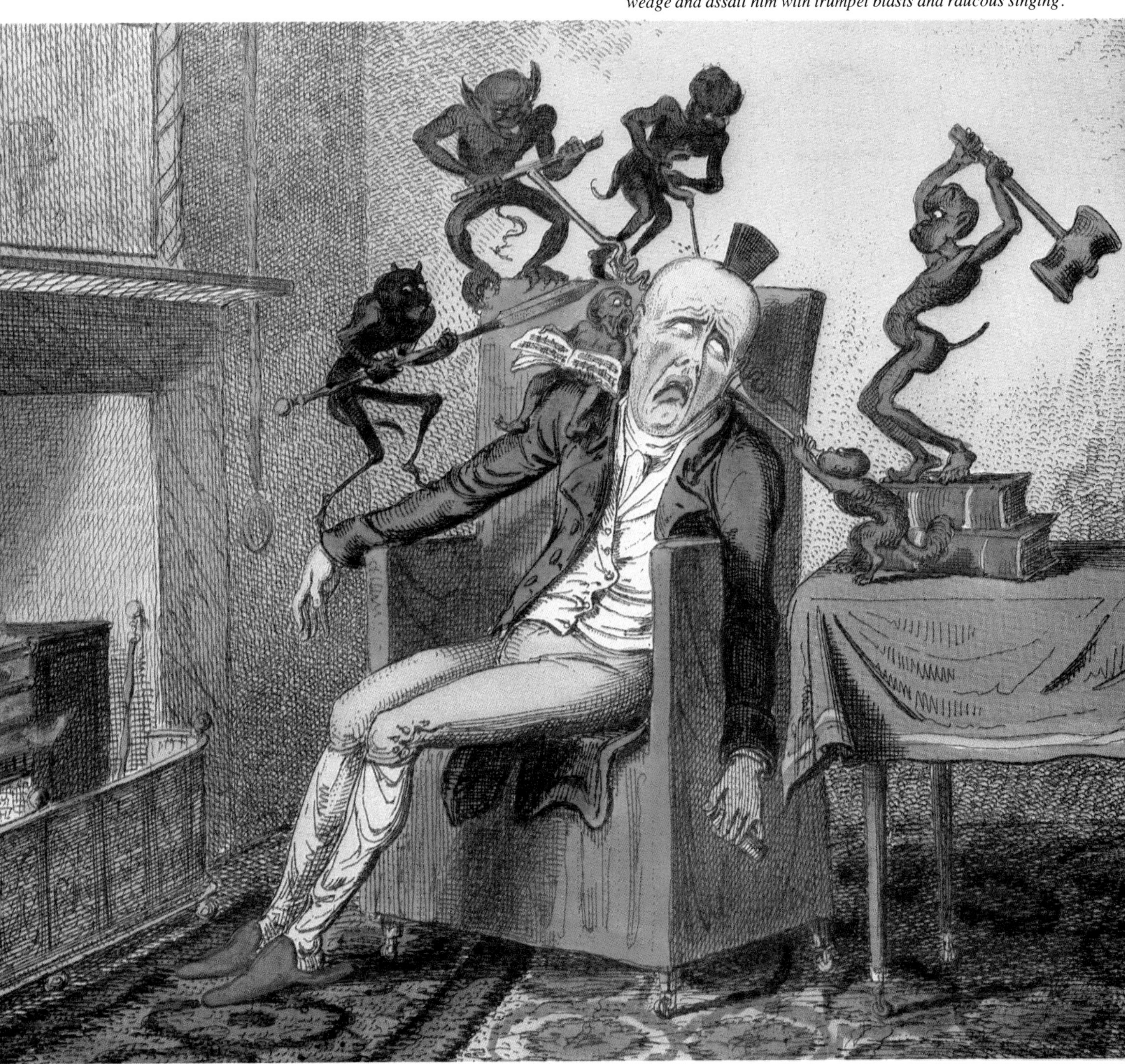

the seemingly healthful step of cutting down on certain excesses can act as a trigger—in some individuals, a return to normal after too much coffee or too many painkilling pills has been shown to be a cause of headaches. Finally, some triggers are primarily psychological—mild depression, anxiety, repressed anger and frustration. By comparison, the illness caused by a single and fully identified type of bacterium or virus is a simple affair.

Warning: a body out of balance

Despite the bewildering diversity of their causes, however, headaches are in one way simple. All of them, as Dr. Wolff suggested, are an effective way of delivering a message. Whatever their causes and symptoms, all headaches are telling the sufferer, very simply, "Your body is out of balance."

For a fortunate minority, such biological signals are mercifully rare: Perhaps as much as 10 per cent of all people never have a headache. These individuals either have constitutions extraordinarily capable of coping with the challenges that produce headaches in others, or they lead lives so moderate and tranquil that the challenges never arise. And most people who suffer headaches do so only occasionally, with minimal disruption of their customary routines. A couple of aspirin, taken at the first sign of trouble, will usually repress the ache.

A survey of headache victims conducted by the National Center for Health Statistics *(chart, opposite)* showed that these occasional sufferers dismissed their headaches as trivial impediments to everyday life—the vast majority of them reported that their headaches bothered them "just a little." Some of them actually enjoy an unexpected physical bonus along with the slight and infrequent pain. When the researchers compared this group with one that had no headaches at all, some surprising facts emerged. One had to do with vision. On the whole, headache sufferers had better vision than nonsufferers, for both near and distant objects. The reason for the difference is unknown—but whatever it is, the gain in visual acuity may well compensate those people, for whom headaches are in any case a matter of little concern.

There is, however, another segment of the population for whom headaches are a matter of central and urgent concern. Perhaps 20 per cent of the people in industrialized nations have headaches that are recurring or severe. Most of these victims are women, and most are stricken in the prime years, between puberty and menopause.

People who know head pain as a chronic condition live anxiously from one bout to the next, never sure when they may suffer the next sick headache, and suffering almost as much in anticipation as during the actual episode itself. They periodically miss days or even weeks of work, avoid social contacts, and become short-tempered or distant with their friends and family members. They may experience such associated symptoms as nausea, visual disturbances, hallucinations and an extreme sensitivity to noise, movement and other sensory stimuli.

Because their troubles are generally poorly understood by those who have never experienced severe or recurring head pain, chronic-headache victims are unjustly regarded by much of society as hypochondriacs and malingerers. And, almost incredibly, some of the victims share this cruel assessment. Investigators have found that chronic-headache sufferers, particularly men, often attempt to deny the experience of recurring, debilitating pain, as though it were a character defect, a sign of weakness.

Taking aspirin almost by the handful, experimenting with more powerful painkillers and with tranquilizers and alcohol in dangerous amounts, succumbing to periods of despair, the chronic sufferers can work themselves into medical problems at least as debilitating as the headache—without attaining much or any relief from the initial pain. Perhaps the only positive thing to be said for such chronic headaches is that their victims learn from long experience that their disorder will not kill them. But as one sufferer grimly commented, for someone deep in an attack, even that can appear "an ambiguous blessing."

People who suddenly and unexpectedly experience extremely severe, unremitting headache are in one important sense even more harshly afflicted. With no prior history of extraordinary head pain, they have no way of knowing what may lie in store for them. Most people struck down in this way immediately assume the worst—a brain tumor, perhaps, or some other equally catastrophic disease—because that kind of possibility, however remote, holds an insidious grip on the human imagination. Even if the pain goes away in a few hours or by the next day, its victim is left with a lingering sense of uneasiness.

Chronic-headache sufferers and those racked with sudden, severe headache pain probably constitute the largest group of patients in the family physician's waiting room. Too often, they are given drugs that mask symptoms and confuse diagnosis, and are told to stop worrying—"Learn to live with it, it's all in your head." No method of handling a chronic or extremely severe headache could be more ill-advised. There is every good reason for continued concern and investigation on the part of doctor and patient, not so much because the disorder may be life-threatening—it almost certainly is not—as because a revolution has taken place in the treatment of headaches.

Today's patient stands an excellent chance of getting substantial relief from the headaches that have taken possession of his life. Old drugs have been improved and new ones discovered; a host of techniques have been developed to stop a headache before it starts, by altering the physical and chemical patterns of muscles, nerves and blood vessels that bring a headache on. Most important, specialized headache clinics now deploy both the drugs and the techniques in complex programs of therapy geared to the specific needs of individual patients *(Chapter 6)*.

From a hole in the head to an aspirin pill

Most of the modern treatments for headache have antecedents reaching back before recorded history *(pages 22-31)*. Plant extracts containing salicylates, chemicals similar to aspirin, were apparently used to relieve pain in every human culture around the world, from Europe to pre-Columbian America to the Pacific Islands. Similarly universal were narcotic extracts of one kind or another, from poppies in the Old World to coca leaves in the New.

Even the skull surgery called trephination was successfully performed by surgeons of prehistoric times; fossil skulls

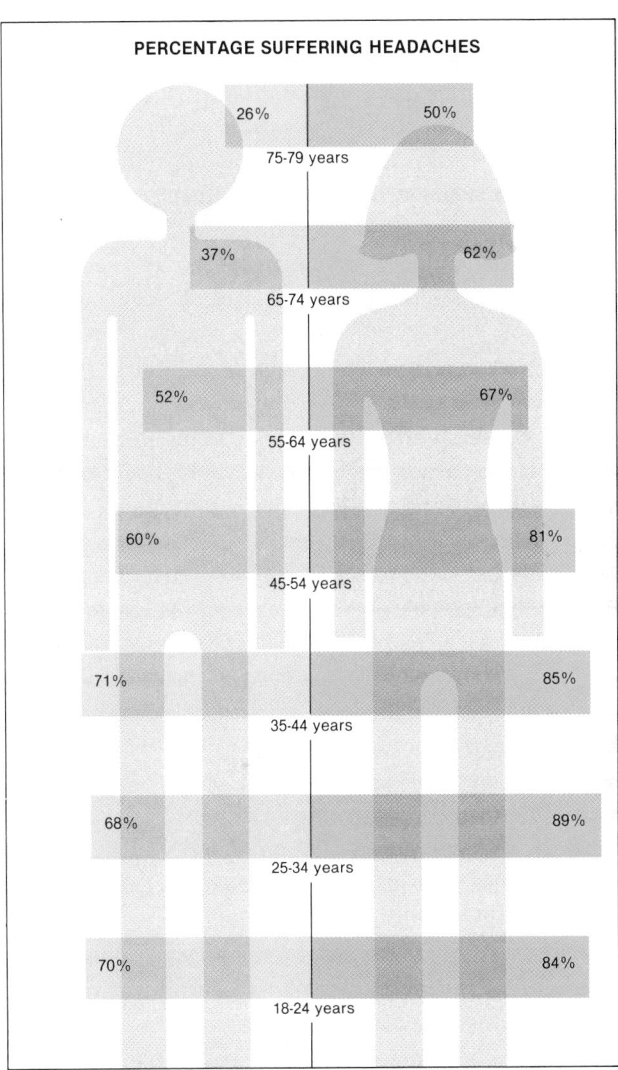

HEADACHES—A WOMAN'S COMPLAINT. *That women have more headaches than men do was confirmed by the National Center for Health Statistics, which surveyed the prevalence of headaches among American adults. The results (above) revealed that women suffered more at every age. More surprisingly, the survey indicated that headaches are most frequent in early to middle years and decrease sharply in later years.*

with the telltale marks of chopped and pierced bone are found almost everywhere. It must have been a fearsome operation then. With the patient's head held firmly in place, perhaps between the practitioner's knees, the medicine man set a sharp stone or flint chisel to the scalp, then drove the tool down with a mallet, cutting through flesh and bone to open a hole. Whatever narcotic was available was used as anesthesia for the operation. In the Andean highlands, for example, the Spanish conquistadors saw practitioners chew a mouthful of coca leaves, the source of the narcotic cocaine, then drip the juice of the leaves from their mouths onto the open wound to produce numbness.

This seemingly outrageous bone-cutting procedure, although dangerous and crudely executed, was and is a rational treatment in some cases: An opening in the skull serves to relieve the pressure of a brain tumor, skull fracture or blood clot, which can cause some of the worst of all headaches. But many early trephining operations must have been performed for headaches that trephination could not remedy: The practitioners possibly believed that the gap in the skull would provide an exit for evil spirits, which were generally blamed for all ailments.

The true causes of headaches are so difficult to divine that sufferers sometimes seek out any treatment, rational or not, that promises relief. Some of the fake remedies and quackery that abounded in the past have continued into modern times. The first court trial under the United States Pure Food and Drugs Act of 1906 was brought against one Robert N. Harper, the purveyor of a product with the wondrous name of Cuforhedake Brane-Fude. The principal ingredient of Harper's concoction was alcohol. Its painkiller was acetanilid, a chemical that can be very toxic. Yet Harper's Brane-Fude competed successfully with aspirin until government scientists established in court that it was not food for the brain and could be poisonous.

One reason good headache remedies were so slow in coming is the difficulty scientists encountered in studying the head—and particularly the mechanisms of its pain. Before the development of modern surgical techniques, the internal parts could be examined without risk to life only in cadavers, where they yielded few secrets as to their activity in health or sickness.

In the living body, headaches posed an additional frustration: They were invisible and could not be detected by established diagnostic methods. The kinds of symptoms that doctors had trained themselves to recognize and interpret—a telltale rash, a swelling, a rattling sound, an infectious organism—simply did not exist. Nor could the pain of a headache be accurately assessed by instruments comparable to a thermometer, stethoscope or blood-pressure gauge. Only the sufferer, notoriously subjective and imprecise in describing his symptoms, could tell the doctor where the pain was, how diffuse, how severe, and of what distinctive texture. No wonder a leading Australian headache specialist, Dr. James Lance, remarked ruefully that "the talents of the great detectives of fiction would not be lost in trying to unravel some of the complexities of headache."

Tracking the causes to nerves and arteries

The specialized study of headaches as a set of unique diseases really dates from 1940. Beginning in that year, Drs. Bronson S. Ray and Harold G. Wolff of New York Hospital reported a series of extraordinary experiments that revolutionized scientific understanding of head pain. The two men complemented each other perfectly in their researches. Dr. Ray, a professor at the Cornell University medical school, was a brilliant surgeon; Dr. Wolff, perhaps the greatest student of headaches in modern times, was director of Cornell's Department of Neurology.

The subjects of the experiment were patients who had come to the hospital for head operations. As the doctors described them, these patients were carefully chosen. They were "intelligent and cooperative, so that not only could pain be reported but its site and nature could be described"; they were "relatively free of apprehension and of preoccupation with pain"; and the "operative procedures were such that the patients were not too prostrate or inarticulate to describe their sensations." In practice, the last criterion meant that the operations were performed under local anesthetics, which did not blot out consciousness or prevent speech.

Outside the area of the anesthetic, with scalp, muscles and bone cut open or lifted away by Dr. Ray and his assistants, Dr. Wolff could study the effects of a wide variety of pain-producing stimuli: heat, irritating chemicals, electric shocks, and such mechanical stimuli as stroking, stretching and crushing. In one series of experiments, the researchers hooked fine silk threads at three points around the wall of an artery; when all three were pulled simultaneously, the artery was, in effect, mechanically distended—and pain was felt. Ultimately, the researchers probed virtually every accessible structure of the head. The subjects responded as sensations were experienced, giving the precise locations of pain (often elsewhere than at the point of stimulation) and telling as best they could what kind of pain they felt—dull or sharp, throbbing, burning, and so on.

By 1945 Drs. Ray and Wolff were able to identify the structures that are pain-sensitive and thus may be headache-related, both extracranial (between the skull and the scalp) and intracranial (within the skull). Externally, the skin of the scalp and its blood-supply network of arteries proved to be pain-sensitive; so were the underlying face, scalp and neck muscles. Skin pain was either pricking or burning, and sharply localized, with the pain sensed at the exact point of stimulation; muscular pain was more often described as aching, deeper and more diffuse. Internally, the tissues between the skull and the brain proper were pain-sensitive, along with several intracranial blood vessels, and each of these parts had a unique combination of sensations as its signature. Also involved, both externally and internally, were specific nerves. On the other hand, the bones of the skull and the soft tissue of the brain were completely insensitive to pain.

How the head is put together

From these elementary observations evolved a series of investigations into the intricate workings of every part of the pain mechanism and the interrelations of each part with

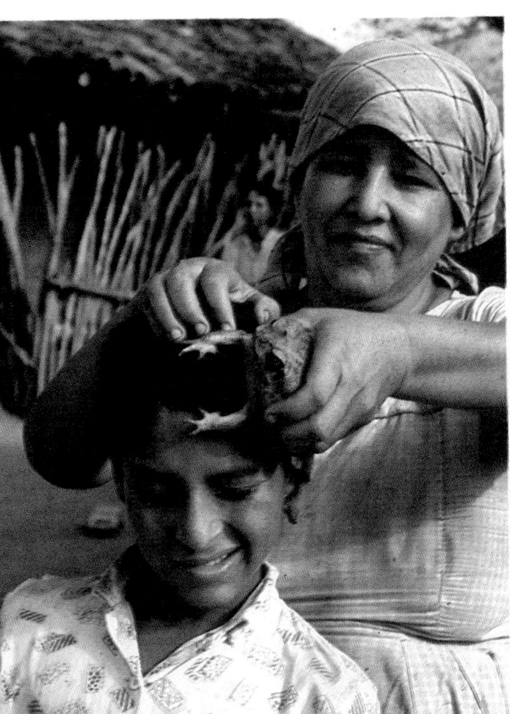

A Mexican woman rubs the head of a squirming young patient with a live toad to relieve his headache. According to one explanation, the toad is expected to absorb the pain—and the amphibian's cool body may indeed ease the ache temporarily.

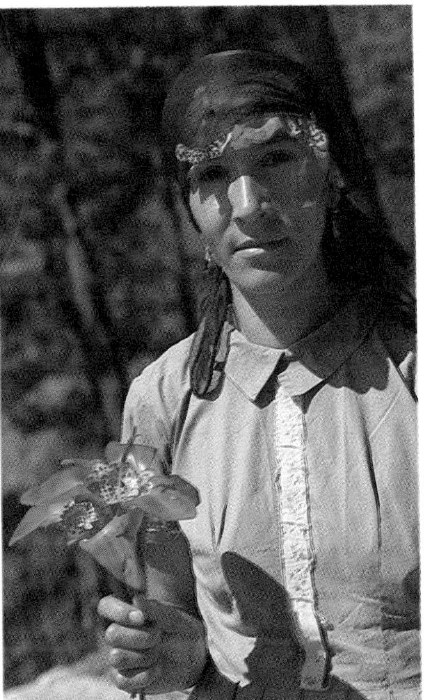

Tiger flowers bound to the forehead is the cure favored by a woman of the Sierra Madre, who holds two more of the flower remedies. Because the petals are cool and moist, they may soothe headache in the manner of a cold compress.

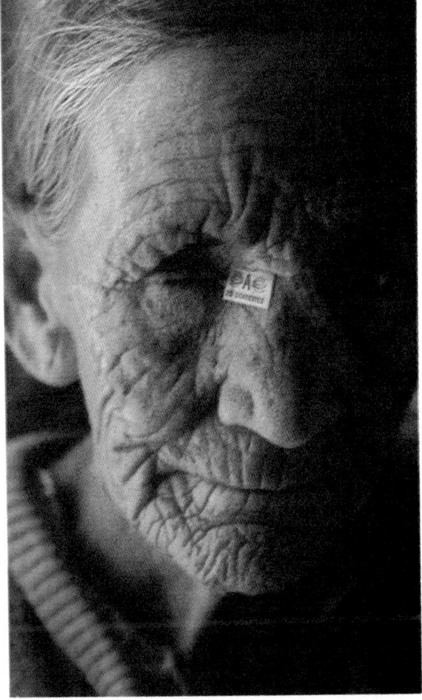

Tax stamps from cigarette packs, applied to the face, are this woman's headache cure. Tobacco's nicotine constricts some blood vessels, and perhaps because the stamps smell of tobacco, devotees credit them with power over vascular headaches.

all the others. But what the researchers discovered, and how their investigations—later greatly expanded—contributed to the understanding and treatment of headaches, form part of a picture that is larger than the study of pain alone. The larger picture, built up over centuries of study by anatomists and physiologists, includes the structure and function of all the myriad parts of the head. Within this picture, the discoveries of Drs. Ray and Wolff fit like the last piece of a jigsaw puzzle, linking head-pain stimuli and responses to the vulnerable parts of the scalp, the skull and the vital contents of the skull.

To begin with, two complex systems—the circulatory or vascular system, and the nervous system—coexist, overlap and impinge upon each other and upon virtually all the tissues in the narrow confines of the head. The circulatory system is, of course, the closed-circuit blood-pumping plant for the entire body. Centered in the heart, it carries fresh, oxygen-laden blood outward, under pressure from a large vessel called the aorta, through progressively smaller arterial conduits to supply all living tissue; at the same time, it returns oxygen-depleted blood to the heart through a similarly diffuse system of veins. Each of the blood vessels in the system is somewhat elastic, permitting minor but constant alterations in diameter and blood flow without the individual sensing any change at all. But, as is now known, changes that exceed the vessels' normal range of expansion and contraction can produce head pain.

The nervous system is the body's far-reaching internal communications network, responsible for collecting, interpreting, storing and responding to a broad range of stimuli that arise both outside and inside the body; nerves are also the receivers and transmitters of the sensation of pain. The head is where the major share of information processing is carried out, and it is also the site of the body's most highly developed sense organs. Consequently, the head is disproportionately rich in nerve tissue, and extremely sensitive to pain stimuli.

Interrelations between these all-pervasive blood vessels and nerves are almost unreckonably complex. They involve not only vessels and nerves alone, but specialized muscles, not under the voluntary control of the mind, that consist of smooth sheets or rings. It is these smooth muscles that cause the constriction and dilation of blood vessels, and thus, indirectly, the pain of a headache. What is more, the muscles themselves are controlled by specialized nerves called motor nerves, and a malfunction in these nerves also plays a part in the mosaic of head pain.

Where it hurts—and where it doesn't

Considerably simpler to examine and unravel are the head's structural parts, which are arranged in relatively tidy layers. Moving from the outside in, the first of these components is the skin of the face and scalp. This apparently simple covering actually consists of two distinct layers, the epidermis at the surface and the dermis directly beneath it. Averaging $^1/_{200}$ inch thick on the face, and slightly thicker at the top and back of the head, the epidermis is perforated by openings for sweat glands, hair shafts and sebaceous, or oil, glands, all of which arise from the underlying dermis. It is the dermis that furnishes the skin with its strength, its elasticity—and its capacity for vascular and nervous pain. This layer of the skin contains vast communities of nerve endings that receive and transmit notice of the stimuli and sensations—heat, cold, touch, pressure, pain—that may constitute threats to the body's security.

In the branches and internal connections of these nerves lie the starting points of a great variety of headache pains. The trigeminal nerve, for example, largest of all the cranial nerves, has sensory endings in the skin of the face. But it also has sensory endings in the delicate membranes that line the mouth, and motor endings in the chewing muscles—and almost all of this web of nerves is sensitive to pain. Finally, the pain-sensitive capillaries—tiny blood vessels—are richly distributed throughout the dermis, where they may respond dramatically to certain stimuli, as anyone given to blushing knows only too well.

Immediately below the skin lies the subcutaneous tissue, which insulates the interior organs, chiefly with a thin cushion of fat cells, and connects the skin to the next-deeper layer, the skeletal muscles. Here, again, both nerves and

	Muscle tension	Classic migraine	Common migraine	Cluster	Sinus	Eyestrain
PAIN						
severe		■	■	■		
dull	■				■	■
aching	■			■	■	■
throbbing		■	■			
nonthrobbing	■			■	■	■
pressure	■				■	
tightness	■					
tingling	■					
LOCATION						
one side		■	■	■		
both sides	■		■			
forehead	■	■	■		■	■
back of head	■	■	■			
top of head	■	■	■			
upper neck	■					
temple		■	■	■		■
cheek					■	
eye				■		

RECOGNIZING HEADACHE TYPES
Healthy heads may all feel alike, but each aching one hurts in its own way. In this table, the most common headache types are listed across the top; the location, intensity and kinds of pain each type displays is indicated below. These characteristics help identify a headache's cause—and may suggest a cure.

blood vessels can produce pain. A skeletal muscle is composed of long, slender, striated cells, or fibers. Each fiber is under the control of a motor nerve, which ends in a nerve-muscle junction at the surface of the muscle. Upon stimulation by a combination of chemical and electrical impulses carried by the nerve, individual muscle fibers thicken and shorten; collectively, the fibers tense the entire muscle to produce movement of skin or bone.

In the process of contracting, especially during prolonged or particularly strenuous activity—constant grimacing, jaw clenching, and the like—the thickened muscles press against neighboring blood vessels, reducing the flow of blood to the tissues of the head. The oxygen-starved tissues then release chemicals that act to stimulate sensations of pain. In addition, constant pulling of the muscles presses on adjacent nerves and results in pain.

Altogether the overlapping muscles of the head provide the individual with a highly expressive, often hard-working form of facial and body language. More than 30 delicate muscles are devoted to facial expression alone. Those in one subgroup, sometimes called "the muscles of attention," raise the eyebrows and eyelids, and widen the eyes in surprise. "Muscles of reflection" knit the brows together. Other teams mobilize the brows into patterns characteristic of distress and delight. Those called risorius, or "grin muscles," pull the corners of the mouth straight back toward the angle of the jawbone, and other muscles extend down from the cheeks to turn that grin into a smile. Still other muscles of expression curl the lip, wrinkle the nose, purse the lips and so on.

More massive are certain other muscles in the face: the masseter, or "chewer muscle," and the temporal, or "temple muscle," which work in coordination to operate the jawbones. They can be felt bunching up at the angles of the jaws and over the temples when the teeth are clenched. And the action of any of these muscles, if carried on for too long a period, can squeeze blood vessels and produce a headache—even a facial expression held for a long time can have that painful effect.

Directly within the skeletal muscles of the head is the skull, a collection of superbly engineered, irregularly shaped bones that protect the brain and neighboring sense organs, and give shape to the face and head. With the exception of the very mobile lower jaw, these bones, when mature, are immovable, held rigidly in place by jagged, interlocking joints. But numerous natural openings provide exits and en-

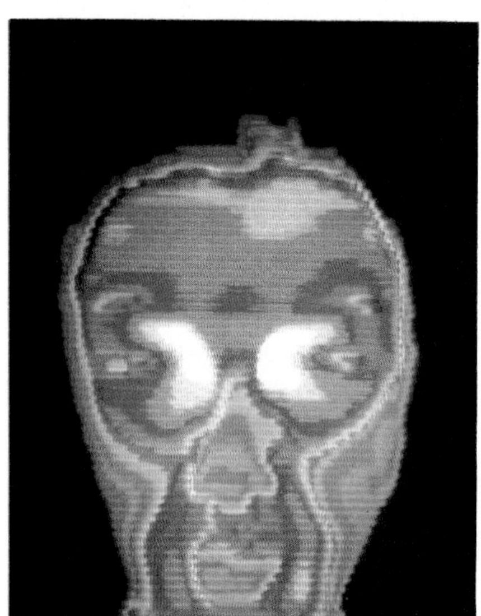

Thermograms, recording the heat of blood as colors (white is hottest, blue coolest, red intermediate), reveal how blood vessels affect headache. A muscle-tension headache (above) has a normal, even pattern, because blood vessels are not involved.

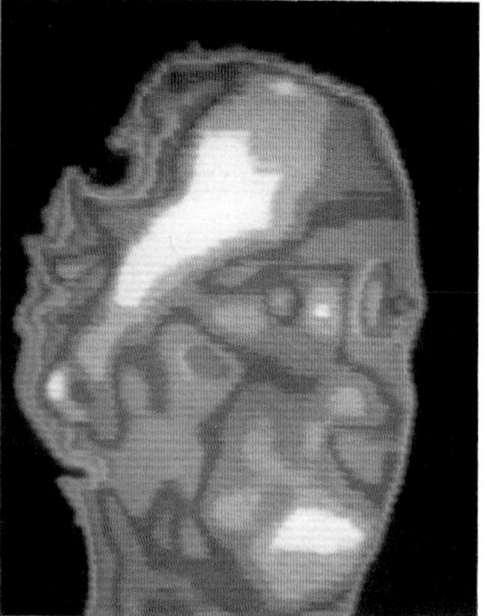

In migraine, blood vessels enlarge, stimulating nerves in vessel walls—usually on one side of the head. The white patch over the right eye is the temporal artery, grown larger and warmer than usual, and contributing to pain on the right side.

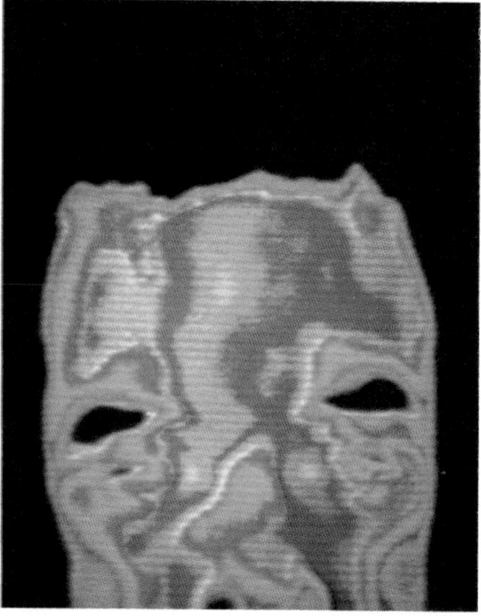

Red colors near the left eye indicate the relatively cool temperatures caused by reduced blood flow on the aching left side in a cluster headache. The condition arises when an artery constricts, limiting blood flow; sharp pain follows.

tries for nerves and vessels. Although the bones themselves are not sensitive to pain, the openings do contain pain-sensitive structures.

The part of the skull that encases the brain, known as the cranium, is made up of eight separate bones. One of them, located at the base of the skull, contains the foramen magnum, an opening less than $^4/_5$ inch wide where the brain and the exquisitely sensitive nerves of the spinal cord merge. The rest of the skull consists of 14 other bones that create the architecture of the eyes, nose, cheeks, mouth and chin. Within these bones, about 20 air cavities, called sinuses, reduce the weight of the skull without diminishing its strength. These cavities have membranous linings that are structurally similar to skin; like skin, the linings are richly supplied with nerve endings and blood vessels, and they are similarly sensitive to pain.

Given the rigidity of the skull and the jelly-like softness of the brain it coddles, the next layer of the head's structure is indispensable. Immediately inside the cranium a series of membranes known as the meninges absorbs shocks and gives gentle support to the brain. The outermost of the meninges is the dura mater, Latin for "hard mother." This stern parent is composed of a tough, fibrous material that fits to the underside of the bones and to some extent smooths over their tough ridges. Next comes a pair of layers containing innumerable intercommunicating channels filled with a clear liquid called cerebrospinal fluid; it cushions the brain from blows to the head, damps the effects of inertia when the head shifts position quickly, and generally provides buoyant support. Finally, the exceedingly soft and forbearing pia mater ("tender mother") lies in intimate contact with the outer surface of the brain, fitting into every fissured contour of that most delicate of organs.

The innermost tissue, the brain itself, is an elaborately folded and fissured material that bears something of a resemblance to the meat of a walnut. The brain does not react in pain to mechanical stimulation, such as the probing of a surgical instrument, because it contains no nerve receptors that are sensitive to pain. However, any changes in the brain's tissue—a tumorous growth or general swelling, for example—may exert pressure upon neighboring arteries and veins that do contain such nerve receptors, thereby producing pain sensations.

The headaches of everyday life

As the anatomy of pain production began to assume sharper outlines, headache researchers realized they were handicapped in talking about their discoveries by inadequate terminology. Mankind's oldest complaint no longer fit into the simple term, headache; there were many kinds, each with its own probable causes and course of treatment. In the early 1960s several professional groups decided independently to establish a comprehensive system of classification.

In the United States, a committee of specialists appointed by the National Institute of Neurological Diseases and Stroke identified no fewer than 15 major categories of headache and a substantial number of minor categories. Soon after, the American Association for the Study of Headache organized all the categories more simply under three main headings. Still used by most physicians in identifying head pains, these broad groupings are muscle-contraction headaches, vascular headaches, and traction and inflammatory headaches. Beyond these physical ailments lies a fourth group, so-called psychogenic headaches, which have no clear physical origins, do not respond to such physical remedies as drugs or surgery, and are mainly treated by psychiatrists.

Headaches associated with muscle contraction *(Chapter 2)* are probably the most common type. Popularly known as tension headaches, they are produced by the unrelieved contraction of the muscles of the head and neck. Typically, this persistent pulling produces a steady dull pain that lasts an hour or two; if the muscle tension becomes a habit, however, the ache may recur over periods of days, weeks, even years. The pain of a muscle-contraction headache is most often felt on both sides of the head, in both temples, at the back of the skull or neck, or along an entire "hatband" around the crown. The trigger, or cause, of the headache can be either physical or emotional—or more often, both—but in every case actual, not imaginary, pain is involved.

The category of vascular headaches is a huge grab bag of

head pains, ranging in consequence from such occasional nuisances as hangover and hunger headaches *(Chapter 3)* to severe and chronic migraine, or sick headaches, and cluster headaches *(Chapter 4)*. All have in common the swelling of blood vessels; the pain of such headaches results from the distention of these vessels and the irritation of pain receptors nearby. Because vascular headaches involve the circulatory system, the pain is typically rhythmic and throbbing, corresponding to the pulsing of the blood from the heart. In migraine the hurt is usually restricted to one side of the head.

The difficulty in treating vascular headaches lies partly in the variety of their triggers. Along with certain foods and drinks, for example, a cold substance taken into the mouth can induce a headache. The so-called ice cream headache, which strikes many people when they eat this sweet, has nothing to do with the chemical composition of ice cream; the trigger is temperature.

According to some authorities, the ice cream headache is vascular; as supporting evidence, they point out that some 95 per cent of the victims of migraine—the worst of all vascular headaches—also suffer ice cream headaches. But other authorities say that a direct irritation of nerves is the real cause *(page 17)*. As they explain it, iced drinks and ice cream irritate the tongue, the palate that divides the mouth from the nasal cavity, and the back of the throat. These tissues contain many sensitive endings of the cranial nerves called trigeminal, glossopharyngeal and vagus, which can carry pain sensations to the forehead, to the area behind the eyes and to the top of the head. The irritation to nerve endings is thus felt as a headache. And the remedy, according to Dr. Joel Saper of the Michigan Headache and Neurological Institute and Dr. Kenneth Magee of the University of Michigan, is not to give up ice cream, but to cool the mouth slowly by "allowing small amounts of ice cream to melt in the mouth before devouring the delicacy in globs or scoop by scoop."

Aches that can kill

Some tension and vascular headaches are dreadful to experience, but none directly shorten a victim's life, nor do they inflict any lasting physical damage. The third broad category, traction and inflammatory headaches, is of a different order. Here, pain is a secondary symptom of disease in or injury to the head, and of complications that, if ignored for any length of time, may result in irreversible and even life-threatening damage. No sufferer should attempt to smother such headaches with painkillers or any other kind of self-administered therapy; prompt medical attention is essential to successful treatment.

Though the secondary headaches are generally lumped together under the terms traction and inflammatory, the two groups differ widely in origin. Traction headaches arise from a mechanical force—it may include not only traction, or pulling, but also pushing—exerted against pain-sensitive structures inside the cranium. The cause of the aggravating pushing or pulling may be an intruding structure, such as a brain tumor, a blood clot or the accumulation of pus called an abscess. As such potentially dangerous structures grow larger, they displace the tissues around them, eventually causing head pain. If growth is slow, pain may at first be misleadingly mild, intermittent and easily relieved in its early stages by aspirin. But the pain will increase progressively, and neither aspirin nor more potent painkillers will get at the root cause of trouble.

A different group of secondary headaches, more appropriately called inflammatory, develop from primary inflammations that are named after the structures they affect in the cranium: meningitis, phlebitis (from the Greek for "vein"), and arteritis. Temporal arteritis, the form doctors see most often, strikes the arteries at the sides of the head, particularly in the elderly, and can lead to loss of sight. Its symptoms, typical of inflammatory headaches, include a persistent, intense, deep-set ache together with tender, even rigid temporal arteries.

In some complex cases, a mild inflammatory headache can develop into a severe one. For example, sinusitis, an inflammation of the membranes that line the sinus cavities, can cause a relatively moderate inflammatory headache—sinus headache. These are rare: Headache specialists estimate that nine out of 10 patients who complain of a sinus headache are actually suffering one of the ordinary muscle-tension variety. But when inflamed sinuses are the cause, they can and sometimes do lead to more serious trouble. Occasionally, channels that normally drain the contents of the sinuses into the nasal cavity are blocked. Then, unless a doctor drains the sinuses artificially by drawing off accumulated pus, a new ailment may develop. Collections of pus backed up in the blocked sinuses can eventually force their way up into the meningeal cavities of the cranium, producing meningitis.

One variety of secondary headache, neuralgia, is dreaded not so much because of its danger but for the terrible intensity of its pain; it does not threaten life but ruins it. The severe pain arises in nerves near the face. The most common forms of the disorder are trigeminal and glossopharyngeal neuralgia, which affect two of the nerves involved in an ordinary ice cream headache.

Trigeminal neuralgia, or *tic douloureux,* a one-sided recurrent pain, generally strikes persons over 40 years of age, most of them women. Its aching, burning, stabbing pain comes in volleys that may last from 15 seconds to four minutes, typically on one side of the face and head. The detonator of the neuralgic attack is often a draft of cold air against a distinctive trigger zone on the face but, depending upon individual sensitivity and the distribution of specific hypersensitive spots, a kiss, the pressure of a make-up brush or a towel, or even such acts as chewing, talking or blowing the nose may also set it off.

Glossopharyngeal neuralgia, often simply called tic, is a rarer condition. The pain and its timing are similar to those of *tic douloureux,* but the sensitive zone is generally located at the back of the throat and tongue; from there, the pain radiates upward and outward to produce nightmarish jabs around one ear. Not surprisingly, swallowing is the primary trigger.

The specific symptoms of all the varieties of traction and inflammatory headache are so numerous and technical that self-diagnosis is neither practical nor prudent. But to assist sufferers, headache authorities at the National Institutes of Health have drawn up a list of alarm signals: Those who experience them should seek medical attention. Some of the items on this list are obvious—it is difficult to imagine, for example, that convulsions would be dismissed lightly—but other signals are so subtle as to be easily missed. Every one of

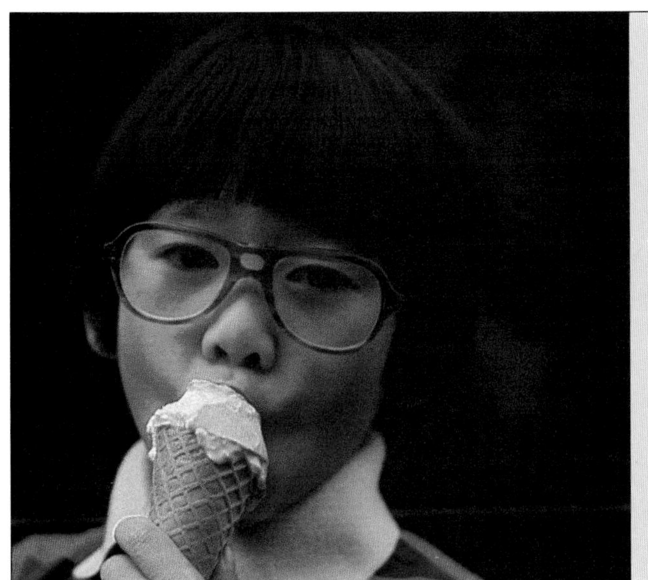

Not everyone gets the pleasure this boy does from eating ice cream. In some people—particularly those who suffer from migraine—the treat brings on a brief but intense headache. The reaction is caused by the cold, which stimulates nerve endings in the mouth and throat as indicated in the drawing at right.

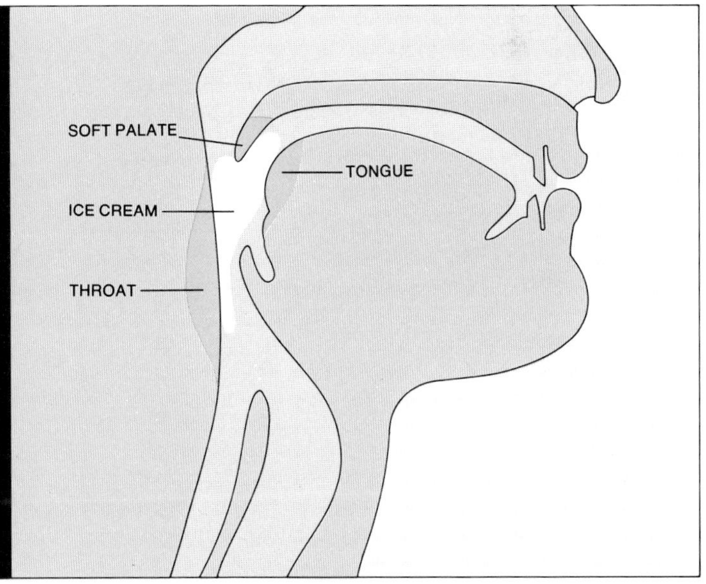

To produce an ice cream headache, a large glob of cold food or drink must strike the blue areas (above)—the back of the throat and tongue, and the soft palate. In these and neighboring areas, sensitive endings of the glossopharyngeal, vagus and trigeminal nerves set off the severe head or face pain of neuralgia.

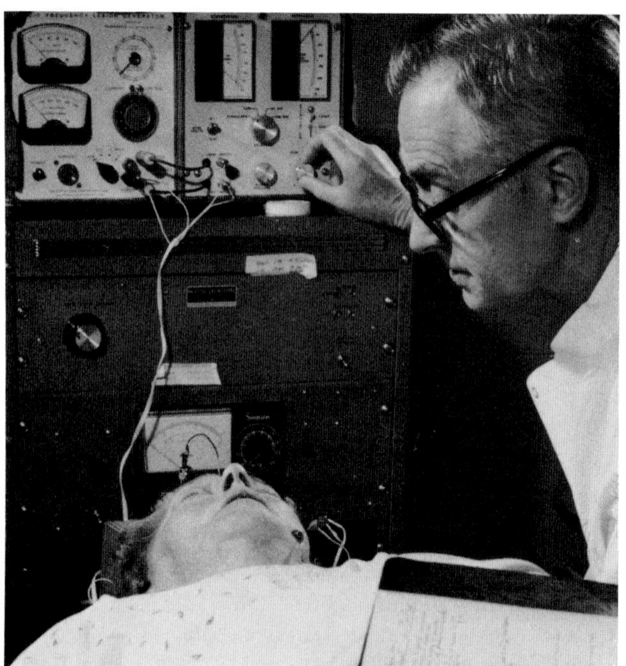

Plagued by the stabbing pain of trigeminal neuralgia, an anesthetized patient undergoes a therapeutic procedure, called thermocoagulation, that seals off offending pain nerves. Dr. William Sweet of Massachusetts General Hospital monitors a machine that beams radio waves through a long electrode needle inserted into the woman's cheek and down to the trigeminal nerve center near the base of the brain. The heat produced by the waves—up to 212° F.—destroys small pain nerves without damaging larger fibers that transmit other sensations. Another electrode is fixed to the woman's scalp for an electrical ground.

them, however, is a possible indication of serious trouble.

- Any headache that comes on suddenly and is marked by excruciating pain.
- Any headache associated with fever. This sign is especially ominous if the fever follows the headache rather than, as in the customary pattern of influenza symptoms, merely accompanying it.
- A headache accompanied by convulsions.
- Headaches of any strength accompanied by mental or neurological abnormalities, such as blurred or double vision, confusion, loss of alertness or consciousness, or loss of bodily function, coordination or sensation.
- A headache following a blow to the head.
- Any pattern of headaches localized in the ear or eye.
- Any pattern of headaches occurring in an older person who has previously been free of frequent headaches.
- Recurring headaches in children.
- A pattern of headaches, at any age, that interferes with routines of living.
- Frequent headaches, especially if they exhibit a change in severity or pattern from routine aches of the past.

Real pains that are only in the mind

One unusual kind of head pain, not dangerous to life but often debilitating, masquerades as the traction type of organic headache. It most often strikes after a head injury and has thus acquired the mouth-filling name of post-traumatic muscle-tension headache. Yet it is not directly caused by such a physiological shock. It has its origins in the sufferer's psychological make-up rather than in physiological, organic ailments.

Although the victim of a post-traumatic headache may be convinced of the organic nature of his pain, the symptoms quickly reveal to a skilled diagnostician that this is not the case. Most individuals can expect to experience a traction headache immediately after they sustain a head or neck injury. Such trauma-induced headaches may last from several days up to a week or maybe even two. After that period, physiological repairs take effect, and the patient gradually becomes free of symptoms. A physician can monitor the course of the repairs, and tell when healing is complete.

By contrast, a post-traumatic muscle-tension headache may appear in the aftermath of head injury or surgery, but may also follow high fever, or even psychological shock. It generally starts later than an organic post-traumatic headache and goes on for months, even years. Physicians treating the complaint can locate no anatomical cause other than the fact that certain muscles are maintained in a constant and painful state of tension. The pain is usually dull and generalized, although localized tender spots may also develop in the area of the original injury.

Certain factors seem to predispose a patient to this kind of reaction after an injury. In a study of 63 patients at New York Hospital, researchers found that patients who were incapable of meeting the demands of their jobs, frustrated by what they regarded as lack of recognition, or in conflict with their associates were especially prone to post-traumatic muscle-tension headaches, with symptoms so severe that it became difficult or impossible for them to work.

The research did not suggest that any large number of unhappy workers with occupationally debilitating headaches were faking their symptoms. The headaches were every bit as real, and frequently as painful, as those produced by migraine or brain tumor. It was the victim's unconscious mind, afflicted by what some doctors call an accident neurosis, that caused the cranial muscles to contract. The neurosis could not, in all likelihood, be controlled, and the injury itself was an almost fortuitous occasion for some deep-seated unhappiness to express itself.

A not-so-surprising factor that seems to play a role in provoking the onset and extending the duration of these headaches is the progress of lawsuits or compensation claims arising out of the initial injury. No one seriously engaged in headache research has suggested that the majority of people suffering from a so-called compensation headache are doing so just to win a large settlement as redress for an injury. But the mind and emotions have extraordinarily strong effects upon the body, and a tendency toward anxiety or depression, coupled with an opportunity to gain financial redress, can be overpowering.

Dr. Steven F. Brena, Director of the Pain Control Center at Emory University in Atlanta, maintained that persons with a tendency toward this kind of psychosomatic expression are encouraged to continue their behavior by social forces around them—the lawyer who dwells upon the injury to ensure convincing testimony, family and friends who want to be sympathetic, courts that draw out proceedings according to a stately pace all their own, the various compensation agencies of government or private insurance that will finally pay the bill.

Not only the pain of compensation headaches, but the effectiveness of drugs used in their treatment can reflect the complexities of this ailment. After treating some 240 victims with antidepressant drugs, Dr. Lee Kudrow, Director of the California Medical Clinic for Headache at Encino, noted a variation in the degree of relief provided by identical doses. Dr. Kudrow then divided his patients into two groups: one consisting of persons who were engaged in current litigation, another of those who were not involved in legal action or had already received compensation. Immediately, the discrepancies were clarified: 57 per cent of those who had no financial interest in preserving pain responded successfully to drugs; among those who still awaited an award, only 21 per cent got any benefit.

A study that was reported in Great Britain found that relatively simple psychological measures produced good results in treating such headaches. Researchers compared two contrasting treatment programs for post-trauma pains. One group of patients received what the researchers called active care, which included daily visits by the doctor for reassurance and discussion; daily encouragement, when appropriate, to get out of bed; and after the hospital stay ended, follow-up treatment by the same doctors who had provided hospital care. A second group received routine treatment: The patient had considerably less personal contact with his doctor and was offered only cursory explanations of his injury or of what he might expect in the next few weeks; the hospital staff did not effectively restrain the patient's instincts to remain in bed, to dwell on his injury and to give in to some measure of dependency. The researchers reported

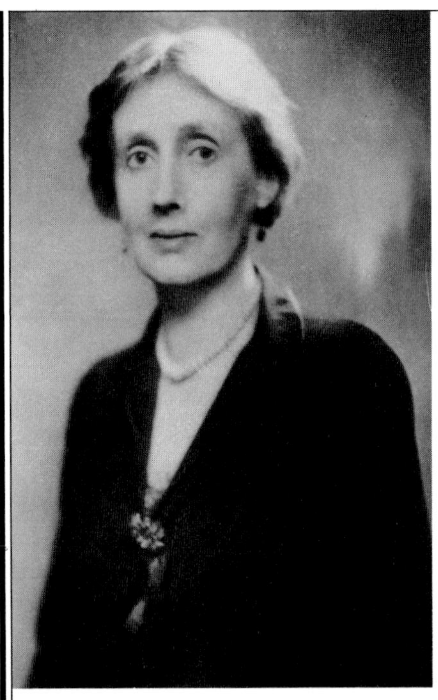

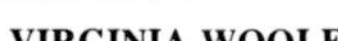

Common aches of uncommon victims

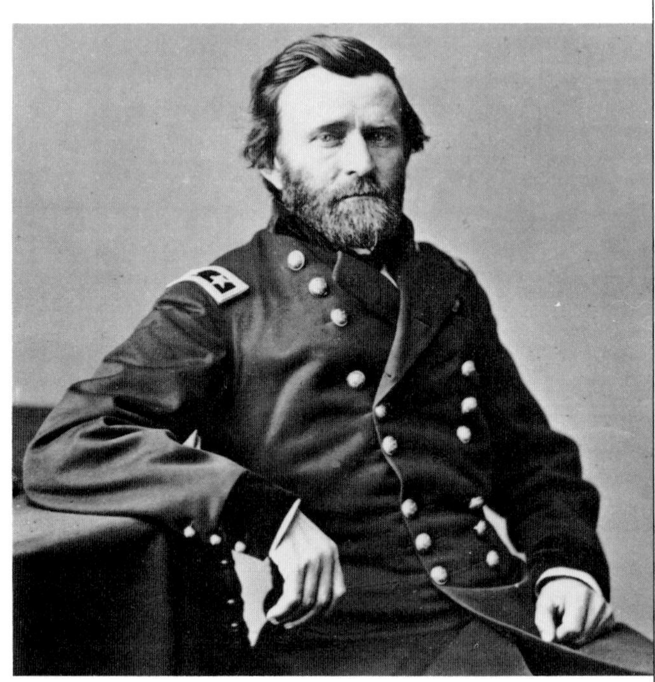

VIRGINIA WOOLF

Novelist Virginia Woolf was plagued by headaches—perhaps a sign of the severe emotional distress that marked her life. She conjured up a vivid image of the pain of "a first rate headache" in a 1929 letter to her writer friend Victoria Sackville-West: "I am being kept quiet today and so am rather grumpy. All my own fault: I insisted on writing a little yesterday and so brought on the headache—or rather—for what it feels like—tempted the rat to gnaw the nerves in my spine—fourth knob from the top."

ULYSSES S. GRANT

General Ulysses S. Grant's headaches were probably migraines—brought on, as migraines sometimes are, by tense, critical situations. "I was suffering very severely with a sick headache," he wrote in his journal for April 8, 1865. "I spent the night in bathing my feet in hot water and mustard, and putting mustard plasters on my wrists and the back of my neck, hoping to be cured by morning." That day he received a letter from General Robert E. Lee surrendering the Confederate forces. "The instant I saw the contents of the note," wrote Grant, "I was cured."

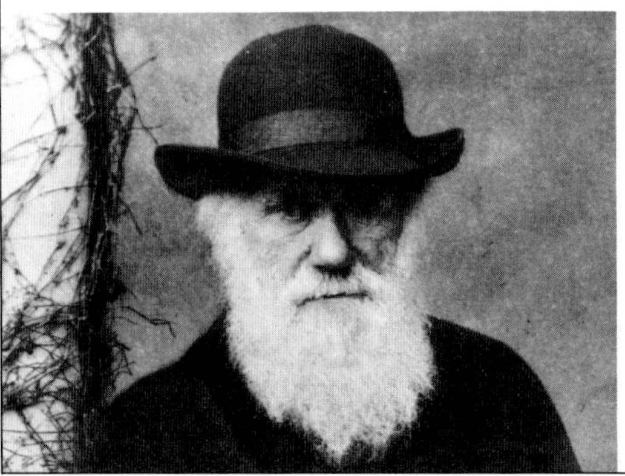

CHARLES DARWIN

The pioneer of evolutionary theory was a shy, worry-ridden man who suffered chronic migraines, often precipitated by stress. A few days before his wedding, Darwin's dread of a formal ceremony overcame him. In a letter from London to his fiancée, Emma Wedgwood, he complained of a "bad headache, which continued two days and two nights, so that I doubted whether it ever meant to allow me to be married."

that those in the active group were back at work in 18 days, on average, while the members of the routine group spent an average of 32 days convalescing.

The mysteries of conversion headaches

Although some post-traumatic headaches are rooted in psychological stresses, the pain itself comes from a physical effect, the stress-related tensing of muscles. Such physical expression of an emotional problem is typical of most psychologically determined headaches. Indeed, mental upsets are behind a great many headaches of all kinds. But one curious type of headache is entirely in the mind. No blood vessels are expanded or contracted, no muscles tensed, no internal or external agents seem to be acting on nerve endings, yet the head hurts, often severely and continually. These are the marks of the mysterious ailments called conversion headaches. They respond little, if at all, to antidepressants or painkillers, and they need no precipitating incident or injury to bring them on.

The term conversion, borrowed from the language of psychoanalysis, refers to the expression of some emotional disturbance—usually sexual conflicts or repressed aggression—in the more socially acceptable terms of a physical illness. Patients suffering conversion headaches are totally convinced of the organic nature of their sickness and sometimes can briefly mislead a physician into believing that some neurological disorder exists. But they often give themselves away by what psychiatrists refer to as *la belle indifference,* or "beautiful indifference," a tranquil facial expression completely inappropriate to the degree of pain reported, and one that medical doctors have come to associate with this psychogenic disorder.

Conversion patients are frequently unable to function in a normal social or work situation. They tend to experiment with every conceivable form of painkiller and tranquilizer, often in massive doses, in an unsuccessful effort to deaden the psychogenic pain. Along with treating the conversion reaction itself, then, the physician and psychiatrist must free the patient from drug dependency. In recent times some physicians have tried various forms of placebo surgery, including such serious—and questionable—operations as cutting nerves and fusing vertebrae, in an effort to bring peace to the sufferer. However, it is now recognized that the victim of conversion headache can obtain lasting relief only through intensive psychotherapy, which helps the patient deal with the emotional tensions that originally triggered the conversion mechanism.

Modern research has made it painfully clear that the causes of headache are as heterogeneous as those of any of the ailments known to mankind. When any headache proves persistent or severe, a physician should always be consulted, and if the family doctor cannot help, then the sufferer should go on to specialists or, best of all, a headache clinic.

If the headaches are of the common muscle-tension variety, the first step is to find out what brings them on; the next step is to work to avoid those mechanisms by changing either internal behavior or external environment. If the headaches are vascular, it is possible to avoid substances that cause some of them. And if they are genetic in origin and thus essentially unavoidable, like the majority of migraines, drugs can make life easier.

How different these options are today from those few available not long ago is revealed in an amusing anecdote about George Bernard Shaw, who suffered a monthly migraine headache for nearly seventy years. At one time Shaw was introduced to the renowned Arctic explorer Fridtjof Nansen of Norway. He asked Nansen whether he had ever discovered a headache cure. "No," said the hero. But Shaw went on: "Have you ever tried to find a cure for headaches?" "No," replied Nansen, now thoroughly puzzled. "Well, that is a most astonishing thing! You have spent your life in trying to discover the North Pole, which nobody on earth cares tuppence about, and you have never attempted to discover a cure for the headache, which every living person is crying aloud for!"

Shaw was wrong, of course, in assuming a single cure existed. There is not, and never will be, one therapy for all headaches. But many cures do exist, tailored to specific headache syndromes, and they are available to the individual willing to pursue them. ❋

An ancient battle against an everyday ailment

To ease headaches, people throughout history have literally left no stone unturned: In Europe in the 16th Century, and probably earlier, operations were performed to remove stony deposits—"head stones"—that some medical practitioners blamed for head pain. The surgery, of course, was pure fakery *(pages 30-31)*, the surgeons quacks.

Indeed, of the thousands of headache cures tried over the ages many, like the supposed removal of head stones, have been utterly worthless. Yet some worked, and still others seemed to—if only because they served as temporary, if occasionally painful, distractions from an ailment that in all likelihood would have disappeared by itself anyway.

Perhaps the oldest treatment for head pain is also the most drastic. Stone Age men used primitive blades and drills to cut holes in the skull *(page 24)*, possibly because they thought the holes offered pain-provoking demons a means of escape, but more likely because they found the treatment sometimes worked. The procedure, called trephination, can relieve pressure inside the skull, thereby eliminating a cause of some severe head pains.

The Greeks practiced a different kind of surgery for head pain. They believed that an excess of a body fluid, or humor, caused many ills, including headaches. To draw off the surplus and relieve the pain, the Greeks advocated bloodletting. The theory and practice survived for millennia, though methods differed. Like Stone Age trephination, bloodletting may have been of help to some sufferers—by lowering the blood pressure of migraine victims, for example.

Other ancient headache remedies relied not on surgery but on physical manipulations *(pages 26-27)*, which doctors now know can occasionally produce relief by loosening tightened muscles and realigning joints that are chronically out of alignment. Also prescribed were poultices, mixtures or brews made from plants or animal parts. One Ninth Century cure from the Loire Valley of France suggested that headache sufferers mix vulture brains "with the best of oil and put it in the nose, and it will expel all ailments of the head." Somewhat more rational was a remedy popular among 17th Century American Indians, a concoction made from the sex glands of male beavers. Once drunk, it quite likely made some headache victims feel better: The glands contain a type of salicylate, the chemical that later became aspirin.

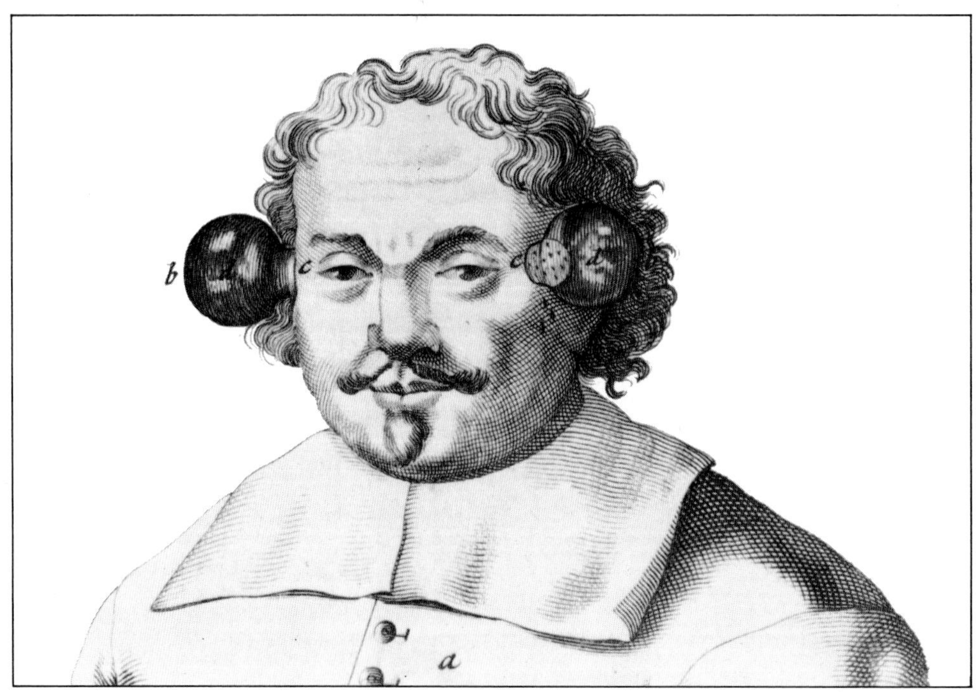

A Dutch illustration (above) details a 17th Century version of an ancient headache treatment—bloodletting. Here, heated cups were placed over incisions in the temples; when the air in the cups cooled, a vacuum drew out blood, perhaps easing head pain. At right, in a Swedish painting of the same period, a barber-surgeon lets blood by slicing into a patient's pate.

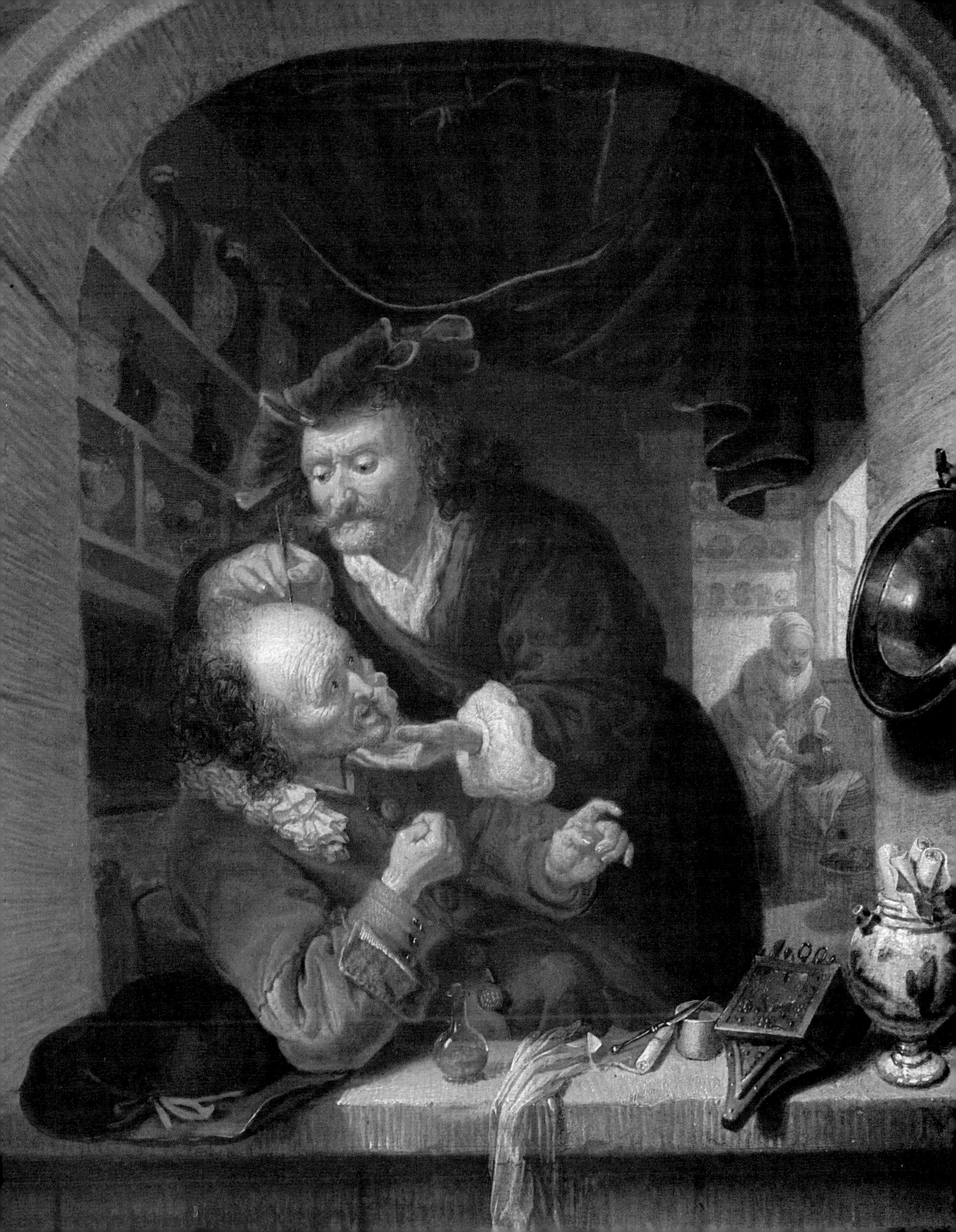

A hole to let pain out

Thousands of Neolithic skulls, like the one below, bear marks of trephination. Seldom performed with anesthesia—except among Peruvian Indians, who employed a type of cocaine—the surgery consisted of cutting through the scalp and into the skull with flint or obsidian tools. The chips of bone were lifted out, leaving a gaping hole.

The practice seems to have been almost universal, for trephined skulls have been found on nearly every continent. Almost half the patients are thought to have survived, if only for a few days: Many trephined skulls show evidence of healing—new bone growth around the holes. One South American man appears to have survived seven such operations.

This drastic procedure was—and is, as performed now with electric drills—a viable way to relieve dangerous pressure on the brain caused by injury or illness. Most trephined fossils bear marks of damage in battle or accident. But some lack any such sign, suggesting that their owners suffered nothing more than severe headaches—until their pains were inappropriately treated by skull-shattering surgery.

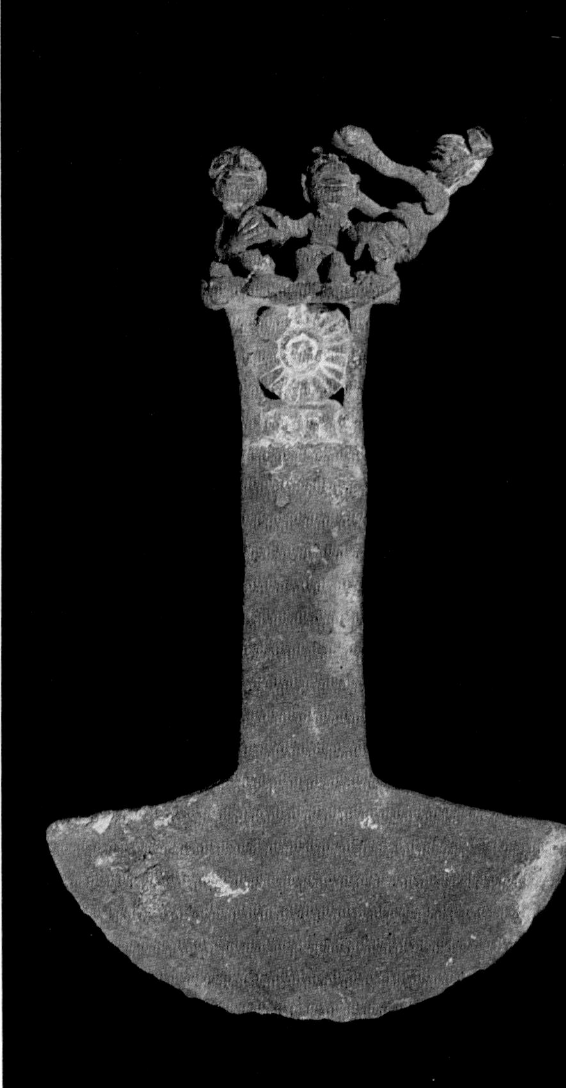

Human figures adorning the handle of a bronze trepan, made by Chimu Indians in Peru, illustrate how the tool was used to make a hole in a patient's skull. An assistant (left) holds the patient as the surgeon (right) cuts through the bone.

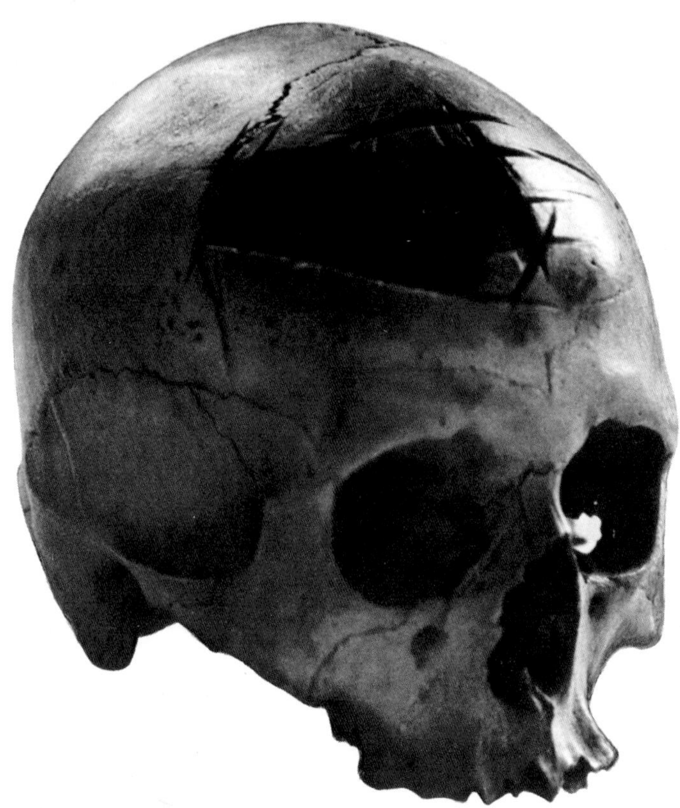

Slash marks, probably made by a trepan like the one above, crisscross a gaping hole in a 12th or 13th Century Peruvian girl's skull. Because the hole shows no signs of bone regrowth the girl very likely died as a result of her operation.

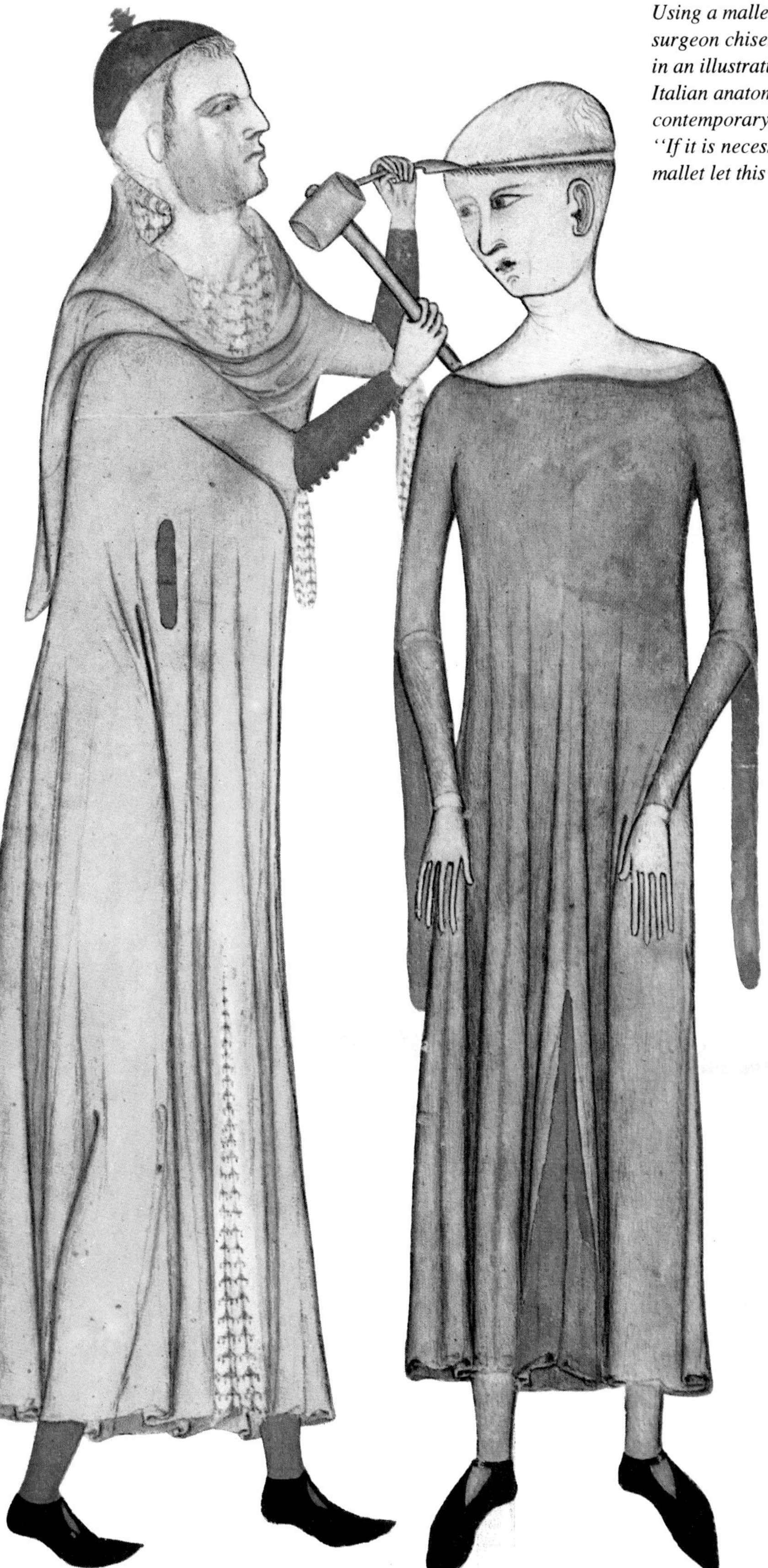

Using a mallet and trepan, a medieval surgeon chisels a hole in his patient's skull, in an illustration from a 14th Century Italian anatomical treatise. One contemporary medical textbook cautioned: "If it is necessary to strike with the mallet let this be done gently."

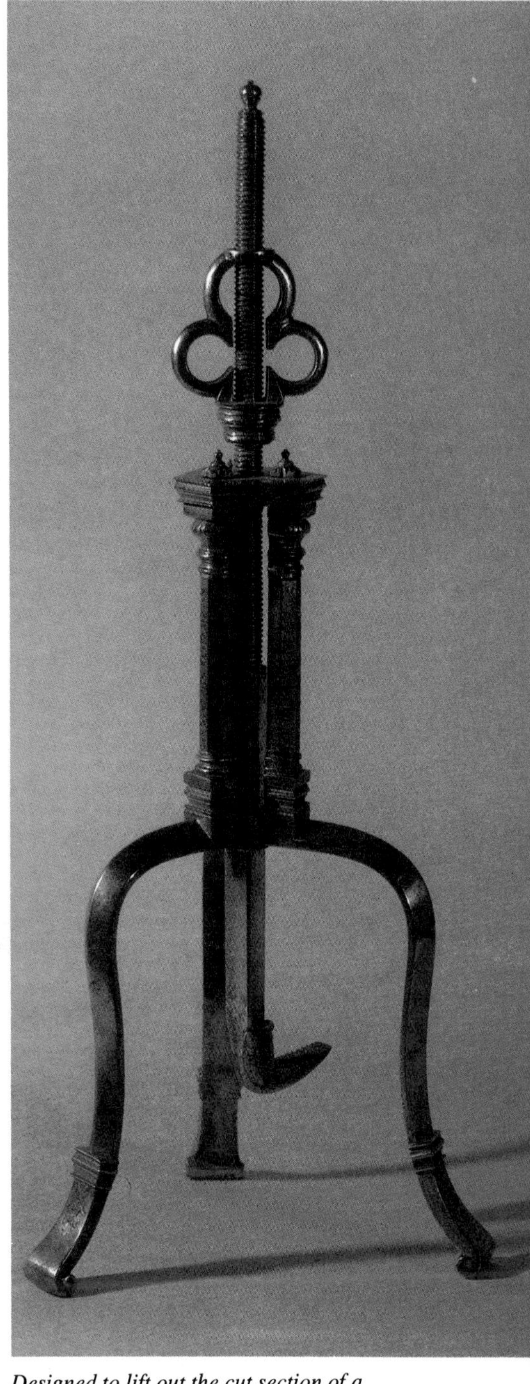

Designed to lift out the cut section of a trepanned skull, this 16th Century bone extractor worked like an automobile jack, prying out the piece—its threaded shaft was screwed upward while the three legs of the frame rested against the patient's head.

Working aches away by hand

Not all head pain originates where the pain is felt. A jaw that pops its hinges out of their sockets—as misaligned jaws are prone to do—can tighten face and head muscles, producing headaches; stiff neck muscles can have a similar effect.

The Aztecs of the 16th Century practiced massage *(below)* to alleviate one important cause of head pain—tight neck muscles. Twenty centuries earlier, the Greeks had perfected a different technique for another source of headaches. To push a jaw back into place, a doctor and his assistant used their bare hands *(right)*. Essentially the same technique is used today for this type of dislocation.

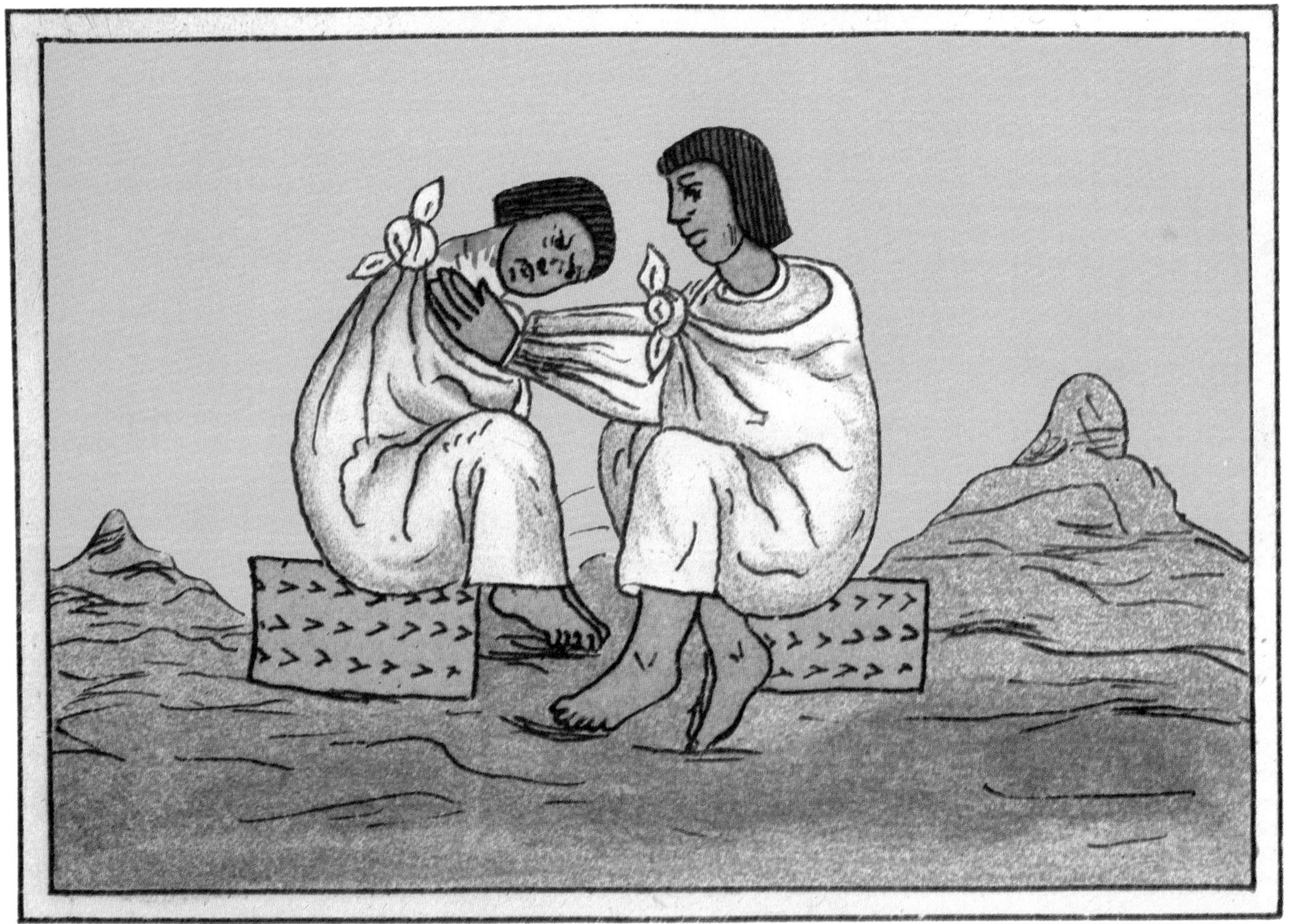

Relieving a wrenched neck, an Aztec physician massages his patient's neck muscles, first relaxing and then stretching them, in a 16th Century illustration. The treatment is effective in soothing headaches caused by tightened neck muscles.

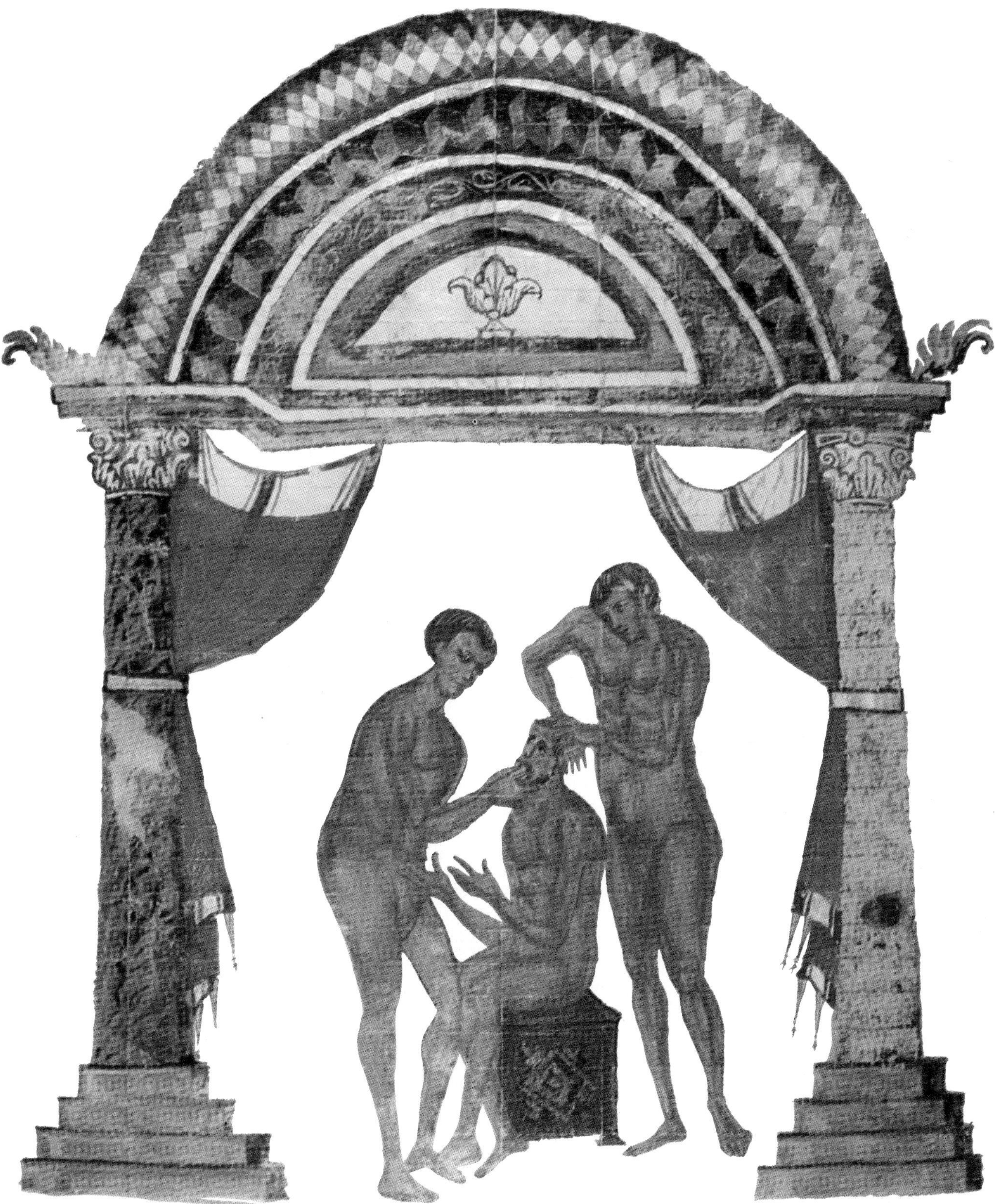

A 10th Century European illustration depicts a Third Century B.C. Greek therapy: While an assistant holds the patient's aching head, a surgeon (left)—his thumbs depressing the patient's jawbone—uses his fingers to guide the bone back into its socket.

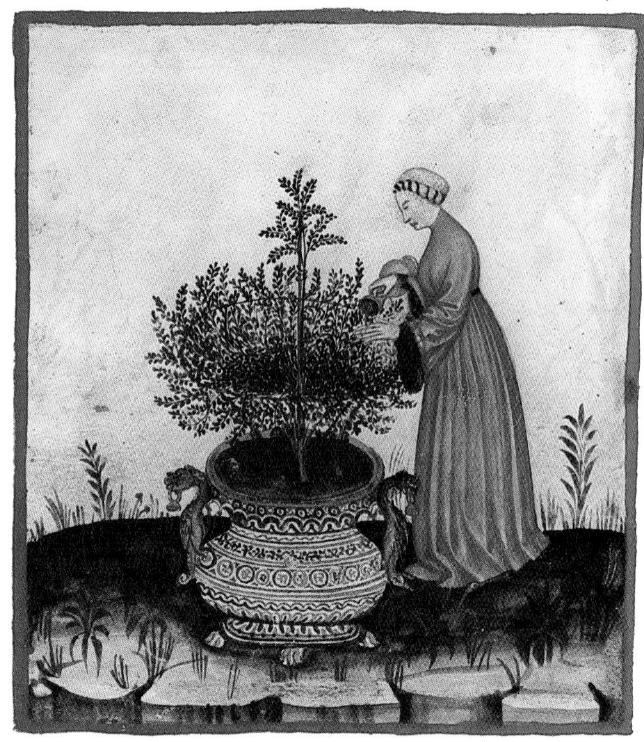

A woman in a 16th Century Italian illustration harvests marjoram for use against headaches from common colds. The herb was placed in the nostrils and inhaled. An aromatic oil in marjoram may have eased head pain by opening sinus passages.

Cures from plants

In about 77 A.D., the Greek physician Dioscorides compiled a list of 600 herbal remedies for various ills. His headache cure may have been one of the best ancient prescriptions. He suggested an extract of the ruta plant, a woody shrub. The plant contains rutin, a chemical that lowers blood pressure. Thus Dioscorides' remedy may indeed have helped relieve the pounding of headaches brought on by the enlargement of blood vessels.

Some herbal remedies were not nearly so helpful—Pliny the Elder, a Roman contemporary of Dioscorides, advocated scraping moss off the head of a statue and wearing it on a red string tied around the neck—but many others were based on successful experience. In most parts of the world, extracts of willow twigs and other plants were providing headache sufferers with curative salicylate compounds long before their modern version, aspirin, was developed.

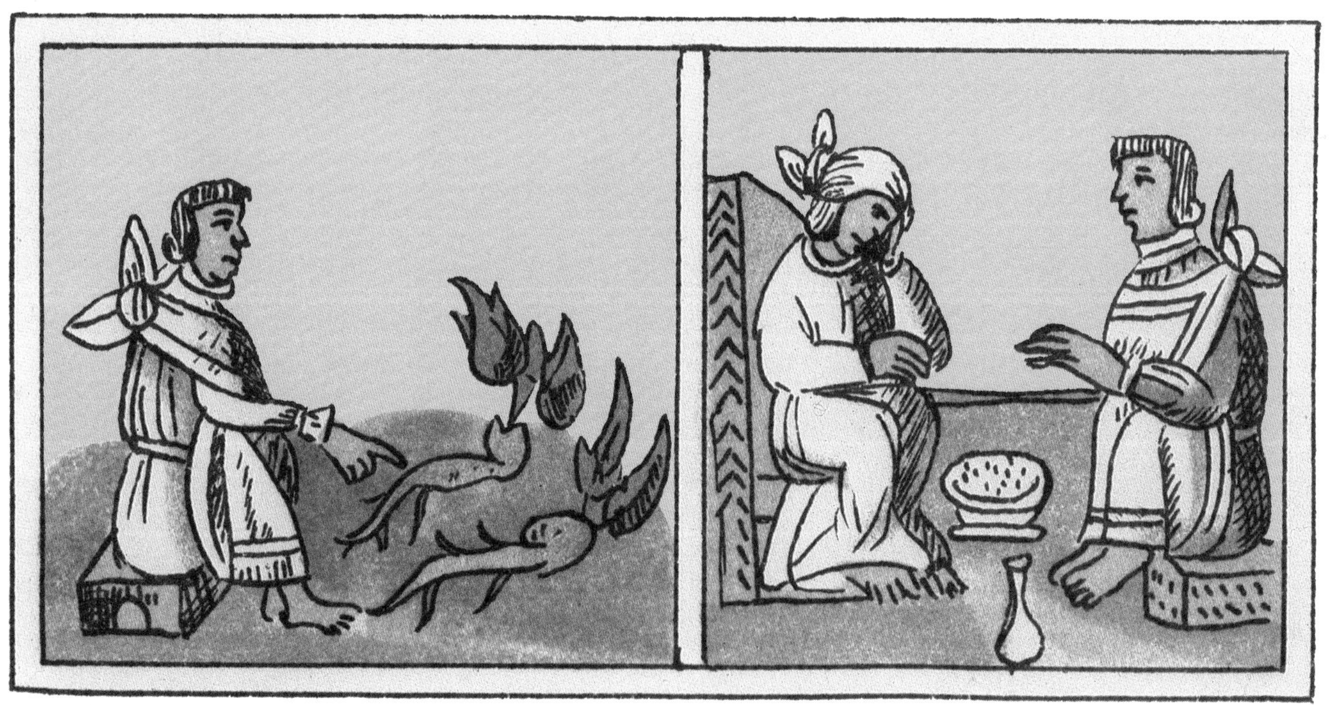

Two 16th Century Aztec illustrations show the stages of a popular headache cure: At left, a medicine man gathers an herb, probably tobacco; at right, he burns its leaves to ease the suffering of a patient, who presses a poultice of leaves to his head. The nicotine in tobacco constricts some blood vessels, perhaps explaining tobacco's relief of vascular headaches.

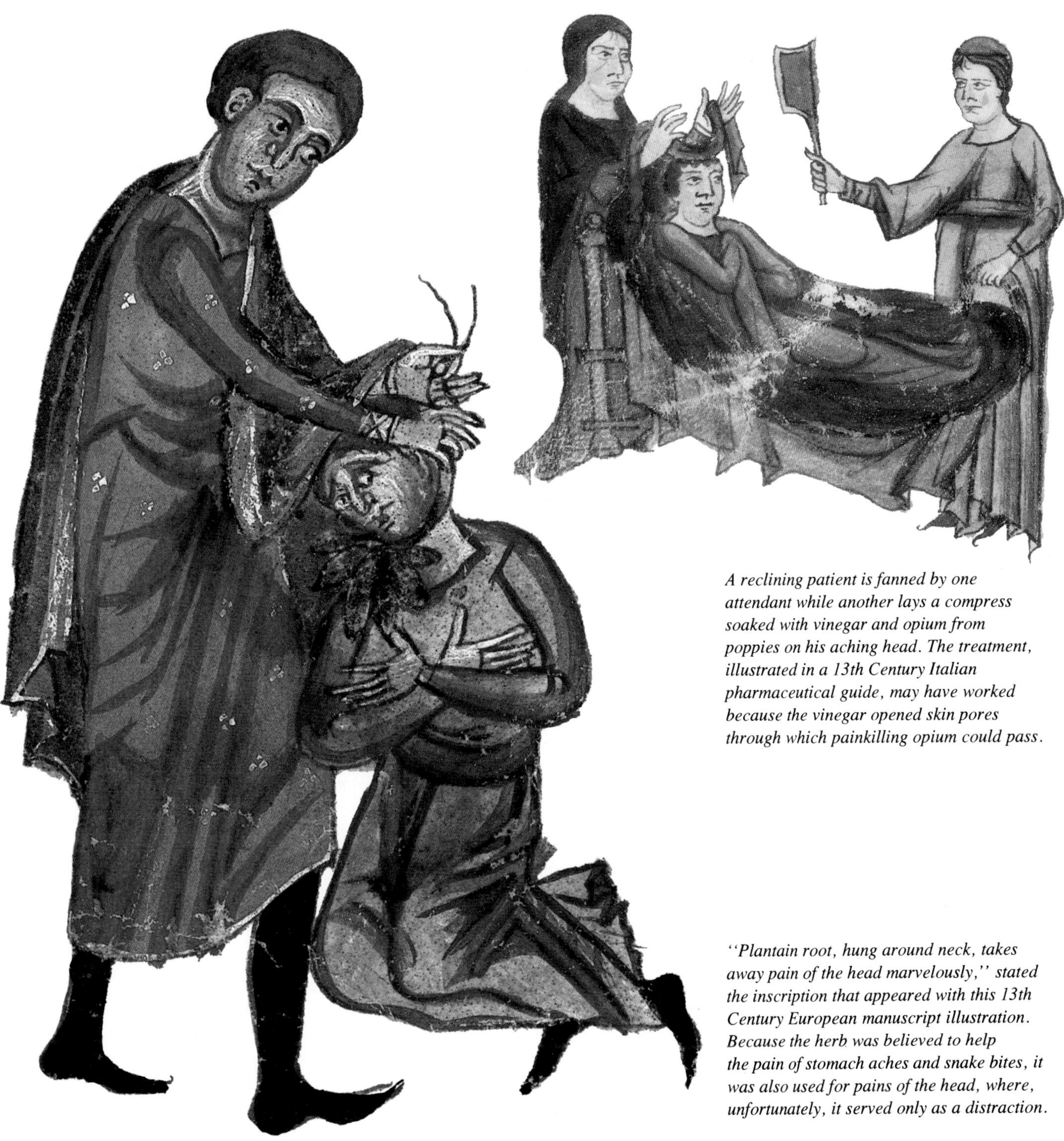

A reclining patient is fanned by one attendant while another lays a compress soaked with vinegar and opium from poppies on his aching head. The treatment, illustrated in a 13th Century Italian pharmaceutical guide, may have worked because the vinegar opened skin pores through which painkilling opium could pass.

"Plantain root, hung around neck, takes away pain of the head marvelously," stated the inscription that appeared with this 13th Century European manuscript illustration. Because the herb was believed to help the pain of stomach aches and snake bites, it was also used for pains of the head, where, unfortunately, it served only as a distraction.

The quack's fake stone

"We see the weakness and credulity of man is such," lamented essayist Francis Bacon in the 17th Century, "that they will prefer the mountebank or witch before a learned physician." Then, as now, headache sufferers unrelieved by standard treatments turned from reputable medical practitioners to the waiting arms of quacks. Holding out hope, these medical mercenaries profited from promises of quick cures.

Their sales pitches almost always were garbed in shreds of medical fact and logic. For hundreds of years before Bacon's day, for instance, people had known that kidney and gall bladder pain frequently was caused by minerals that accumulated in those organs. Thus, playing on an unwitting victim's scanty medical knowledge, quacks diagnosed "head stones" as a cause of headache. For a fee, the stone could be removed. There was no stone, of course, but the quack would provide one *(right)*. In the meantime, the medical razzle-dazzle—and the pain of the operation—may at least have made the victim's original headache disappear.

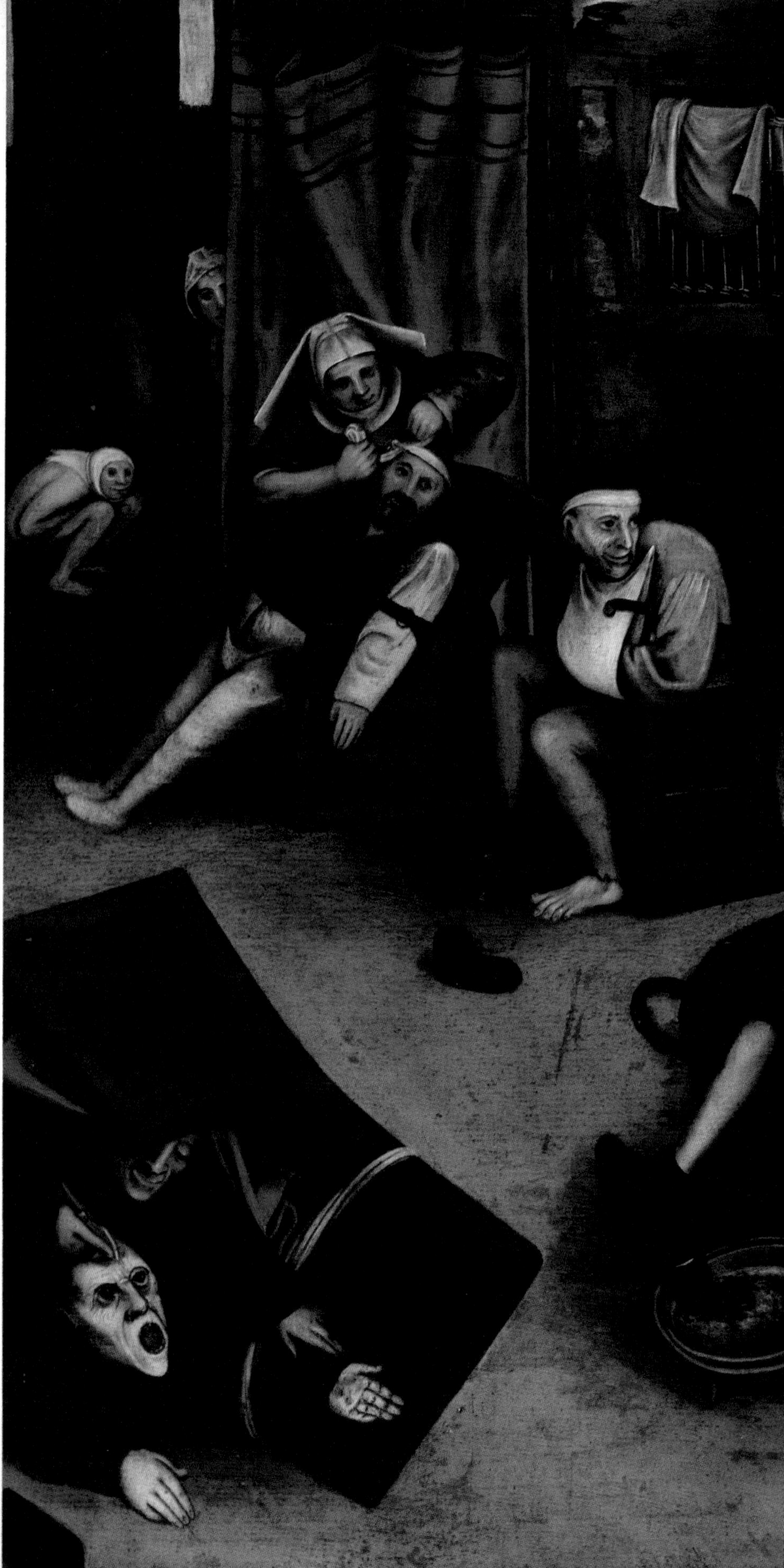

In a 16th Century painting after the Flemish master Pieter Bruegel, four quacks in a clinic perform bogus operations to remove head stones, a reputed cause of pain. At center, one practitioner pretends to extract a stone—it was slipped to him by his assistant—from his unsuspecting patient's head. At lower left, a groaning patient who has overturned his chair in agony holds his head stone as another of the surgeons finishes the operation.

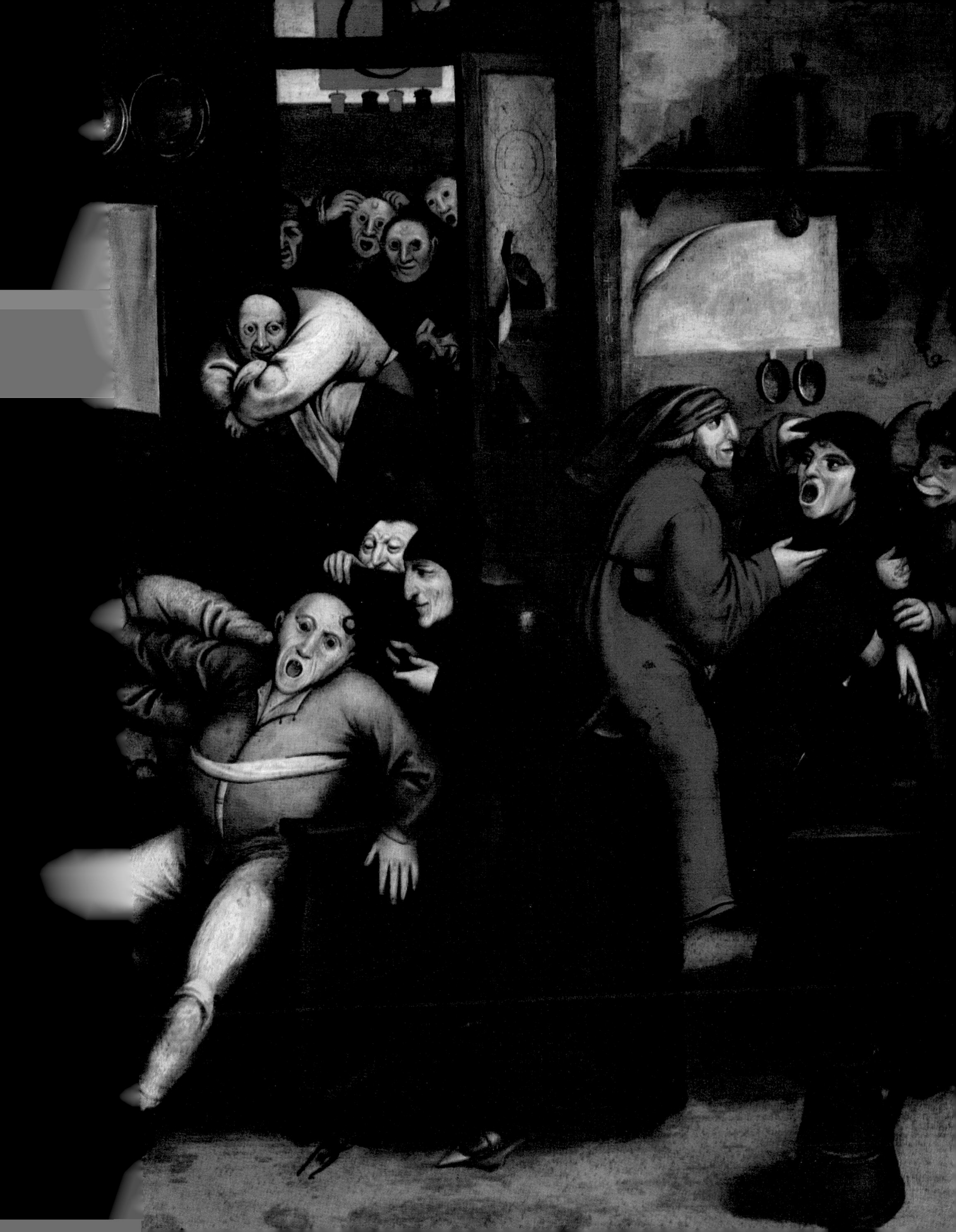

CHAPTER 2

The viselike grip of tension

Do women suffer most?
Hunting for hidden triggers
Exercising the body to help the head
First aid for tight muscles
Psychological causes, physical effects
Strategies for fighting chronic pain

The most common headache is often caused by an evolutionary leftover. Human beings share with other animals a wondrous mechanism designed to help them survive threats to their existence—the fight-or-flight response, a reaction preparing them to confront an enemy or take to their heels, whichever seems prudent. This defense mechanism tenses muscles, slows digestion, speeds the heart, and constricts some blood vessels while dilating others. The physiological changes serve a purpose, increasing energy and sharpening the senses for emergency action. When the action is completed, energy is used up, tension is released, and the threatened individual feels relieved whether his response to the challenge has been heroic or not.

But physical dangers no longer threaten human life at every turn; more often the threat that arises is psychological—from deadlines, budgets, promotions, school grades, health concerns, social pressures. For such stresses, the tensed muscles of the fight-or-flight response are actually counterproductive. Energies are summoned up only to go unspent; the wound-up muscles of the individual under pressure remain tightened. One painful outcome is the muscle-contraction, or tension, headache.

Although psychological stress is properly blamed for most such headaches, these common maladies can result from purely physical—if not life-threatening—stress. If certain muscles in the body are subjected to prolonged tension—from reading slumped in a chair, driving in night traffic, stretching to paint a ceiling, or straining to see in harsh light—head pains may result, sometimes in areas removed from the tensed muscles.

However the muscle tension arises, it hurts because the contracted muscles cut off the supply of oxygen to muscle cells, temporarily damaging them. The affected cells release chemicals that transmit to the brain warning signals of pain *(Chapter 5)*.

Muscle-tension headaches can be relatively infrequent or daily occurrences; but in either case they are controllable and not dangerous. In most instances it is a simple task to sort out tension headaches from other kinds, thanks to the well-defined character of their symptoms. Treatments and prevention strategies may also be fairly obvious if the causes can be identified; many of the remedies are of the self-help and home first-aid variety.

The classic indicator of muscle-tension headaches is the quality of the pain its victims experience. The sensation tends to be dull, as contrasted with the sharp, stabbing pulsations of common vascular headaches *(Chapter 3)*. The pain is also typically mild to moderate, as distinct from the more severe distress of migraine or cluster headaches *(Chapter 4)*. Tension headaches also differ from more serious head pains in developing without such warning signs as visual abnormalities and nausea.

Patients in the grips of such headaches have variously described the sensations as "viselike," "crushing," "sore all over," and "like a too tight headband." A tender, stiff neck, indicative of muscle tension in the neck and shoulders,

The classic gesture of a headache sufferer, hands to head, fingers rubbing the temples, can help ease the tight muscles of a tension headache. Stress and overwork are frequent causes: Sitting hunched at a desk and reading with inadequate light contracts muscles in the head, neck and face so that they hurt.

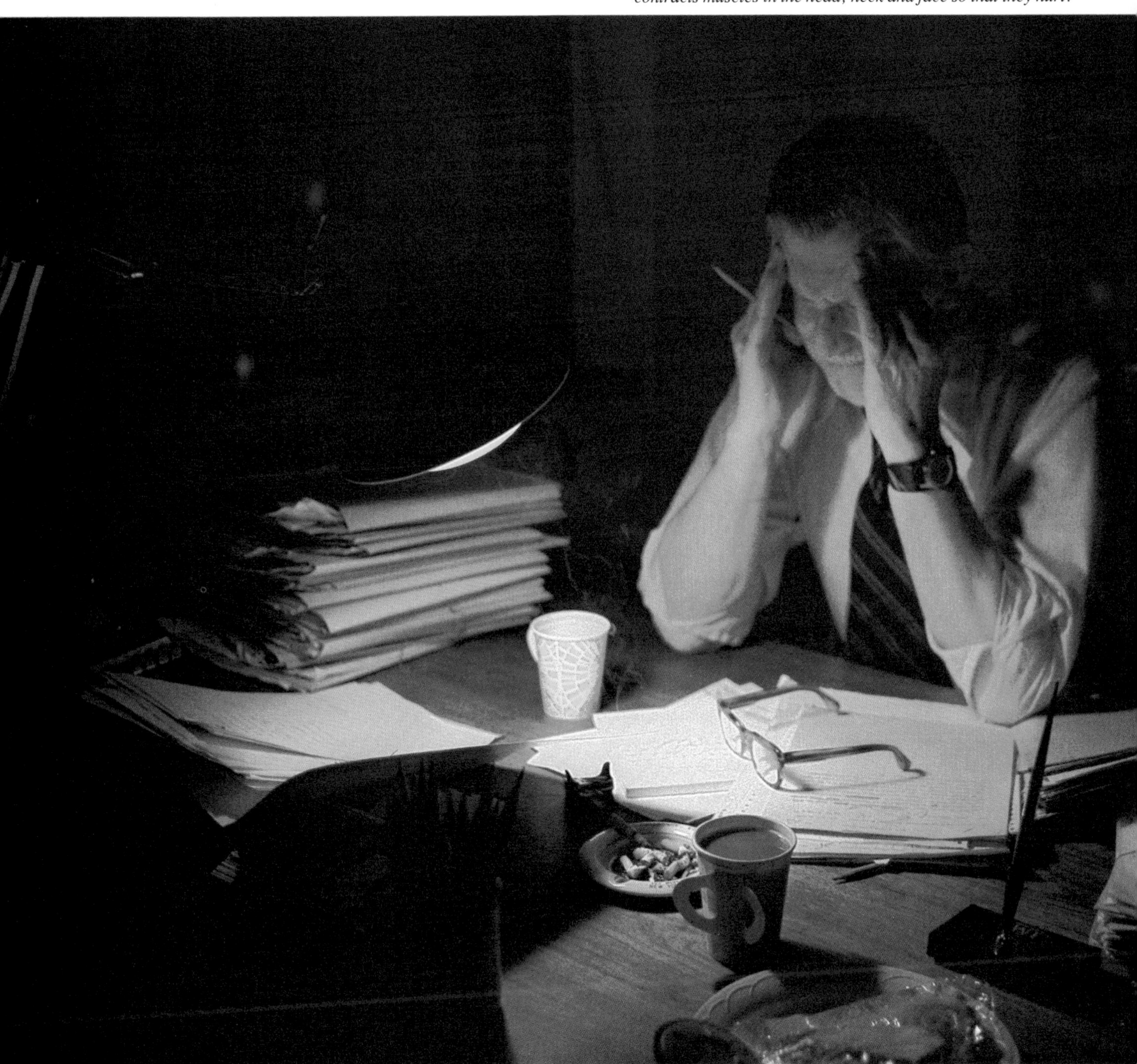

is another common symptom. Some people report that their scalp becomes so sensitized as to prevent them from brushing their hair.

The second most prominent characteristic distinguishing muscle-tension headaches is location. In nine out of 10 cases, they are bilateral; that is, the head hurts more or less equally on both sides. Sometimes the pain will involve virtually every head muscle from the back of the skull forward to the brow. Only in a small minority of muscle-tension headaches is the pain one-sided; in such a case the pain is usually localized near the adjacent temple or ear, and the immediate cause is likely to be associated with some abnormality of the sufferer's teeth or jaw.

The location of the pain, however, does not necessarily correspond to its point of origin. Muscles that are tensed in one part of the body may create an ache that is felt somewhere else, a phenomenon called referred pain. The nerves that carry pain signals from the neck and shoulder muscles meet the pain-signaling nerves from the muscles of the head and face at a common point in the upper neck—in effect, creating a sort of electrical junction box. At this junction signals can cross over, or jump, from one circuit to another, causing referred pain.

Researchers have identified several of these circuits whose pain signals—originating at certain muscles in the head, neck and shoulders—are consistently switched to other parts of the head and neck. Thus the trapezius, the large flat muscle on either side of the upper back, transmits pain to the neck and temples; the temporalis, or temple muscle, sends pain to areas adjacent to the mouth and over the eyes; the masseter, or chewing muscle, can cause pain in the mouth or ears; the sternocleidomastoid muscle on either side of the neck may generate pain in the forehead, ear, face or chin; and the splenius capitis, at the back of the neck, transmits pain to the top of the head.

Muscle-tension headaches as a whole account for an estimated 80 per cent of the head-pain disorders that beset those in modern industrialized societies. Although thought of by many as an adult affliction, they are found not infrequently in children. Studies conducted in Australia and the United States, for example, found that about 15 per cent of the victims recalled their attacks beginning before they were 10 years of age.

Do women suffer most?

In most pain clinics, women with chronic muscle-tension headaches outnumber men by a substantial margin, though whether this indicates an actual preponderance of women sufferers in the general population or simply more women patients seeking relief remains to be determined. Dr. James W. Lance of the University of New South Wales in Sydney, Australia, estimated a 3-to-1 ratio of women patients over men. Despite statistics such as these, few experts believe that women suffer more tension headaches than men. Dr. Adrian M. Ostfeld of the University of Illinois College of Medicine maintained that Western societies have stereotyped headache as a woman's disease, associated with frailty, menstruation and frequent complaining. "Men," he said, "usually do not admit to headache unless they are frightened or incapacitated by it."

Nor is there any evidence that modern industrialized societies have a monopoly on muscle-tension head pain. "Headaches just don't know races, creeds or geographic distribution," said Dr. David R. Coddon of New York's Mount Sinai Medical Center Headache Clinic.

Within modern societies, however, a number of authorities claim that tension headaches strike city-dwellers more frequently than their country cousins. A city, by its very nature, is a crowded, anxious, pressure-producing environment, less likely to provide support and reassurance than a smaller, closely knit rural community. Indeed, city folks not only suffer more headaches, but the intensity of the headache may well be directly related to the size of the city. "The common garden variety headache," explained one New York City specialist, "is a symptom of a harried organism—and New Yorkers are harried."

City or country, the majority of people experience occasional muscle-contraction headaches. Whether they arise from psychological stress or physical exertion, they seldom last long and, if they occur only infrequently and without any significant pattern, they can reasonably be dismissed as of no consequence beyond the moment. Some people, unfortunately, find their systems responding with tension headaches several times a week. Certain patterns in the events surrounding the headache and the timing of its onset may be apparent to the sufferer and his family—the headache that comes on every afternoon on a high-pressure job, for example—but often the cause-and-effect relationship is so subtle as to escape notice by those close to the situation. The victims are in the grip of chronic muscle-tension headache, which has a major psychological component.

Because the causes of chronic headaches are likely to be hidden in the psyche, they may prove difficult to treat. But the occasional ones not only are readily relieved by simple measures but often can be prevented. Their immediate causes frequently are trivial, and because the pain arises only on occasion, its arrival generally can be linked to some triggering event. Once you have marked the cause of a common headache, you may be able to avoid it.

Among the most common precipitating factors are the physical stresses of awkward posture or eyestrain, mental stresses such as prolonged concentration or boredom, and emotional stresses such as excitement or anxiety, repressed anger or feelings of rejection. The trigger may bring on a headache only occasionally, as when infrequently used neck and shoulder muscles are held tense during gardening; or it may bring on a headache every day, as can occur among those who hunch up their shoulder to hold the telephone to their ear during the workday and then leave the office with a tension headache.

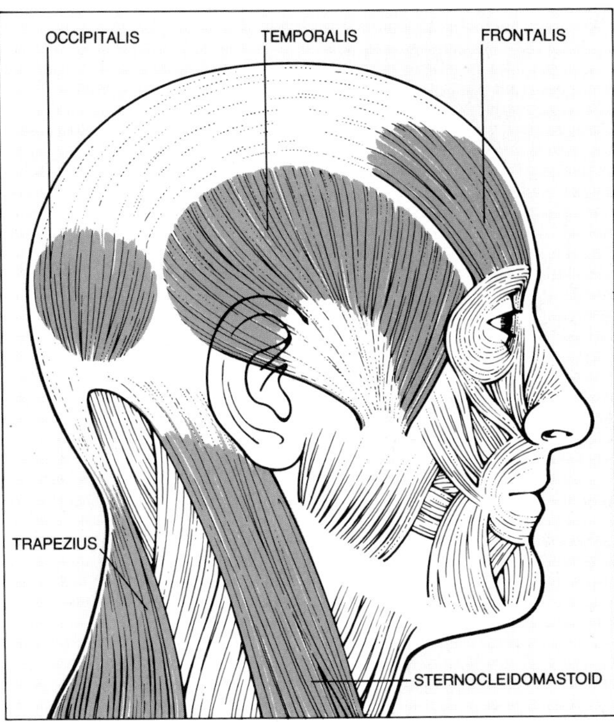

The head muscles that are most likely to tighten and cause a muscle-tension headache (reddish color above) can be affected by either physical or emotional stresses. A headache at the front of the head need not originate there: A tense trapezius muscle can set off a chain reaction, causing other muscles to seize, and producing pain in the forehead.

Hunting for hidden triggers

Isolating the trigger of a muscle-contraction headache usually requires that you make a dispassionate examination of the physical, mental and emotional habits of your daily life, whether at work, at home or at play. In taking this inventory, take into account the phenomenon of referred pain, for the trigger may well be located at some distance from the head. Because tension in back, shoulder and neck muscles can be referred to the head, the way you hold your body while

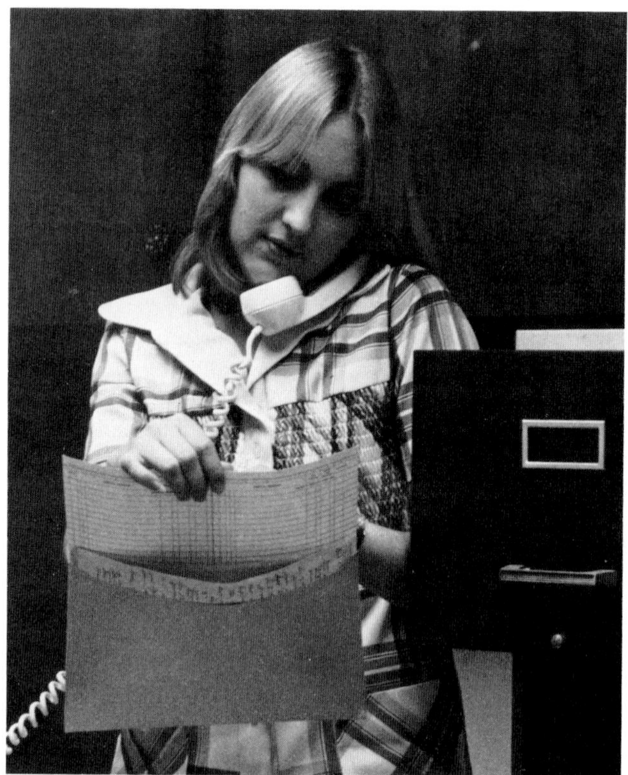

Chinning a telephone against her shoulder to free her hands, a busy secretary invites a so-called telephone headache—actually caused by muscle tension. The pain may be felt across the forehead, but it arises in neck and shoulder muscles kept in tension as head and shoulder are pressed together. The remedy is a change in telephone habits: Sit in a straight but relaxed position, hold the phone by hand, and breathe slowly to ease tension.

sitting, standing, working, driving or sleeping may cause a headache more often than you might expect.

Neck muscles, particularly, contract under stress. According to Dr. Marilyn Moffat of New York University, people under physical or emotional stress move their heads forward, tensing their neck muscles. The greater the stress, the farther forward the head moves. This tendency is often observed among drivers who, when caught in traffic or bad weather, sit anxiously with necks jutting forward, teeth clenched and hands tightly gripping the wheel.

The daily work of many people also tends to promote the neck posture that brings on headache. Office workers and students sit hunched over a desk, head forward, for long periods. Factory workers bend forward to perform precision assembly or machine work.

Even relaxation may lead the unwary into neck-tensing postures that cause headaches. At the end of the day, many people flop into a soft chair to read. The chair may feel comfortable, but its very softness forces a chin-on-chest posture that tenses neck muscles. Equally stressful is watching television while lying in bed, with the head propped on a pillow at right angles to the rest of the body. Dr. Joel R. Saper of the Michigan Headache and Neurological Institute was able to trace the muscle-contraction headaches of one patient to her weekly bridge game. Persistent questioning elicited the fact that she held her cards in her lap, straining her head and neck to look down at them. Finally Dr. Saper ordered her fitted with a cervical collar—the kind used to treat people who have injured their necks in automobile accidents—so that she had to hold her head upright. "To the patient's delight, and to ours as well," he wrote, "her headaches lessened."

Such measures are rarely necessary to prevent tension headaches caused by posture. Generally you can avoid these head pains by paying attention to the way you hold your body, whether you are reading in bed or driving a car, and by choosing equipment and furniture designed to keep the strains of body weight distributed naturally. Chairs and beds cause many muscle pains, including some of those that afflict the head.

Most experts recommend an orthopedic mattress firm enough not to sag under the sleeper's weight but sufficiently pliant to conform to the body's contours, particularly the weight-bearing hips and shoulders. The best sleeping posture is on the side, with the legs bent, the arms down and the head and neck supported by a pillow in their normal vertical alignment with the rest of the body.

If you can get to sleep only on your back, position the pillow so that it supports your neck as well as your head and place another pillow under your knees to relieve strain on your lower back. One specially designed therapeutic pillow, developed by Dr. Lionel A. Walpin of Cedars-Sinai Medical Center in Los Angeles, provides four different combinations of head and neck support. The central part of the pillow, where the head rests, is soft on one side and medium-firm on the other; on each side, the upper border offers a narrow, firm support for the neck while the opposite border provides a wider, firm neck support. Simply by turning the pillow around or flipping it over, the user can combine either a wide or narrow neck support with either a soft or firm headrest. Such pillows and similar cervical support devices are available at surgical- and orthopedic-supply houses.

Because many people now spend most of their days sitting down, well-designed seats are important in preventing muscle tension. A good chair should support your lower back, should enable you to shift position readily and should hold your body so that its load is borne primarily by the bony protuberances, called ischial tuberosities, located at the bottom of the pelvis.

Many modern easy chairs and sofas violate all three principles. Overstuffed seats, in particular, encourage poor posture by forcing body weight backward off the built-in supports of the pelvis. Most experts recommend harder chairs with relatively straight backs and armrests. The hard seats distribute the weight properly; the straight backs support lower, and sometimes upper, back muscles; and the armrests relieve tension on neck muscles by supporting the weight of the forearms. Rocking chairs are considered particularly good because their straight, high backs provide support for both the lower and upper spine while their rhythmic rocking action moves and stretches tensed muscles and induces an overall sense of relaxation.

The height of a chair seat should coincide with the fold at the back of your knees when your feet are comfortably planted on the floor. It should suit the height of a work surface, which should be at the level of the bottom of the elbows when the arms are straight below the shoulders. If a chair cannot be set to comfortable height, the relative heights of the seat and work surface can be adjusted by placing the chair on a platform or by sliding boards under the legs of the desk or work table.

These height standards are not met by automobile seats, which are very low. To lessen muscle fatigue and tension while driving, adjust the position of the seat so that your lower back is firmly supported by the seat. Your legs should be within easy reach of the floor pedals while remaining bent at the knees, and your hands should be able to hold the steering wheel while the upper arms fall comfortably onto the rib cage. Hold your head as erect as possible, centered over the torso with chin up.

Office seating also contributes to muscular tension and headache. It is an adage among orthopedists that the chairs executives give their secretaries are better than the swivel chairs they allow themselves. The movable backs of many such chairs are too loosely sprung to provide adequate support for the back, the seats are too soft for proper weight distribution and the armrests sometimes prevent the occupant from pulling the chair close enough to a desk to keep from craning the neck.

The typing chair, on the other hand, has none of these problems. But it must be properly adjusted: The small, lightly padded backrest should provide firm support from the small of the back to just below the shoulder blades. And the height of the seat should be adjusted to the user's height as well as to the task at hand. Typewriter keys should be located at waist height so the typist does not stress neck and shoulder muscles by reaching upward or by stooping downward toward the typewriter.

Sometimes headache-producing postural habits can be changed with the aid of inexpensive devices available at

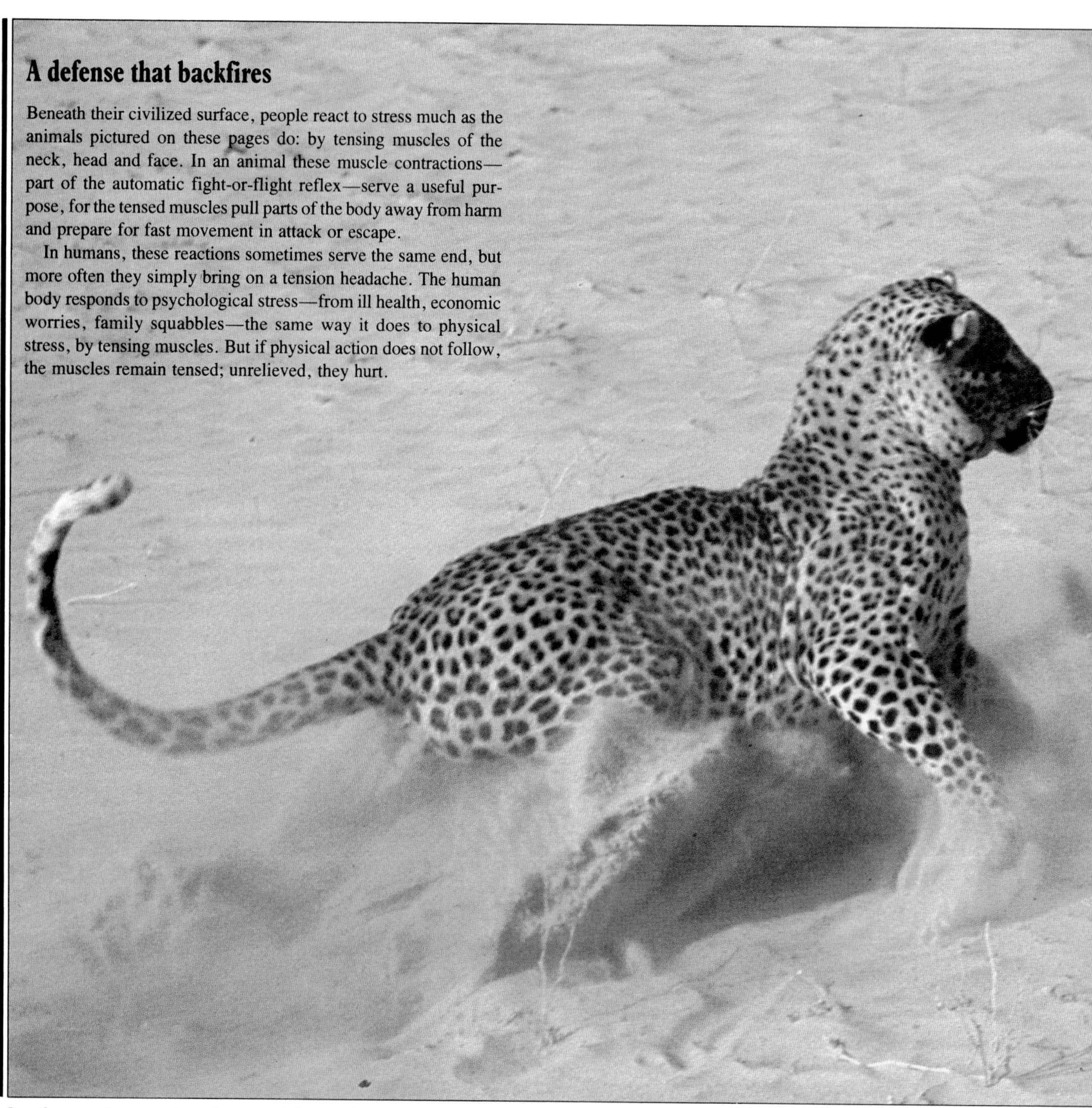

A defense that backfires

Beneath their civilized surface, people react to stress much as the animals pictured on these pages do: by tensing muscles of the neck, head and face. In an animal these muscle contractions—part of the automatic fight-or-flight reflex—serve a useful purpose, for the tensed muscles pull parts of the body away from harm and prepare for fast movement in attack or escape.

In humans, these reactions sometimes serve the same end, but more often they simply bring on a tension headache. The human body responds to psychological stress—from ill health, economic worries, family squabbles—the same way it does to physical stress, by tensing muscles. But if physical action does not follow, the muscles remain tensed; unrelieved, they hurt.

In a famous photograph by John Dominis, a baboon attacked by a leopard leaps back in typical fighting posture: mouth open wide, teeth bared, head drawn into shoulders, back arched, hair raised to increase apparent size. When a human being responds to stress this way, the muscular tension often cannot be released in physical action, and a headache results.

A wolf, tail between legs, assumes its fight-or-flight pose as it defends its turf with fangs displayed in a snarl, back arched and ears flattened. Defensive reactions such as an arched back and pulled-down head are used by many creatures, including humans. Tensed back and neck muscles signal muscles in the front of the head to tighten, causing the typical tension headache.

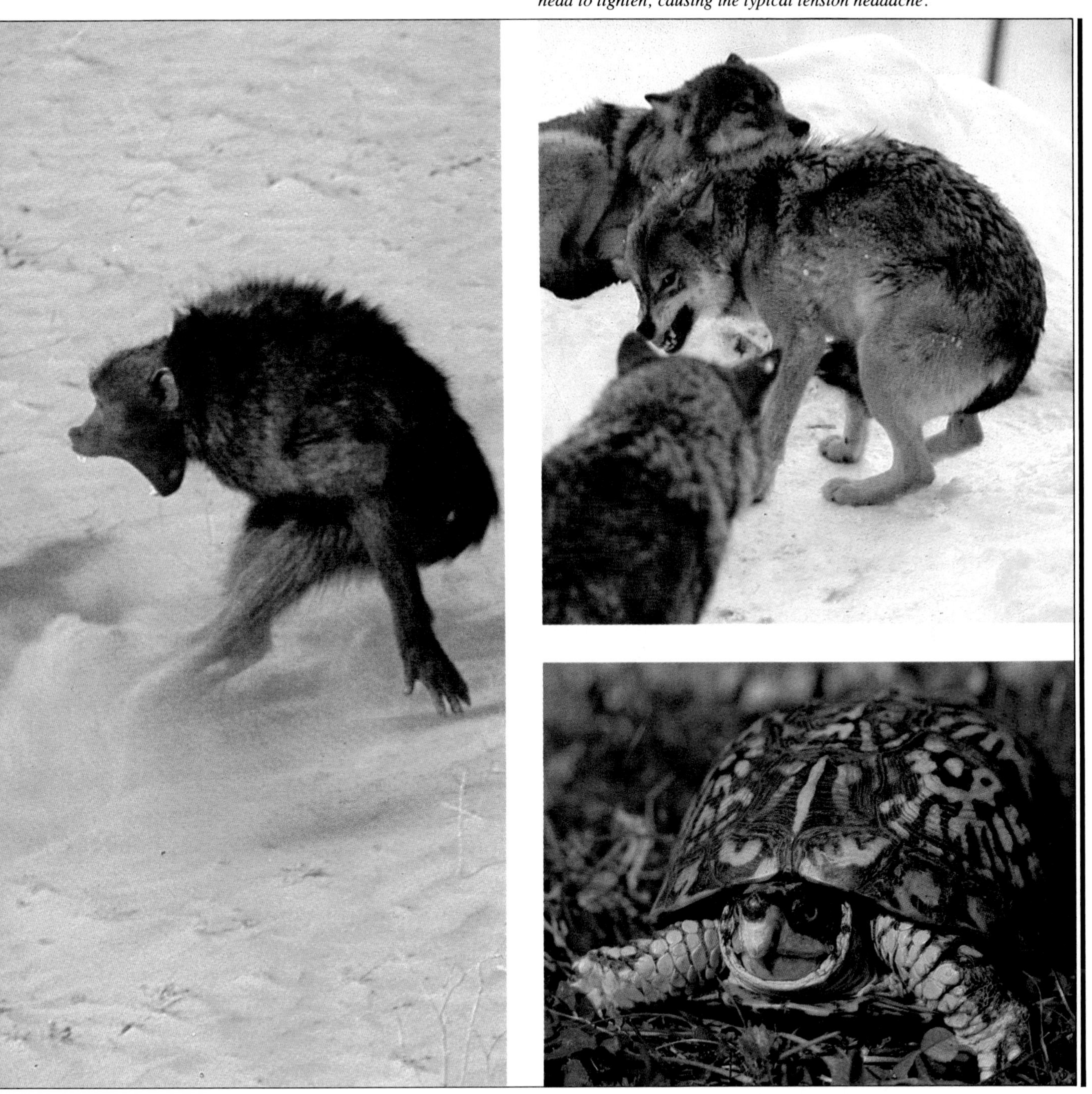

The ultimate example of tense neck muscles as a defensive reaction is the turtle: at the first sign of danger, its strong muscles automatically contract and pull its head into the protective shell.

office-supply stores. Book or paper stands, for example, can help prevent neck tension by raising written material from a horizontal desk top to a more accessible viewing angle. Special holsters for telephones, which balance the receiver on the shoulder while leaving the hands free for other work, allow office workers to avoid hunching up their shoulder to hold the phone—a common source of tension headache among secretaries and salespeople.

Even the best-designed equipment and the most careful attention to posture cannot prevent a strain on muscles if you are forced to sustain one position for long periods of time. Rest breaks are thus essential to preventing headache, whether you are driving a car, working at a desk or reading a book in an easy chair. The most important step is frequent shifts in position. Stand up, walk around and move as many parts of your body as you can.

Exercising the body to help the head

Some exercises are designed especially to relieve tension not only in head muscles but also in the neck, shoulder and back muscles linked to headaches *(pages 50-59)*. A few of these routines, such as the neck roll described on page 56, can be done while you are sitting at a desk. To relieve neck tension while driving, drop your shoulders down as far as possible while simultaneously reaching upward with your head—in effect, making a longer neck. During rest stops, rotate your arms and shoulders, perform some deep-knee bends and take a brisk walk.

In addition to headaches traced to posture, head pains may arise from eyestrain—although most authorities think this cause is much overrated. Students and office workers often complain of eyestrain headaches, for example, but many such pains are triggered during intensive study or other close-up work, suggesting that poor neck posture is as likely a cause as eyestrain. And Dr. Maurice J. Martin of the Mayo Clinic pointed out that "the necessity to perform unpleasant work, or to continue an involvement in an emotionally repugnant situation" may be more important than eyestrain in these cases.

Eyestrain can often be ruled out by noting the time of the headache's onset—if your head hurts when you wake up in the morning, eyestrain is hardly likely to be at fault. Among susceptible individuals, the headache usually develops in the afternoon or evening. The pain may be felt only around the eyes, or may be referred to the forehead, temple or back of the head. If it recurs regularly after a day's intensive close work, visit an ophthalmologist, for true eyestrain most often bothers those whose vision needs correction with eyeglasses—and those who already wear them may need further corrections over the years.

Eyestrain headache can be set off by any of a variety of triggers. One source is, again, muscles—in this case, the special ones that focus the eye lens by altering its shape. When you look at distant objects, these muscles are essentially relaxed, but when you focus on something close, as in reading a book, the muscles contract to squeeze the lens into a more convex shape. If you read or do other close work steadily for a long period, the muscles involved tire and may cause pain. This headache-producing effect, termed by one doctor "freezing in focus," is easily countered by interrupting the close work every once in a while to allow the lens to relax and refocus on a distant object—looking out the window is a good way.

However, continual refocusing of the eyes can also hurt. Repeated shifting of view up and down, as occurs when museums' visitors look from guidebooks to exhibits, or when students repeatedly glance from desks to chalkboards, sometimes triggers what is referred to as academic headache. Part of the problem is refocusing, part movement. Eye muscles are accustomed to continual side-to-side shifting, but not to continual up-and-down movements, which fatigue them easily. To prevent or relieve this type of headache, raise the reading material closer to eye level, thus reducing the up-and-down shift in gaze.

Improper lighting conditions are likely to aggravate eyestrain headaches. The fault may be working with too little light or with rapidly flickering light, such as may appear on television screens and computer display terminals. Glare, or extreme contrasts of light within the field of vision, may trigger a headache by causing a protective contraction, or squinting, of eye muscles. This is a problem for nighttime drivers facing the bright headlights of oncoming traffic and is common at beaches and ski areas, where sunlight reflects off snow and sand. But glare can also be encountered indoors, from reflections off a glossy printed page, from watching television in a room that otherwise is dark, or even from reading in a spot of bright light surrounded by darkness. To prevent the aggravating effects of glare, arrange lamps indoors for even, modulated illumination *(pages 42-43)*, wear sunglasses and a brimmed hat outdoors, and when driving at night, shift your gaze to the right side of the lane as an oncoming car goes by.

First aid for tight muscles

Acute muscle-tension headaches, no matter how they are triggered, typically go away in a few hours even if you do nothing more for them than get some rest. By lying down and closing your eyes for a few minutes, you provide your body with an opportunity to unwind taut muscles; at the same time, you remove yourself from the environment where the tension erupted. Allowing yourself this brief time out may also change your perception of the events that set off the pain: Mountains frequently shrink back to molehills after a little reflection.

However, if you require ''fast, fast, fast'' relief, then one of the mild over-the-counter analgesics such as aspirin or acetaminophen should prove nearly as effective as the advertisements for those products promise. Analgesics do not of themselves transform muscle tension into muscle relaxation; rather, by a series of chemical interventions *(Chapter 5)*, they simply buy time by reducing the sensation of pain. If, at the end of three or four hours when the drug's effects diminish, the stresses underlying the headache have not been resolved and the muscles repaired, then the pain will only surface again.

Taking specific measures to counter tight muscles is, then, an excellent adjunct to aspirin therapy. A gentle massage of shoulder, neck and head muscles is one dependably effective measure. There are many manuals offering detailed descriptions of how to apply massage, but in truth, any laying on of hands that combines tender rubbing, kneading and warming of skin and muscles will have a therapeutic effect. During the massage, keep your eyes closed and try to concentrate on the sensations being elicited rather than on the day's concerns.

Ideally, have someone else gently rub, knead and warm your muscles; if this is not convenient, self-massage will work almost as well. Begin by relaxing the ''worry muscles'' of your forehead and temple: Place your hands across the forehead, with your fingertips touching, and gently smooth the skin from the center toward the temples. Then smooth the brow upward toward the hair line, gently sliding one hand after the other.

For the neck and shoulders, grab handfuls of the tense muscles between your thumb and fingertips, in the same way that you would grab a kitten by the scruff of the neck; squeeze gently but firmly and let go. Repeat this squeezing action over the entire surface of the muscles. When you find hard areas that seem particularly tender, press these knots with firm, circular motions of the fingertips.

Taking a few judicious sips of wine can also bring muscle relaxation and with it relief, provided the headache is in fact a muscle-tension headache and not a vascular type, such as those produced by food, air pollution or high altitude—alcohol will make them worse. And more than one drink can serve as a trigger to bring on a vascular headache.

Exercise of the sort recommended to prevent tension headaches can also cure them. Often a pleasant walk will do as well. Walking uses and thus stretches many tensed muscles, gives you an opportunity to get away from whatever is bothering you, and if you choose your route with care, may also reward with delights of its own—a stroll in the park, along a riverbank, up an attractive city street, can do wonders for routine pressures and worries.

Another excellent remedy for the occasional headache is heat treatment. Warmth increases the blood supply to taut muscles, making them more pliable; at the same time, it increases circulation, helping to carry away pain-inducing toxins that accumulate in strained muscle tissue. A heating pad, a not-too-hot water bottle or a hot, moist compress placed at the back of the neck are all trusted home remedies with proved physiological benefits. A comfortably hot bath will do even better because it treats the whole body. Fill the tub so that you can submerge up to the chin, and stay there for 15 to 20 minutes. (You can maintain a fairly consistent temperature if you permit a trickle of hot water to run from the faucet while you soak.)

Psychological causes, physical effects

Although acute muscle-tension headaches are triggered by both physical and emotional stresses, chronic muscle-tension headaches are almost always associated with emotional problems. Just why some people should succumb to chronic muscle-tension headaches while others do not is still far from being established, but a number of explanations are offered. Some psychiatrists believe that everyone exercises a certain amount of unconscious choice in the disorder developed under stress. Some individuals develop nervous stomach, others backache. The majority hurt in the head, which is the center of thought and feeling and consequently the most susceptible part of the anatomy. The choice of headache may also be suggested, at a subconscious level, by the example of a parent who suffered headaches during the individual's formative years. Headaches thus become a familiar complaint, appearing to be hereditary but, in fact, arising in response to conditioning.

Even more varied are the characteristics that seem to identify the victims of chronic headaches. According to headache specialist Dr. James W. Lance, likely candidates for chronic tension headaches can sometimes be recognized by telltale physical and postural characteristics. "The outward appearance of a patient with tension headaches," writes Dr. Lance, "may clearly show the lifetime habit of muscle contraction in

Lighting to avoid eyestrain

According to lighting experts, fewer than one home in 10 is properly illuminated for the everyday tasks—such as reading and television viewing—that can bring on eyestrain headaches. Fortunately, once lighting problems are recognized they are usually easily remedied *(right)*.

The two lighting conditions often blamed for eyestrain—too little light or too great a contrast between dim and bright areas of a room—can overtax eye muscles and cause tension pain. To avoid these faults, fill each room with diffuse background light and illuminate special areas with bright "key" light. Either fill or key illumination can be provided by natural, incandescent or fluorescent sources, although fluorescents are usually preferred for fine work because they give bright but even, glare-free and almost shadow-free light.

More important than the type of light source is its location and its shade. Every source should be shaded so that it cannot be seen directly. Translucent shades are better than opaque because they add to general fill illumination and reduce contrast; for the same reason, experts recommend shades that throw light up as well as down. It is easy to control brightness by moving lamps or changing bulbs. The best locations keep sources (and their reflections) out of direct view and cast no shadows in work areas.

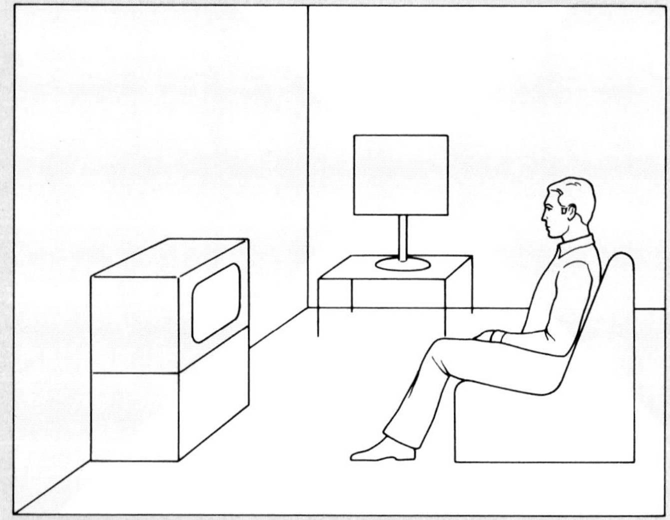

WATCHING TELEVISION
Illuminate the entire room—particularly around the TV set—with soft, indirect light from lamps or fixtures placed where they cannot be seen either directly or as reflections in the screen. Never watch television in a dark room; the contrast between screen and surroundings is a severe strain.

a furrowed brow and deep-set facial lines." Not only are the exaggerated muscle contractions that etch those lines sufficient cause by themselves for periodic headaches, but the anxiety and discomfort they denote suggest a personality given to excessive psychological tension. Other telltale signs are a clenched jaw, a twitching scalp, hands that even in a nominally resting state are often folded into tight fists, feet or legs always twisted or crossed—all fair indicators of an individual who is under emotional stress and whose muscles do not readily relax.

To check the connection between headaches and an inability to relax, Dr. Lance and his colleagues conducted an armchair test. The subject was seated in an ordinary armless chair and asked to extend an arm. The investigator, supporting the extended arm by placing his own hand under the wrist, told the individual to let his arm go completely loose as if it were being held there by an imaginary armrest of the chair. The investigator then removed his hand. Dr. Lance found that the majority of chronic muscle-tension sufferers were unable to relax at will and that their arms remained suspended in air for several moments, held there by muscles that remained tense.

In a similar pillow test, each individual was asked to lie down on a couch. As the investigator placed his hands under the head, the subject was told to relax as though being supported by a pillow. As before, the muscles of chronic tension sufferers remained active, holding the head airborne even after the investigator removed his hands.

To see if you are similarly subject to headache-producing tension, try these tests with the help of a friend. Your results may be influenced by knowledge of what the tests are designed to prove, but extreme states of muscle tension will show through nonetheless.

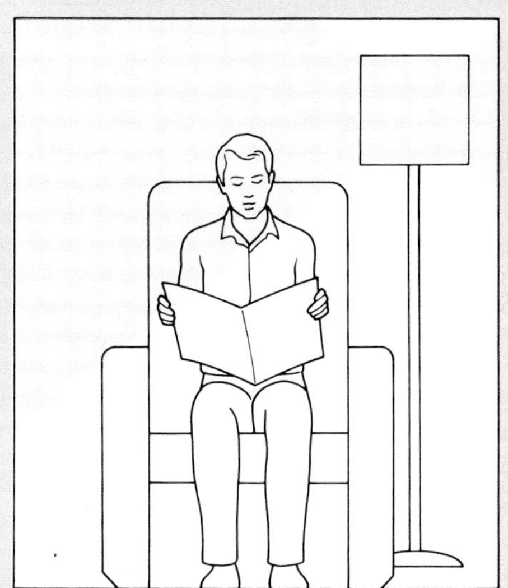

READING IN A CHAIR
Put a lamp with a 100-watt incandescent bulb behind your reading chair so that the light shines over your shoulder. If the lamp must be beside you, the lower edge of its shade should be just below eye level.

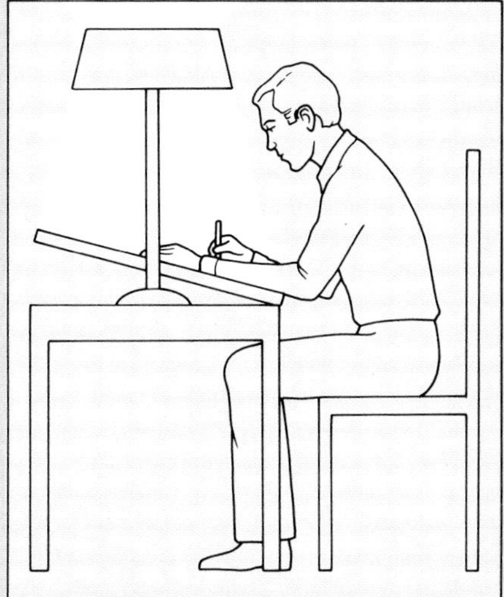

WRITING AT A DESK
Place a lamp 12 to 18 inches tall on the desk, 15 inches from the paper and opposite your writing hand. This will keep shadows off your writing. Use a 100-watt incandescent or 20-watt fluorescent bulb.

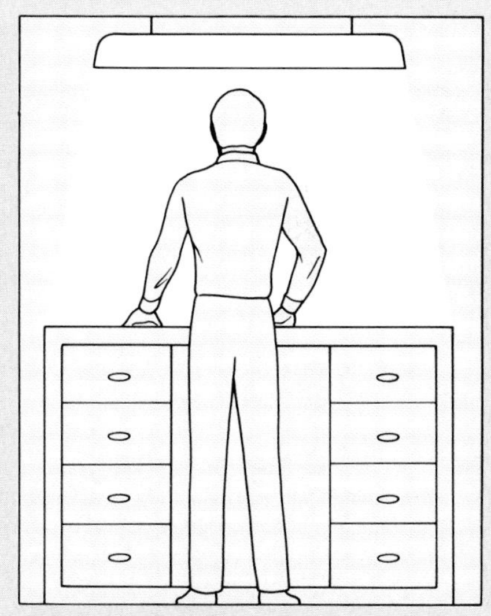

WORKING IN A SHOP
Light the workbench with a shielded overhead fluorescent lamp about as long as the bench. Use a fixture that holds two 40-watt bulbs. If necessary, illuminate very fine detail with a small incandescent lamp.

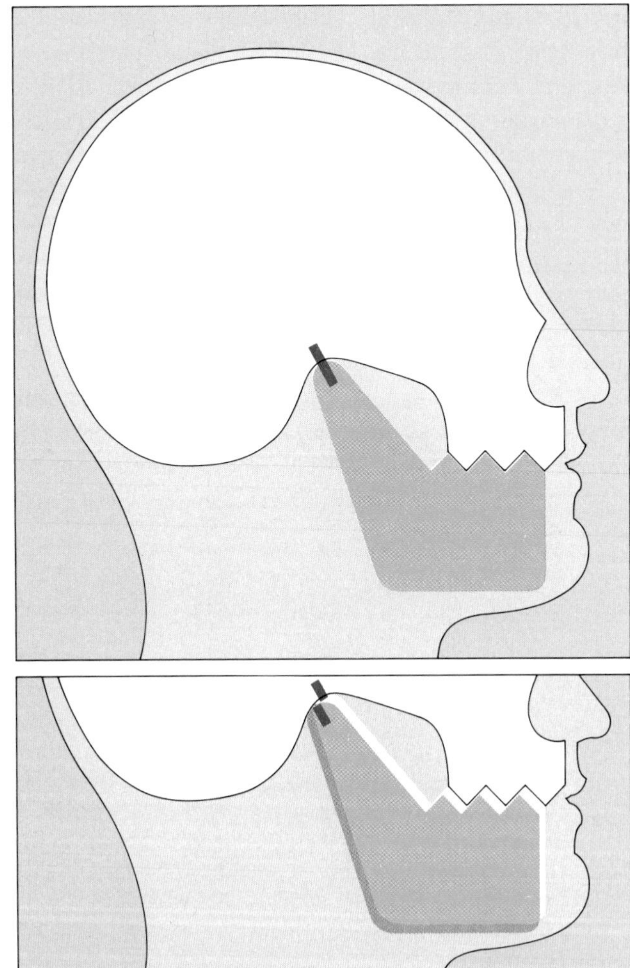

Physicians and dentists disagree about how many headaches are caused by a jaw misalignment called temporomandibular joint syndrome, or TMJ, which is diagramed above along with a normal jaw (top). Ordinarily, the jaw joint lines up (heavy red lines) so that teeth mesh. But if jaw and teeth are offset (lower drawing), jaw muscles strain to compensate, causing symptoms such as those listed opposite. According to dental specialists, this stress causes pain in eight headache victims out of 10; headache physicians think it a less common cause of head pain.

Probing deeper into the psyche, Drs. A. P. Friedman, T.J.C. von Storch, and H. H. Merritt of the Headache Clinic of Montefiore Hospital and Columbia University in New York City, analyzed 1,000 patients who suffered from recurring tension headaches and found them unable to cope with various economic, social, physical or intellectual demands placed on them. Circumstances that might seem manageable, even positively stimulating, to other individuals, seemed highly stressful to the chronic headache victim. The investigators found that the most frequent source of anxiety and tension was hostile impulses toward members of the family or to some authority figure outside the family, such as an employer or a colleague.

Internal conflict was also cited as a factor contributing to chronic tension headaches by three researchers from the Mayo Clinic: Dr. M. J. Martin, Dr. H. P. Rome and W. M. Swenson. They defined three problem areas: vacillating feelings of dependency and aggression toward parents, spouse or work associates; feelings of inadequacy or uncertainty relating to sexuality; and control or repression of the overt expression of those emotions, chiefly anger, that are in some manner socially unacceptable.

Dr. Martin and others in the field have found chronic tension-headache sufferers to be typically sensitive, perfectionistic and apprehensive, with associated problems of insomnia, irritability, restlessness, inability to concentrate and poor memory. Virtually every researcher also cites depression as a distinctive characteristic, although it is not clear whether the depression leads to chronic headaches or the other way around. Dr. Fred Sheftell of The New England Center for Headache reported that many of his patients, when asked if they are depressed, will say with assurance that they are not and then give a recitation of classic physical symptoms of depression: sleep disturbances, constipation, lack of appetite, weakness and fatigue, heart palpitations and sexual disturbances.

Dr. Sheftell said that, as a practical matter, it is not really important to determine whether the depression or the chronic muscle-tension headaches come first, only to recognize that when both are present, both must be treated. "Anyone with a chronic pain problem," he said, "is going to be somewhat depressed; that person is bound to feel a sense of debilitation, a sense of betrayal of his own body." And because depression serves to lessen tolerance for pain, an individual burdened with chronic muscle-tension headache and depression is caught up in a cycle of pain in which the two disorders feed off one another.

Some psychological causes of chronic headaches express themselves in recognizable actions that ultimately bring on the pain. Facial mannerisms, such as frequent frowning or squinting, can provoke a muscle-contraction headache. Even smiling, ordinarily beneficial, can hurt if prolonged. The nervous habits of clenching the jaws and grinding the teeth during sleep are other potential triggers; Dr. R. G. Every, a dental surgeon in New Zealand, thinks that nocturnal tooth grinding is "fang-sharpening," an evolutionary relic that he interprets as a form of repressed aggression. Headaches have also been triggered by day-long gum chewing, often a nervous habit.

Susceptibility to these types of headache is greatly increased by any abnormality or disease of the jaw joint, such as arthritis or the subtle imbalance of the bite referred to as temporomandibular joint syndrome *(left)*. Anyone whose bite is misaligned can strain his head muscles. When he chews, he bears down on a set of teeth whose hundreds of tiny peaked and indented surfaces fail to mesh as nature intended. The jaws shift their relative positions until some less stressful position, or occlusion, is arrived at, and the temporomandibular muscles must accommodate themselves as best they can.

The complications of a poor bite may take years to develop, depending on the degree of misalignment and the sensitivity of the individual. It is not unusual to find the problems appearing in young adulthood, a decade or more after extensive teeth straightening. Or they may appear in later life soon after the loss of teeth, particularly back teeth, to cavities or gum disease.

Specialists differ widely on the importance of temporomandibular problems in headaches. Dr. Sheftell estimated that, although bite imbalances exist in as much as 20 per cent

Clues to TMJ—the jaw headache

To help determine whether patients' headaches are caused by the jaw misalignment of TMJ syndrome *(drawings, opposite)*, one specialist in this ailment, Dr. Brendon Stack, asks them a series of questions like the 12 below. If you suffer frequent headaches and answer yes to six or more of these questions, TMJ might contribute; consult your dentist.

1. Do you hear a grating, clicking or popping sound in your jaw when you chew? Does chewing give you a headache?

2. Do you experience stuffiness, pressure, blockage, ringing, hissing or buzzing in your ears?

3. Are you often unaccountably tired, dizzy or nauseated?

4. Is your jaw painful or locked when you awaken, or do you sometimes wake up with a headache?

5. Do you have pain or soreness in your jaw joints, jawbones or teeth, forehead, temples, tongue, chewing muscles, the side of your neck, back of your head or behind your eyes?

6. Is it difficult to move your jaw from side to side or front to back, or is it painful to press on your jaw joints or on the cheeks just below them?

7. Do you gulp your food or have difficulty chewing?

8. Are you missing back teeth, or have you had extensive dental crowns or bridges put in as dental repairs?

9. Do you clench or grind your teeth?

10. Have you had whiplash, or a blow to the head? Have you ever been treated with a cervical collar or neck traction?

11. Do drugs no longer relieve your headaches?

12. Does your jaw deviate to the left or right when you open your mouth wide? When your mouth is wide open, is it difficult to insert three fingers vertically?

of the population, they are a primary cause of headaches in no more than 2 to 3 per cent of The New England Center's patients. At the other extreme, Dr. Harold Gelb of the College of Medicine and Dentistry in New Jersey estimated that 75 per cent of all muscle-contraction headaches are triggered by temporomandibular joint syndrome.

A special mouthpiece or simple dental repairs can realign the jaw for a normal bite, but may not eliminate head pain, according to Dr. Arthur S. Freese, a British dental surgeon who studied the connection between headache and problems of the teeth and jaw. He concluded that the jaw misalignment can indicate "deep-seated emotional problems that must be treated with care, difficulties to be solved by a psychiatrist rather than a dentist."

Strategies for fighting chronic pain

Because the blame for a chronic tension headache is so difficult to trace, prevention and treatment present complex challenges. Permanent relief may come only through changes in outlook and daily living habits. Some people find it relatively easy to reprogram themselves so that they can avoid headache-producing stress—or so that they can cope without painful consequences; others ultimately decide that the guidance of professional counselors is needed.

Most of the rules for dealing comfortably with everyday tensions sound like the advice a grandmother might give for healthful living:

- Keep your daily routine at a comfortable level. If you are trying to fit more events and responsibilities into your day than you can handle without strain, winnow out some of the nonessentials. You may have to keep track of the time devoted to certain activities and limit them.
- Get enough sleep.
- Eat a balanced, adequate diet, at meals that are reasonably scheduled. Try to keep meals unhurried, pleasurable occasions, free of pressure from business discussions, family disputes or forced sociability.
- Exercise regularly. The kind of physical exertion is not particularly important unless it involves stresses like those you are trying to alleviate. If you tend to play everything

Can faulty jaws affect strength?

Some dentists who attribute headaches to jaws thrown out of line in the so-called temporomandibular joint (TMJ) syndrome also speculate that the condition has more far-reaching consequences. They believe that TMJ may be responsible for a general decrease of physical strength.

These authorities suggest that misalignment of the jaw joint overburdens jaw muscles. When they try to pull the joint back into line, a kind of chain reaction makes other muscles tense as if to compensate—first those nearby in the head, neck and upper back, then those farther away. The result may be that muscles far removed from the jaw can be robbed of strength. Relieving TMJ syndrome, adherents believe, may restore strength to the affected muscles—a matter that could be of vital importance to athletes.

Evidence supporting this idea is scanty, but several athletes who have worn special plastic and metal mouthpieces designed to correct TMJ have benefitted from improved performance. Joe Tyler, an Olympic bobsledder for the United States, found that when he wore a corrective mouthpiece he could lift more weight with his legs, raising 135 pounds 20 times instead of four. He credited the mouthpiece and his increased leg strength with lowering his "push off" time—the time it takes to cover the first 50 meters of a bobsled run—to less than five seconds, a goal he had been pursuing for six years.

A similar mouthpiece was worn by American discus thrower Al Oerter *(right, bottom),* a TMJ sufferer, during qualification trials for the 1980 Olympics. Oerter, who had won the event at four successive Olympiads between 1956 and 1968, was attempting a comeback at the age of 43. He finished fourth—the top three qualified—but he heaved the discus nearly 228 feet, for the longest throw of his career.

Demonstrating with a model of a skull, Dr. Richard Kaufman, a New York orthodontist, inserts a plastic-and-wire mouthpiece that brings jawbones into line. In a real skull, the mouthpiece would fill gaps between improperly meshing teeth to eliminate misalignment that is blamed for some headaches.

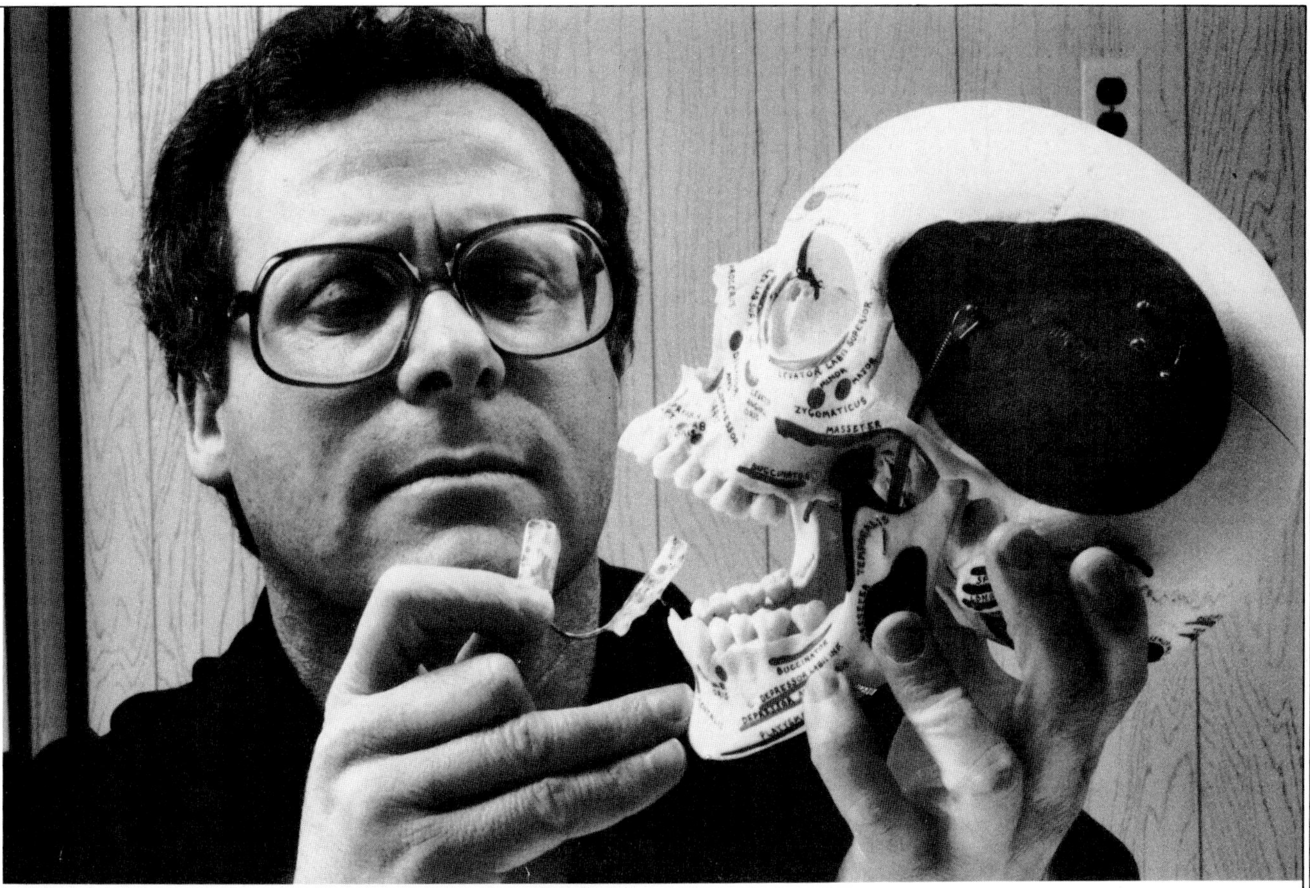

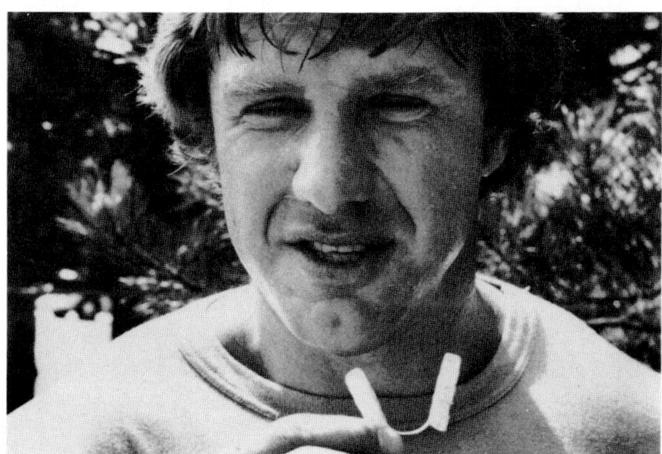

Discus champion Al Oerter shows off a mouthpiece custom-made for him by Dr. Kaufman to correct his jaw misalignment and keep him from overburdening his jaw muscles. The mouthpiece hooks to Oerter's back teeth and is easy to insert and remove.

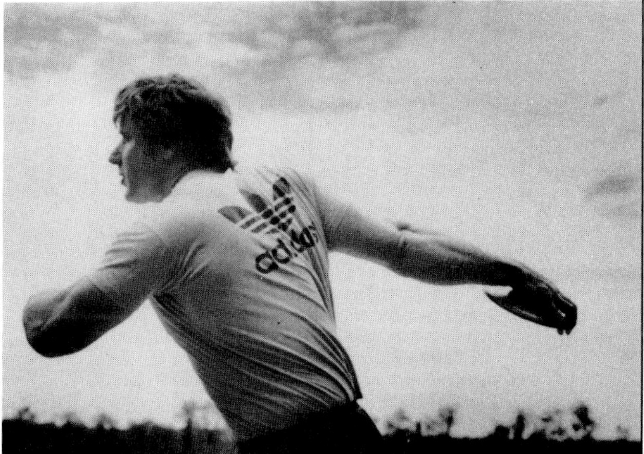

His mouthpiece in place, his jaw problems temporarily forgotten, Al Oerter hurls the discus. He credited the mouthpiece with increasing his strength and lengthening his throw by three to five feet. The device, said Oerter, works only when he bites down on it.

to win, then competitive sports such as tennis or golf are less likely to prove beneficial than swimming or hiking.

• Allot time for recreation—reading, socializing or anything else that is enjoyable, different from your full-time concerns and free of tension.

The idyllic existence prescribed by Grandmother is rarely attainable. Tension and stress, despite the best efforts to avoid them, are inevitable consequences of modern life. They can be reduced before they bring on a headache, however, by applying well-established techniques for relaxation. Simple rest is one—lying down for a while or stretching out in a chair will help. Exercise is another; joggers report that relief from tension is one of the major benefits of running. There are also several forms of mind-body control that induce relaxation, including yoga, transcendental meditation and biofeedback *(Chapter 6);* all have antecedents in ancient meditative practices of the Orient.

One scheme, known generally as the relaxation response, has proved particularly effective in helping some muscle-tension headache sufferers to help themselves. The technique was devised in the 1970s by Dr. Herbert Benson and his associates at Harvard University, based on studies that confirmed the ability of traditional meditative practices such as yoga to bring physiological benefits, including decreased heart rate and decreased production of body chemicals associated with stress. Benson proposed that the ability to slow down such processes was the body's protective mechanism against the fight-or-flight response, the reaction blamed for many headaches.

The relaxation response, unlike the automatic fight-or-flight response, must be evoked by an act of will under prescribed conditions. These Dr. Benson listed as an environment that is quiet and without distraction; a comfortable position in which to practice; a word, phrase or sound that can be repeated over and over again (the equivalent of the *mantra* in transcendental meditation); and, most important of all, a passive attitude. Once these requirements are satisfied, he asserted, an individual can learn to relax every muscle in the body.

Dr. Benson's method has since been modified by other researchers, some of whom use filmstrips and recordings of instructions delivered in a soothing voice to teach relaxation. The script for one such program, prepared in collaboration by Dr. J. M. Ferguson of the University of California at San Diego, J. N. Marquis of Stanford University and Dr. C. B. Taylor of the University of Utah, begins by explaining how to release tension in each of the major muscle groups.

"Put the palms of your hands together in front of you," the script directs, "and push them together as hard as you can. This will stretch the biceps muscles in both of your arms. Keep pushing until your arms begin to fatigue, until they are quivering with tenseness, and quickly let go. Let your arms flop back on the chair and study the wave of relaxation, the lack of tension in them, as they relax. Notice the contrast between how the muscles feel when they are tensed and relaxed. It is this difference between tension, being uptight, and relaxation, that you want to learn to control. The feeling of letting go is the feeling of relaxing. You will soon be able to tell your whole body to let go, to relax in the same way."

Turning to the muscles most often involved in tension headaches, the script says, "Check your forehead. Let it smooth out. Let the furrows in your brow flatten out and the tensions leave that part of your face. Feel the lack of tension in your eyebrows. Let this feeling spread to the muscles around your eyes, to your eyelids, and eye muscles, and then flow down into your cheeks, lips and tongue. Let your jaw hang slack and allow the relaxed feeling to spread up into your temples." The program concludes with instructions for deep-breathing exercises, accompanied by repetitions of the word "relax." The authors assert that, with practice, an individual can learn to use the breathing and word-repetition exercises alone to achieve the desired state of relaxation.

When preventive measures fail, then nonprescription analgesics such as aspirin or acetaminophen may temporarily relieve the pain of a chronic headache, as they do most others. However, people suffering from recurrent bouts of tension headache sometimes overuse analgesics, taking 10 to 20 tablets daily. In those quantities, according to Dr. Joel Saper, analgesics are "unquestionably hazardous to mind and body." The excessive doses somehow lower the pain threshold, requiring the use of larger and larger quantities to achieve relief. And although analgesics are among the safest medicines, they can cause harm *(pages 158-163)*. Alternatively, some doctors are able to relieve chronic tension headache by locating tender spots in the neck or shoulder muscles that trigger pain in the head. These pain centers are then either sprayed or injected with a local anesthetic to numb them and buy time for the muscle to unknot.

Analgesics block the transmission of pain but do not relieve the muscle tension or the psychological stresses behind a chronic headache. More direct action is offered by prescription minor tranquilizers such as diazepam and chlordiazepoxide. Unlike analgesics, tranquilizers reduce both the emotional and physical reactions to stress, relieving anxiety and relaxing muscles at the same time.

These minor tranquilizers may prove counterproductive, however. In some patients they bring on depression—itself often implicated in chronic headaches. For such people, more powerful drugs called antidepressants are often prescribed. They are thought to counter chronic headaches by increasing the availability of norepinephrine and serotonin, body chemicals that regulate moods. Antidepressants have also proved effective in preventing chronic headaches in which depression is not a significant factor; this unforeseen benefit may be linked to the drugs' complex and as yet poorly understood role in raising the body's tolerance of pain.

Tranquilizers and antidepressants can be useful in relieving or preventing intractable tension headaches. But Dr. Arnold P. Friedman, formerly professor of neurology at Columbia University, warned that drugs of any sort are not sufficient. "It is vital," wrote Dr. Friedman, "that the person who suffers from recurrent muscle-contraction headache recognize the necessity of tracking down the 'trigger' or provoking factor, if prevention of repeated episodes of pain is the goal."

In the most serious cases, tracking down the trigger is a lengthy process, requiring the temporary relief provided by drugs, the insight and understanding of a family doctor, neurologist or psychiatrist, and the patience and perseverance of the patient in facing and fighting the pain. ❋

Common aches for the young, severe ones for the old

The most common headaches—muscle-tension, toxic vascular and migraine—are predominantly afflictions of young adulthood. Many begin during childhood: Among 9,000 Swedish schoolchildren under 15 years of age, 58 per cent had already suffered headaches. The frequency and severity of the head pains peak during the young-adult years, and then, for mysterious reasons, taper off between the ages of 40 and 50. In the case of muscle-tension headaches, it may be that older people have learned to cope with the stresses that formerly triggered their attacks.

The relief that comes with age often is costly. For many middle-aged and old people, the common head pains are replaced by more serious headaches: temporal arteritis, trigeminal neuralgia or cluster headache. All cause severe, even excruciating, pain on one side of the face or head. Untreated, all can lead to dire consequences. Temporal arteritis can cause blindness, and the agony of cluster and neuralgia headaches drives some victims to thoughts of suicide.

Because these severe, one-sided headaches are often hard to tell apart, specialists have devised several guides for identifying them. Temporal arteritis causes a persistent, burning pain in one temple, where the affected artery is often visibly inflamed. Attacks occur at random. Trigeminal neuralgia and cluster headaches may occur in patterns of several per day, then vanish for months or years at a time. But the pain of true cluster headaches is boring, as if caused by a drill bit, while the pain of trigeminal neuralgia is razor-sharp. Neuralgic attacks are jabs of pain lasting 20 to 30 seconds, and rarely occur during the night; cluster headaches typically last half an hour or more, often waking their victims from sleep.

All three headaches can be relieved, sometimes permanently, by drugs or surgery. Prompt treatment of temporal arteritis is essential before vision is lost. A sample of arterial tissue is used to confirm the diagnosis, then hormonal drugs such as cortisone and prednisone are given. Severe cases of trigeminal neuralgia are treated with injections of alcohol to give temporary relief, or with surgery to cut the responsible nerve. Drugs can suppress the pain of cluster headaches, but living longer may provide permanent relief: Cluster headaches often disappear after the patient reaches the age of 60.

Exercises to ease strain

The most effective treatment for muscle-tension headaches is simple to prescribe: Relax the muscles that produce the grip of pain. But for those people who suffer from chronic muscle-tension headaches, simple relaxation is quite often maddeningly elusive. Many suffer, headache experts point out, because they have unconsciously trained certain headache-causing muscles to remain tense: When muscles are tensed frequently, they become habitually tight.

Muscles can be trained to relax the same way they are strengthened—through exercise. Like strengthening exercises, the anti-headache exercises are widely varied. Most concentrate on neck and face muscles—the gentle neck-stretching movements pictured below and described in detail on pages 56 and 57 are but one type. Other routines aim at different muscles throughout the body. Even the action of breathing is important; breathing the right way lessens the fatigue that contributes to headache.

None of these exercises are strenuous. However, anyone who is suffering from a circulatory disorder or bone or muscle ailment should check with a doctor before beginning the exercises. Some routines pictured are variants of a type called isometric, in which muscles are exerted but remain stationary. In the process blood pressure may be sharply raised and the heart strained. When isometric exercises are used for relaxation, however, exertion is only momentary.

People who have mastered the routines become sensitive to the signals of approaching tension and can often ward off an impending headache through a special technique known as focusing. For a minute or two they imagine the exercises, thus signaling the muscles to relax—and stopping head pain before it can get under way.

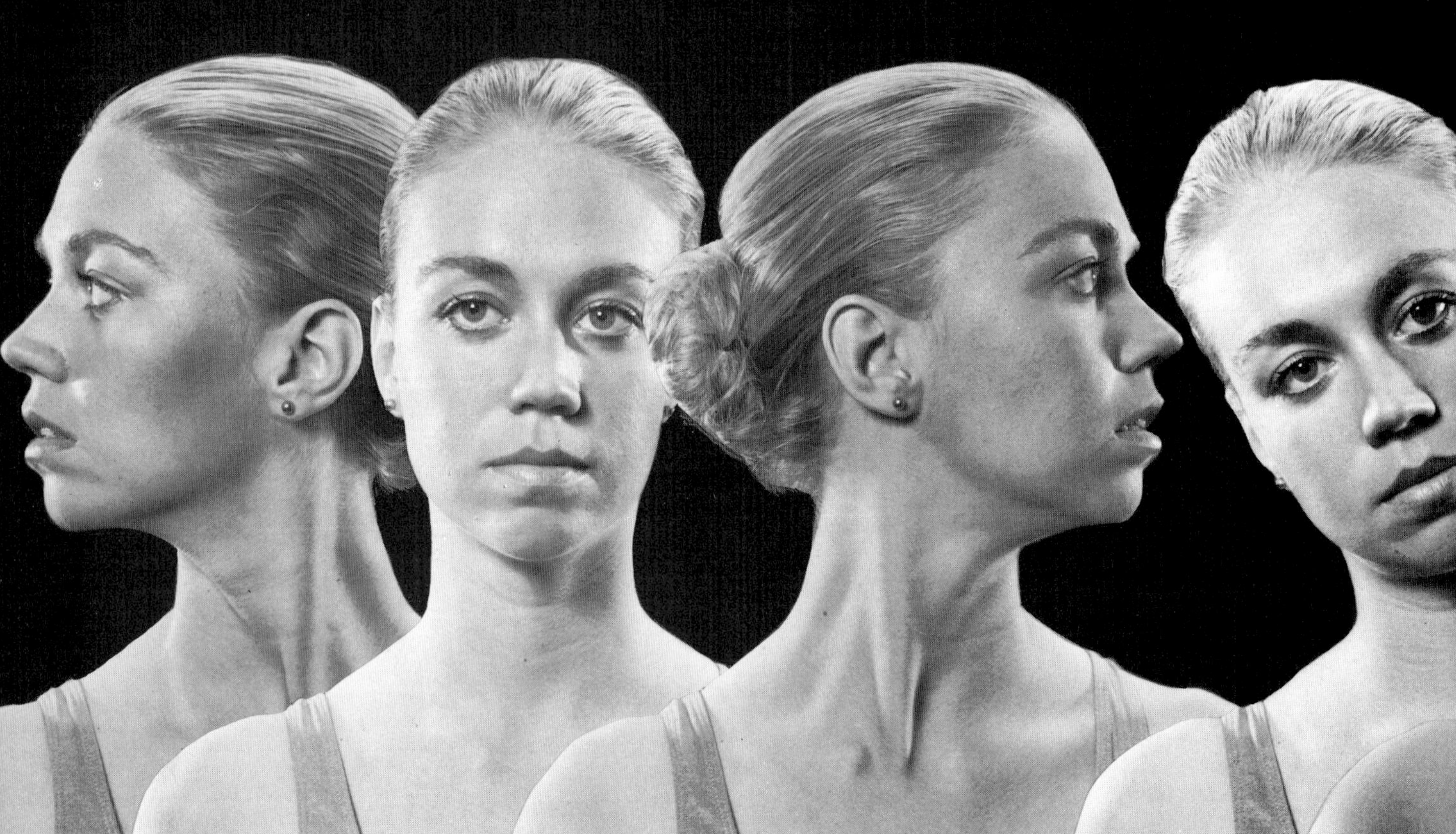

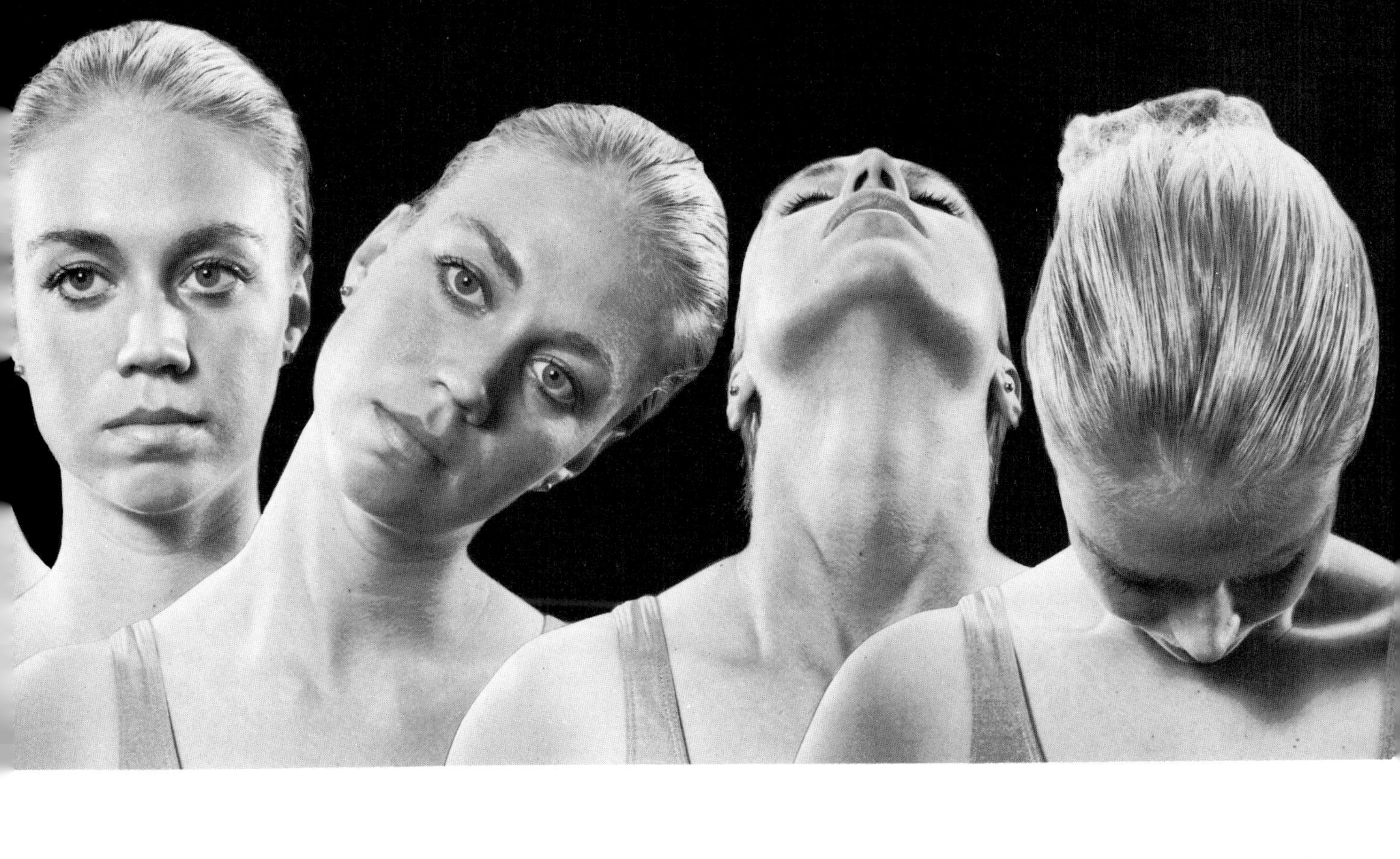

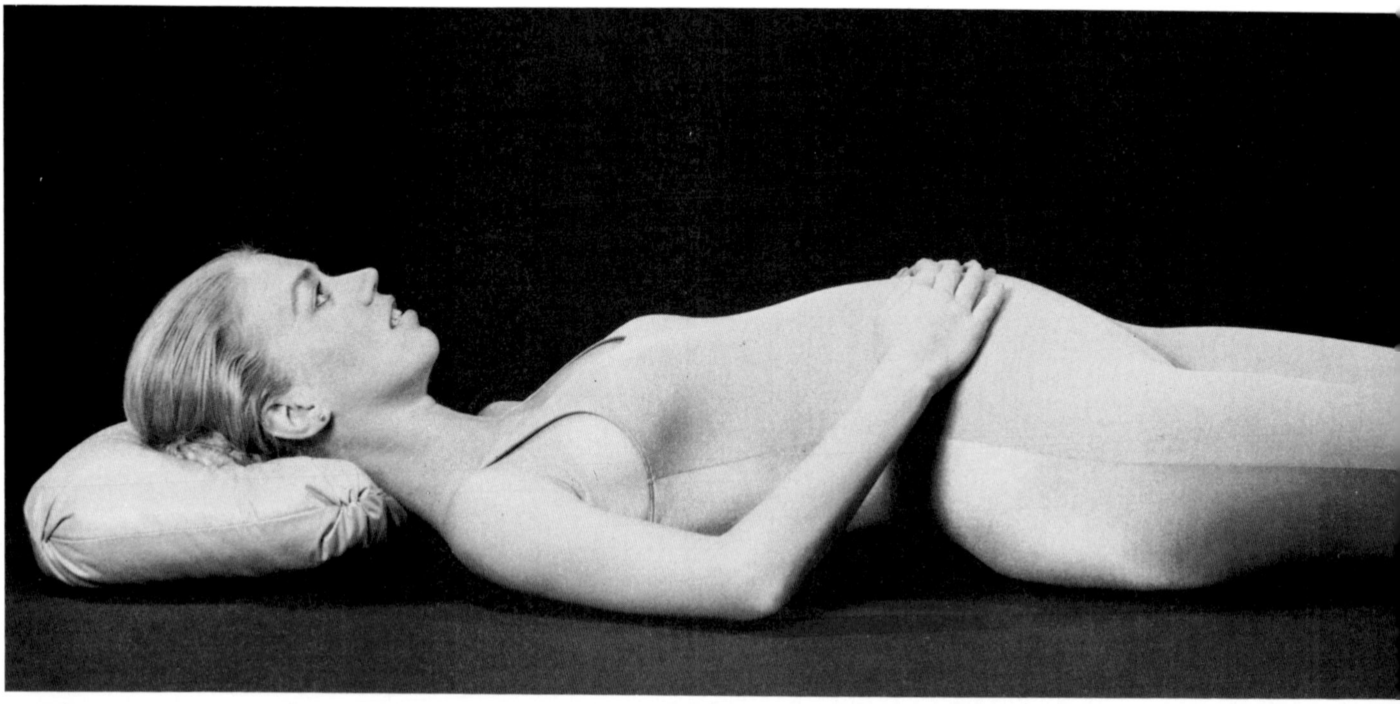

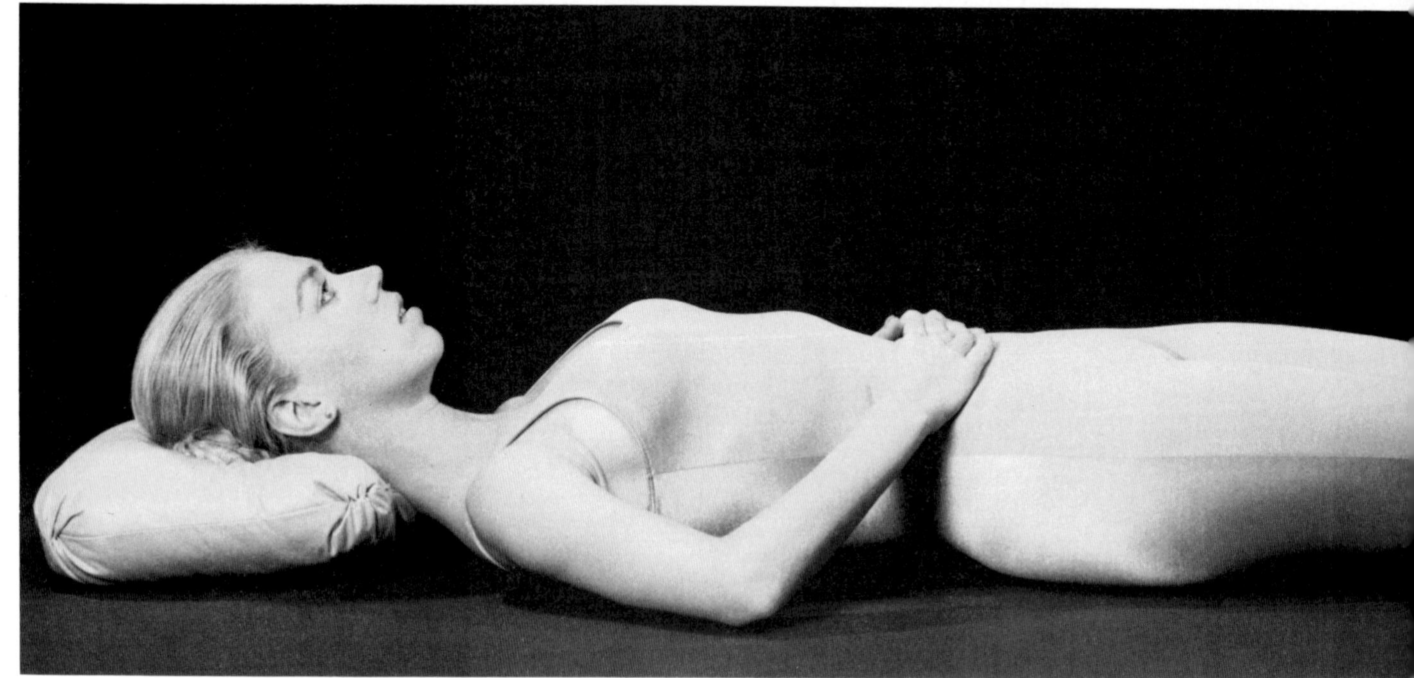

The first step: learning to breathe

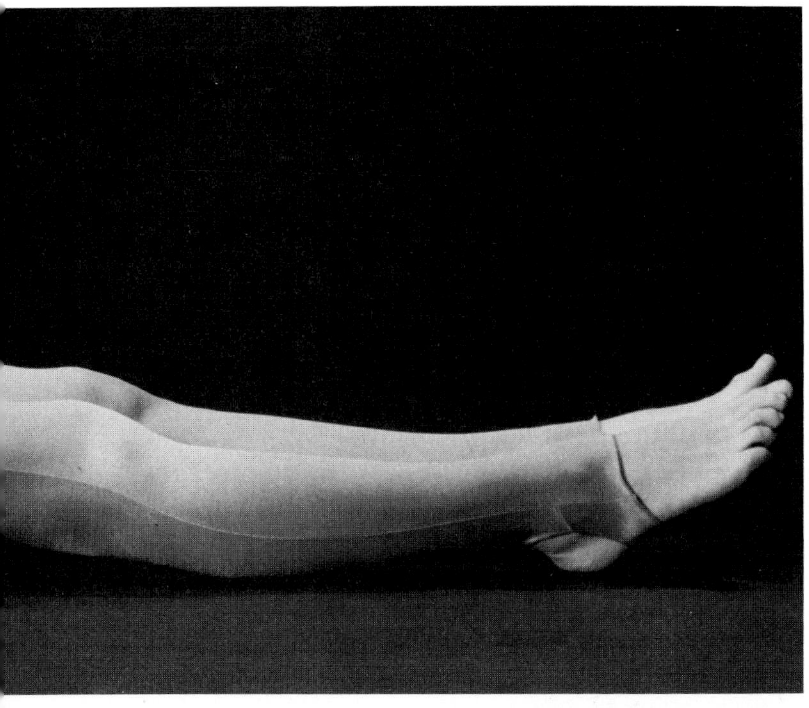

People who are headache-prone customarily take short, shallow breaths that shortchange their muscles of oxygen and do not completely rid body cells of the carbon dioxide they produce. The muscles tire readily, tighten up further and contribute to headache-provoking tensions. Learning to breathe deeply and rhythmically is the crucial first step in dispelling tension and putting muscles fully at ease.

Many people mistakenly believe they are taking a deep breath when they suck in their bellies and fling back their shoulders to expand their upper chests. But pulling in the abdomen pushes up the diaphragm—the broad flat muscle that stretches horizontally across the chest cavity just above the stomach—and thus cramps the lower part of the lungs.

To take a truly effective breath, breathe as if you were trying to take a bellyful of air rather than a chestful. Expanding your abdomen will pull your diaphragm down and allow your lungs to fill to capacity. The time to pull in your stomach is when you exhale: This will force air out of the lower lungs.

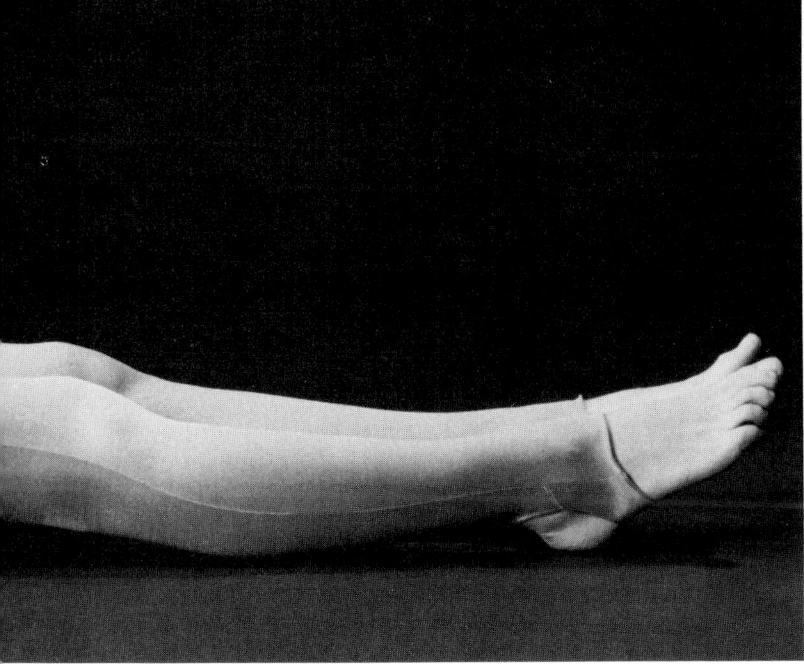

GETTING A BELLYFUL OF AIR
Lie flat on your back with a small pillow under your head. Rest your hands on your abdomen and keep your shoulders, arms and legs limp. Without consciously moving your chest, inhale deeply through your nose, expanding your abdomen as fully as possible—it should feel as if it is ballooning under your hands (upper left). Exhale slowly, contracting the abdominal muscles to squeeze most of the air from your lungs. Repeat five times.

Relaxing the body, muscle by muscle

The exercises pictured here train all of the major muscles in the body to relax by systematically tensing and releasing them. To do the exercises most effectively, tense the muscles as rigidly as possible but only briefly—longer rigid exertion can be harmful. The muscles will relax all the more readily when released.

The relaxation routine, which continues through page 59, is done in sequence, beginning with the resting position at right. Do the exercises in a quiet room and wear loose, comfortable clothing. If the movements seem difficult at first, tighten each group of muscles only as much as you can without feeling uncomfortable. You will soon limber up.

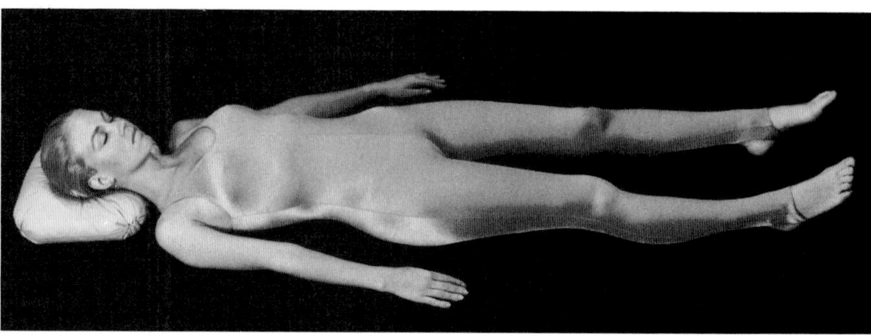

TAKING A COMFORTABLE POSITION
Lie on a firm surface with your head on a small pillow, your arms and legs spread slightly. Allow your arms to lie limp, your feet to droop outward. Take several deep breaths (preceding pages).

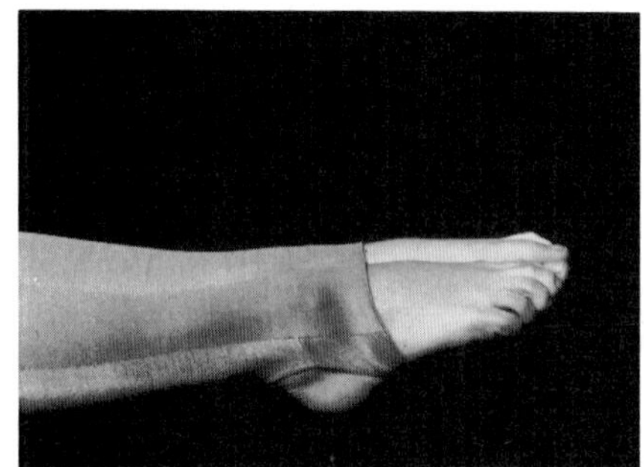

LOOSENING THE LOWER LEGS
Tense calves and feet by pointing the toes straight out (far left). Count to three, allow the feet to go limp for a count of three and repeat. Next, tense the muscles at the front of the legs by flexing both feet toward the head (near left). Count to three, let the feet go limp for a count of three and repeat.

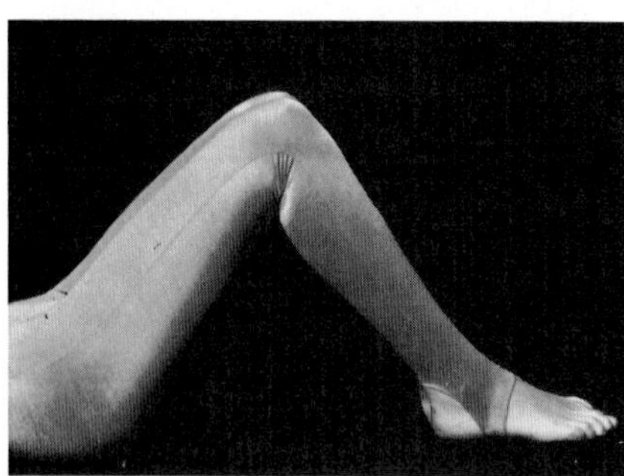

RELAXING THE THIGHS AND ABDOMEN
Bend both legs at the knees and press your feet hard against the floor (far left), tensing the thighs and contracting the abdomen. Count three, then release. Repeat and relax. Next, draw your heels up to your buttocks (near left) and tense the buttocks briefly. Release and repeat, then return to the original position.

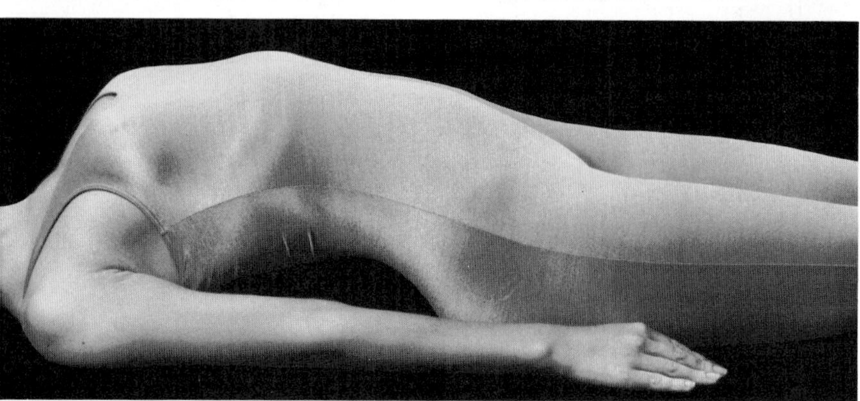

LOOSENING THE TORSO
Keeping your arms and legs lax, arch your torso upward, bringing your back as high off the floor as you comfortably can. Hold for a count of three, then sink back to the floor —raising your knees slightly if necessary— so that your spine is flat on the floor. Rest for a count of three and repeat.

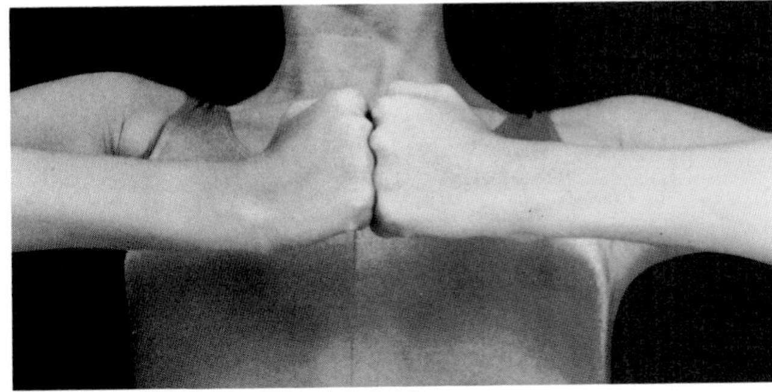

PUSHING AND PULLING TENSION FROM THE ARMS
Press your fists together above your chest (above, left) for a count of no more than three, drop your arms, then repeat. Hook your fingers together, pull briefly, release and repeat.

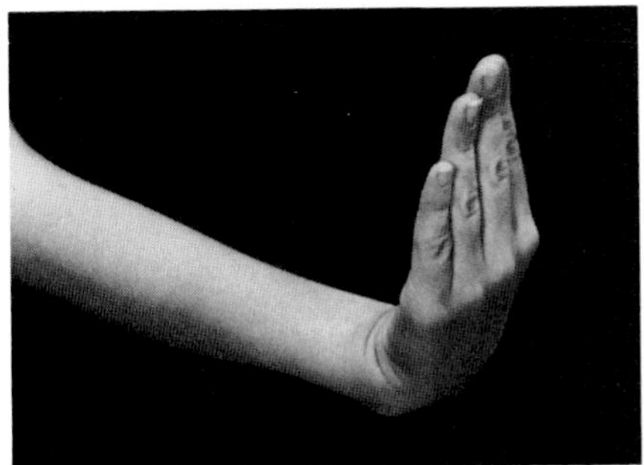

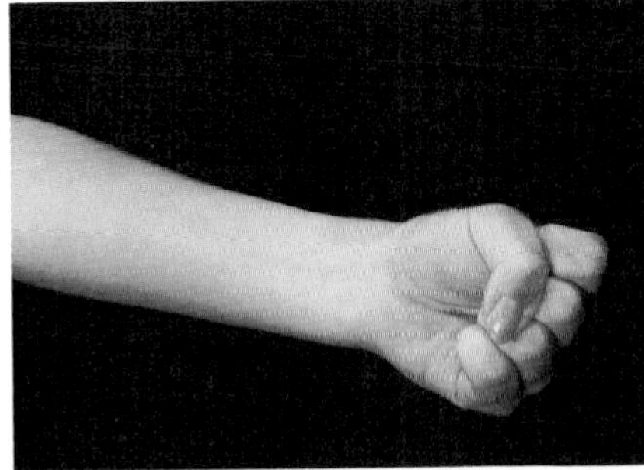

ZEROING IN ON THE LOWER ARMS
With your arms at your sides, your palms upward, bend both hands and point the fingers rigidly toward the ceiling (far left). Hold for a count of three, then let your hands flop to the floor. Repeat. Next, clench both hands tightly for no more than a count of three; release and repeat.

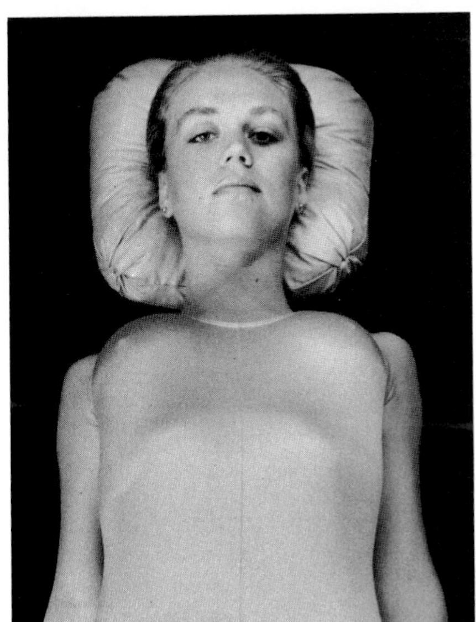

RELAXING THE UPPER BACK
With arms loose at your sides, draw your shoulder blades back against the floor and toward each other, tensing the upper back. Go limp, count three and repeat.

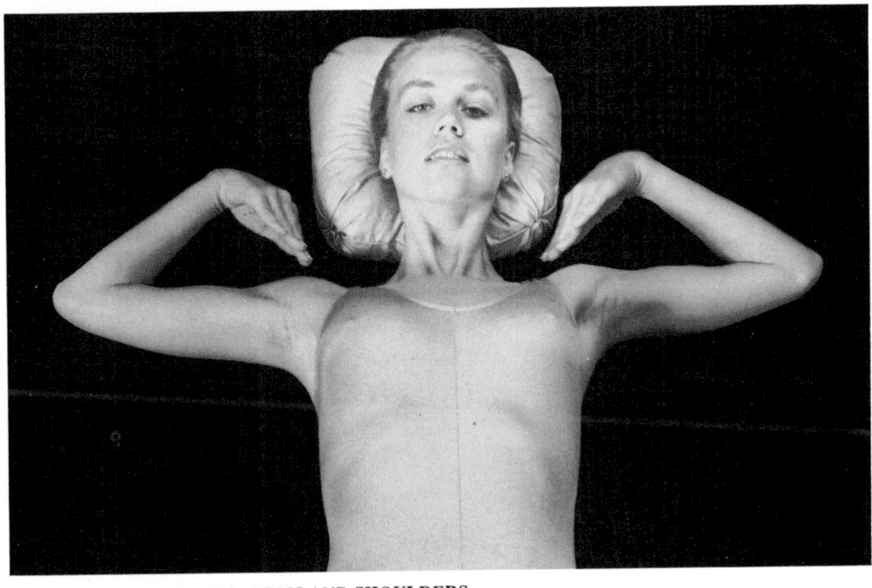

RELEASING THE HANDS, ARMS AND SHOULDERS
Bend your arms out and up at the elbows and raise them until your fingers almost touch your shoulders. Hold both limbs rigid from the shoulders to the fingertips for a count of three, then let them go limp and lower them to your sides. Count to three and repeat.

Stretching out the kinks in a stiff neck

The exercises pictured here are designed to relax the neck, where tightened muscles frequently cause headaches. With the exception of the shoulder-shrugging movements at right, these are all stretching exercises that loosen tight muscles by gently pulling them to their full, uncontracted length.

Such stretching movements can be called into play at almost any time—even during a few minutes' break on the job—to unknot a cramped neck and head off a threatening headache.

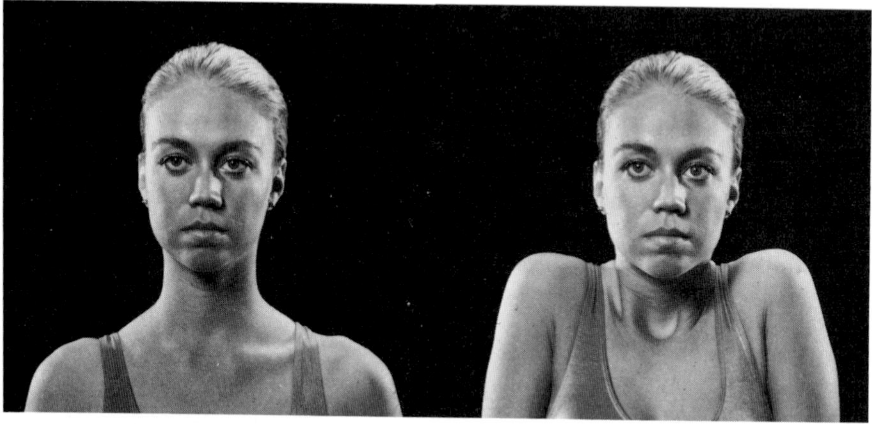

SHRUGGING OFF STIFF SHOULDERS
Slowly draw shoulders up toward the ears. Breathe deeply, then return to the original position. Relax and repeat.

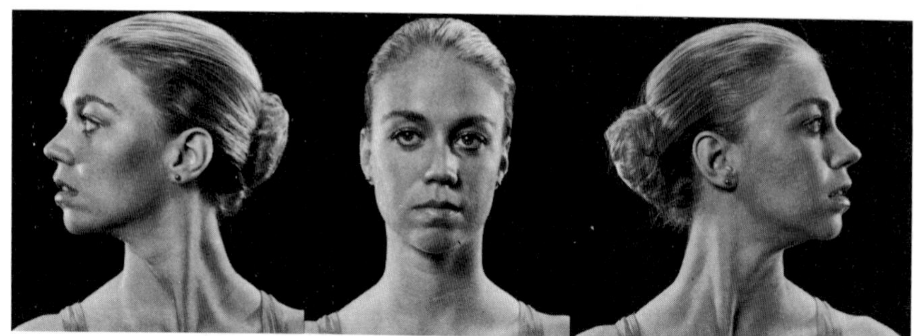

HEAD-TURNING STRETCHES
From a face-forward position, slowly turn your head as far as possible to the right without moving your shoulders. Hold briefly, turn slowly to face forward, then to the left. Hold and return to face forward.

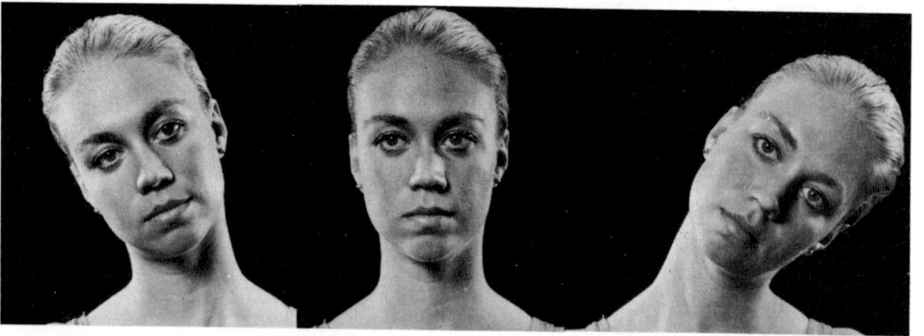

TILTING THE HEAD
Facing forward, with your shoulders held level, tilt your head slowly to the right, reaching for your shoulder with your ear. Hold the stretch for a few seconds, then slowly tilt upright. Hold, tilt left, and then raise your head upright.

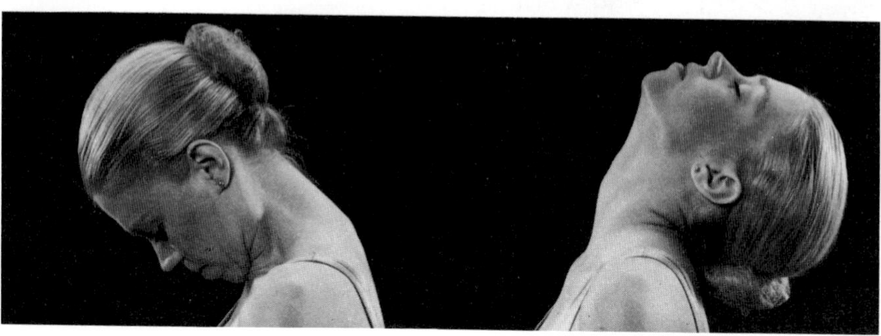

A DEEP, GENTLE NOD
Slowly drop your head forward, bringing your chin toward your chest to stretch the muscles at the back of the neck. Then lift your head and slowly roll it back, pointing your chin toward the ceiling. Bring your head upright and repeat.

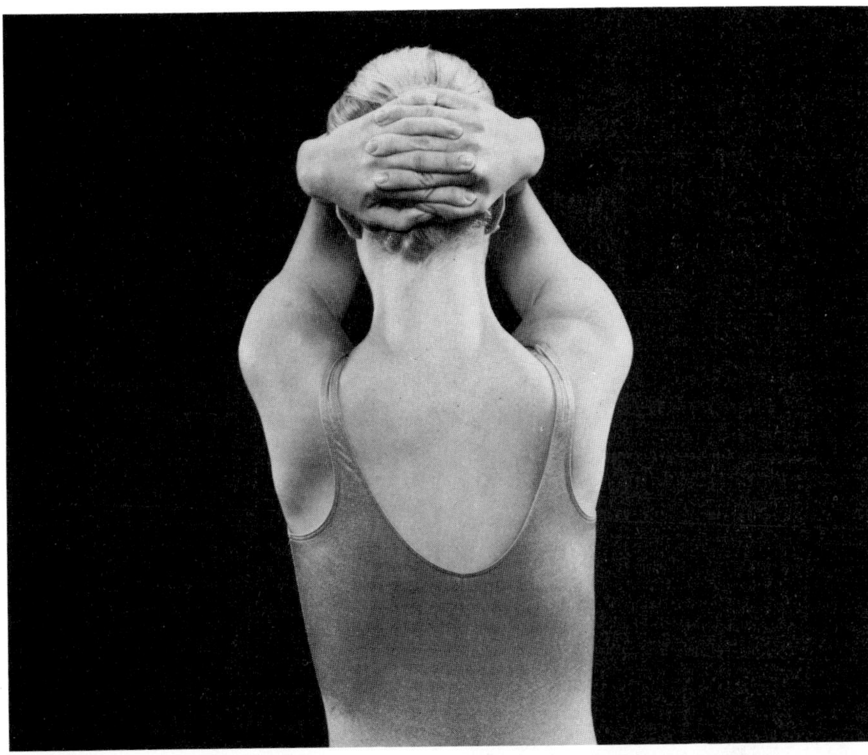

THE TRAPEZIUS STRETCH
Lock your hands together behind your head. Keeping your back straight and your abdominal muscles tight, bring your elbows together in front of your face to stretch the two large trapezius muscles, which extend from the base of the skull, across the shoulders and down to the middle of the back on both sides of the spine.

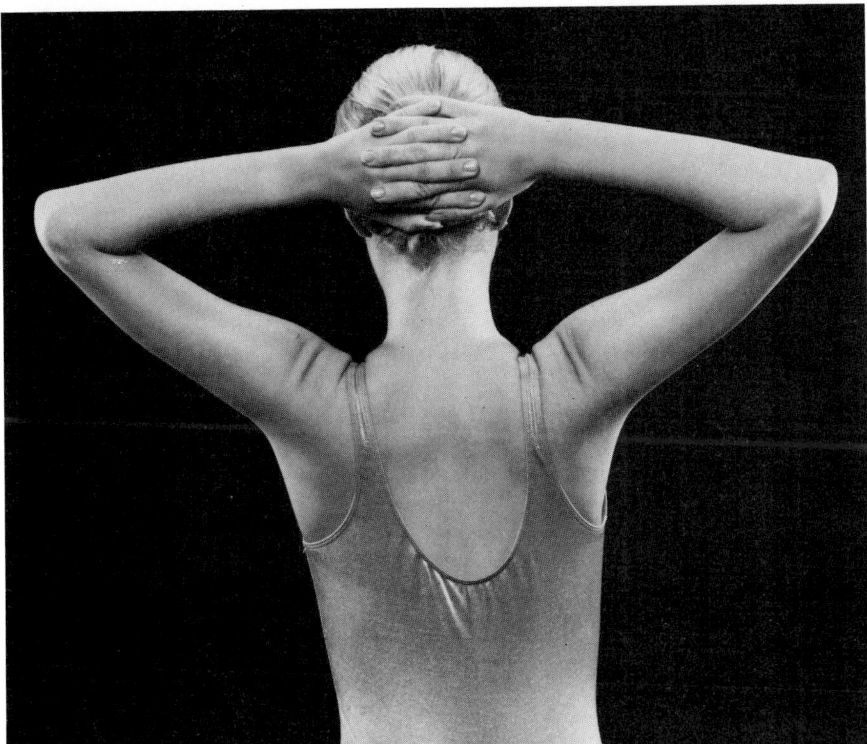

REVERSING THE STRETCH
With your hands still behind your head, pull your elbows back as far as possible— your shoulder blades will move toward one another. Then draw the elbows forward once more and back again. Drop your hands to your sides and relax, breathing deeply.

Working your way to a happy face

A sparkling smile like the one on the face of the model on the opposite page is sometimes hard to muster when you have a headache. But a smile is an excellent antidote for headache. And its opposite—a deep frown—may make things worse. Headache sufferers whose tense faces, in the words of stress expert Dr. Charles Stroebel, take on "the grim posture of a dog going into battle," not only reflect their distress but contribute to it.

A furrowed brow, clenched jaw and tight lips produce muscular tension that can spread up over the head. To unlock those muscles, first tighten them a bit more, exaggerating the grimaces. Then follow the steps as shown; between each, release tension by letting your face go blank and your jaw droop slightly.

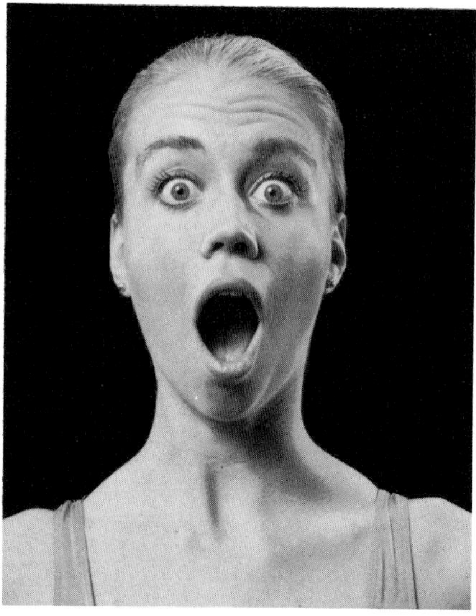

A FULL STRETCH FOR THE FACE
Open your mouth and eyes as wide as possible, raising your eyebrows at the same time. Hold briefly, relax and repeat.

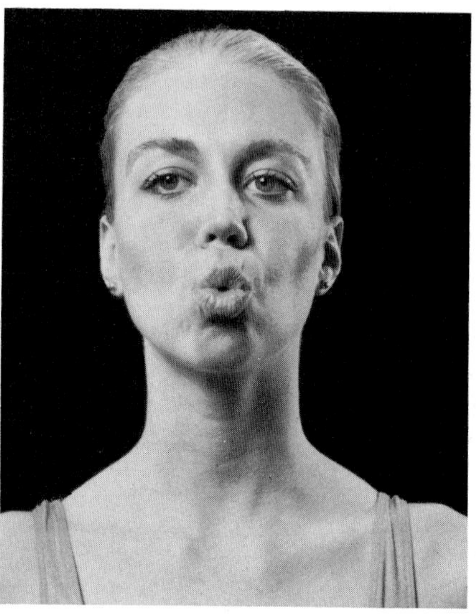

KISSING OFF TENSION AROUND THE MOUTH
Keeping your head still, purse your lips tightly and extend them as if trying to kiss someone just out of reach. Relax and repeat.

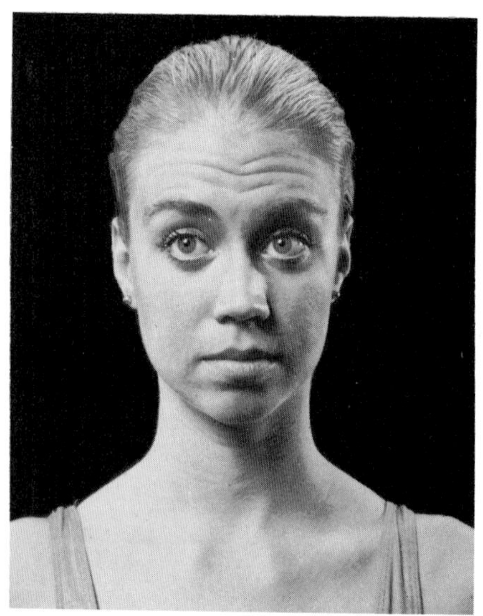

A FURROWED BROW
Raise your eyebrows as far as possible, feeling the stretch in the muscles around your ears. Hold, then let the brows come down to smooth the forehead.

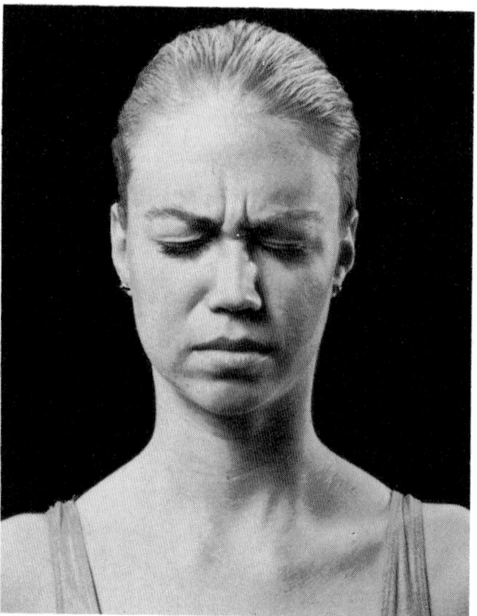

FROWNING—AND WORKING THE SCALP
Bring your brows into a deep frown; hold, relax and repeat. Next, raise your eyebrows high, then frown, alternating several times quickly to move your scalp.

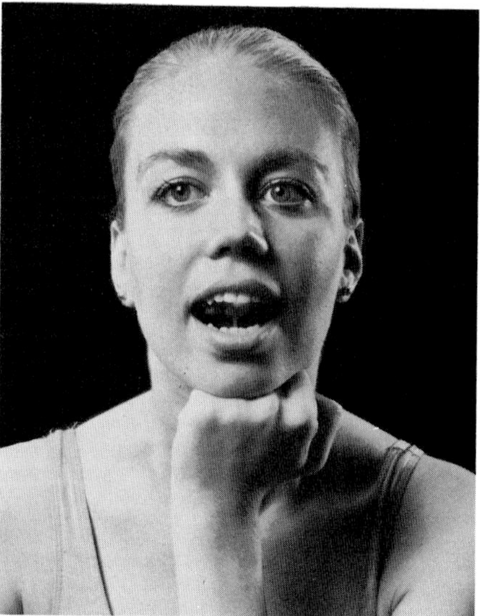

UNLOCKING THE JAW
Plant your chin on your fist, the tip of your tongue against the roof of your mouth, and press your jaw down hard while opening your mouth. Hold, release and repeat.

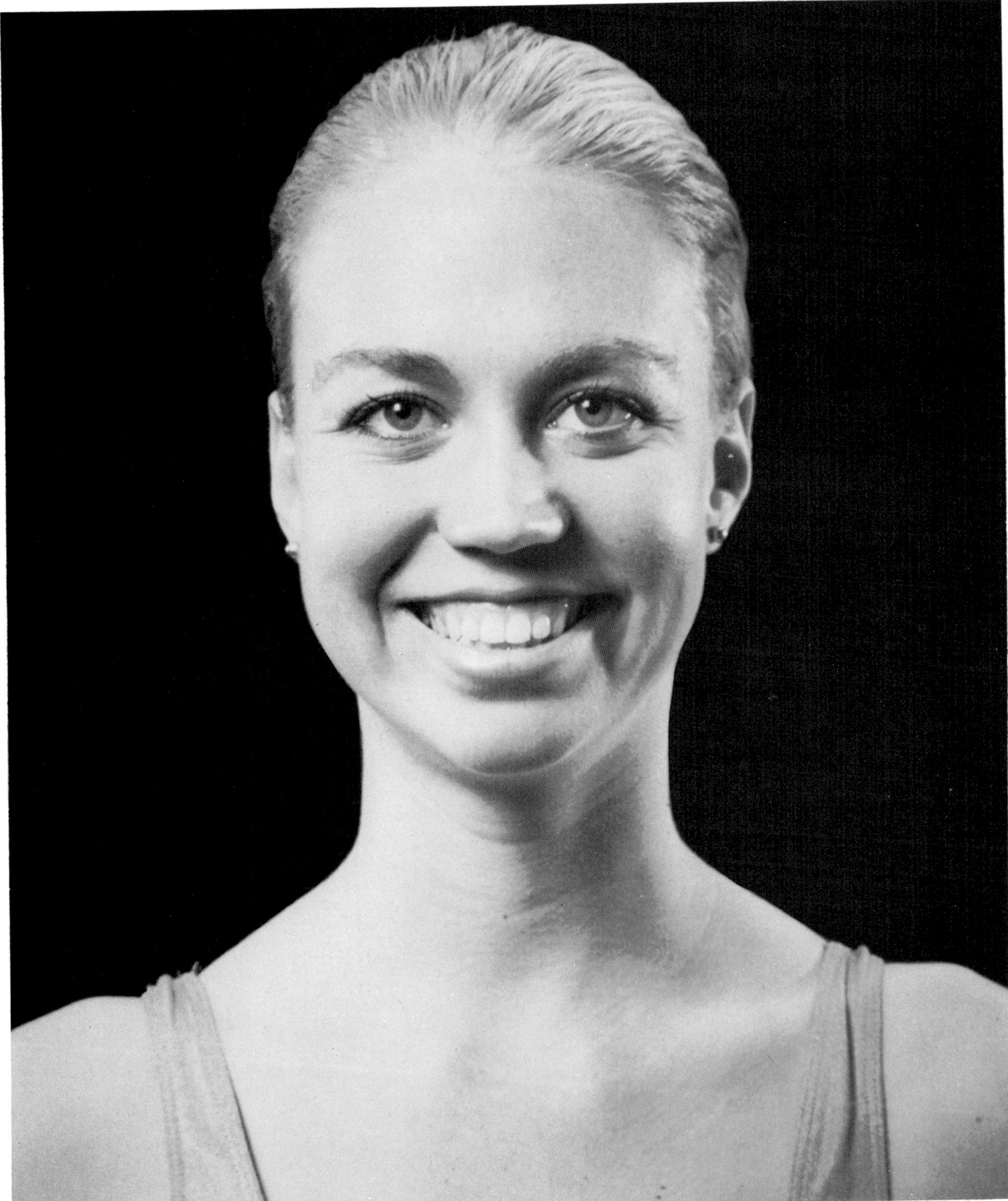

SMILING AWAY THE PAIN
Finally, smile broadly—and do so whenever you feel tension coming on. Using muscles that make you smile releases the ones that produce a pain-provoking frown.

CHAPTER 3

The throb of stretched arteries

The aches in wines and spirits
Coffee: a cause and a cure
The Chinese-restaurant syndrome
Aches in the air you breathe
The right foods for hunger headache
Keeping fever pains out of your head

The hungover head is a stereotype of comic art: Its miserable owner, ice bag to brow, shields himself from light, noise and the prospect of food. The stereotype is accurate if unfeeling. The hangover headache is one type of vascular headache, a broad class of head pains arising from the distention of the vessels supplying scalp and brain with blood. Headaches much like it afflict many people who have never touched a drop of alcohol.

Vascular headaches may be very severe—the incapacitating migraine and cluster headaches *(Chapter 4)* are vascular, for example—but a large number are, like hangovers, of a simpler, less severe and fortunately transient variety called toxic. They involve mainly the arteries supplying blood to the brain rather than those near the surface of the head, as in a migraine attack.

Most toxic headaches signal an acute chemical imbalance in the body, an imbalance generally caused by some substance that gets into the body because it is swallowed, inhaled or absorbed through the skin. But a number of similar headaches arise in other ways; a chemical toxin need not be the cause, and many authorities would define a toxic headache as any vascular headache that is not of the migraine or cluster variety.

These disorders may begin as a reaction to food or drink—not only liquor but hot dogs, Chinese food and frozen dinners—to air pollution, or to the fever of an infectious disease such as influenza. All such stimuli affect the pressure-controlling muscles that form the outer part of the blood vessel, relaxing those muscles and allowing the smooth walls of the vessel to expand. The blood vessel increases in diameter, or dilates. (Physicians, who generally prefer longer words, use the technical term "dilatate," which means exactly the same as "dilate.")

Dilation affects nerve endings that respond to pressure. Embedded in the walls of blood vessels, they assist the brain in maintaining and monitoring its automatic control over blood pressure. When the vessel expands, these nerve endings are stretched, and changes occur in their electrical voltage. If the stretching is sufficient to cause a considerable voltage change, this electrical effect becomes a nerve message that travels to the brain, where it is received and interpreted as pain. It is a kind of pain message unique to vascular headaches, distinctly different from the pain signals of muscle-tension headaches *(Chapter 2)*.

You can generally distinguish a toxic headache from an acute muscle-tension headache by a number of well-defined characteristics. Toxic headaches have a pulsating, throbbing quality, related to the pumping of blood through swollen, stretched vessels. Toxic headaches also hurt all over, in contrast to some muscle-tension headaches, which tend to be bandlike or localized in the forehead or the back of the head. The pain is likely to be increased by straining, stooping or sudden movement.

Some toxic headaches are readily treated. Aspirin and acetaminophen help, as they do in muscle-tension headaches. The ice bag of comic art also provides relief, contract-

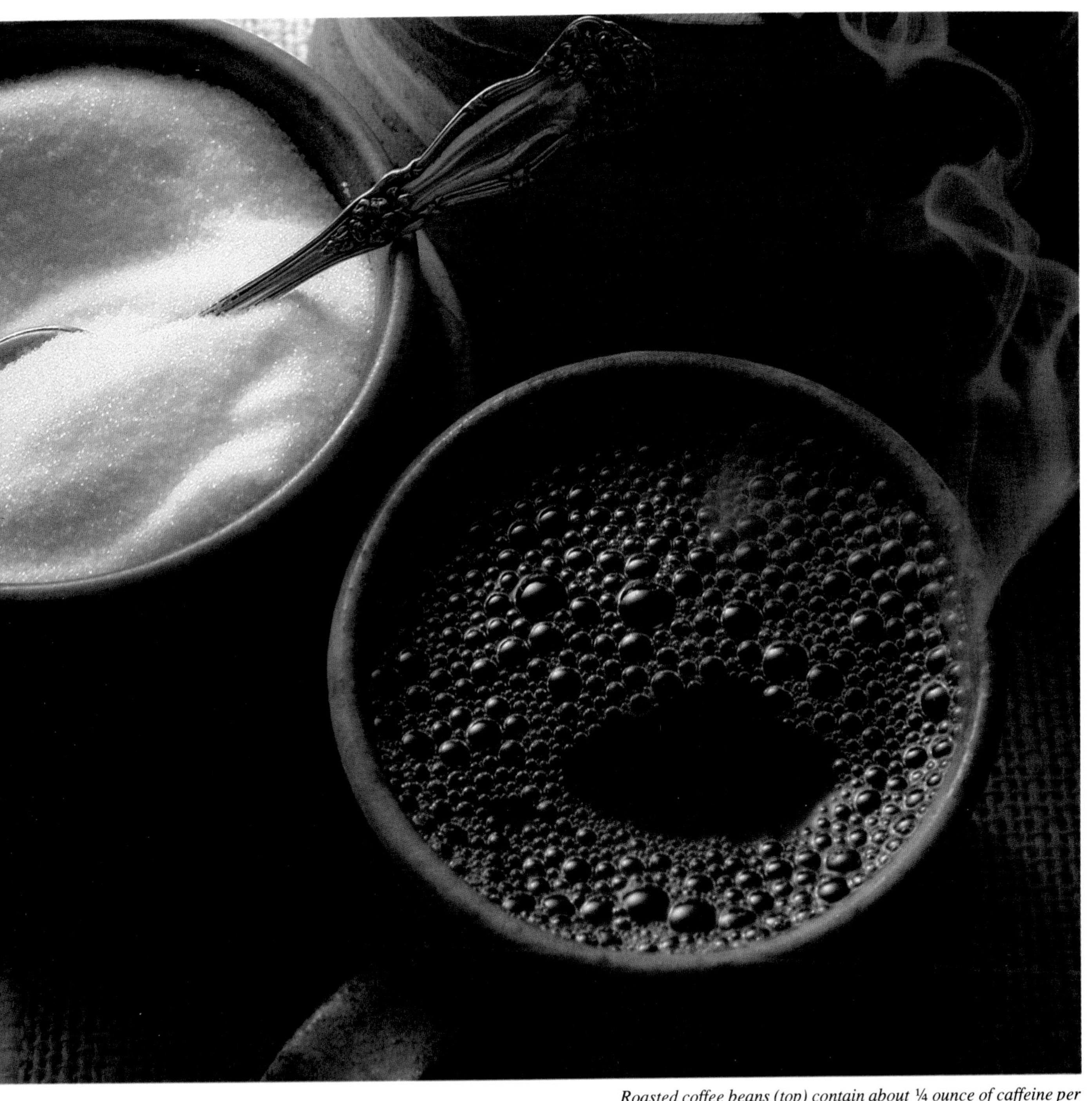

Roasted coffee beans (top) contain about ¼ ounce of caffeine per pound. About ³/₁,₀₀₀ ounce is present in an average 5-ounce cup, and it can cure or cause headache. Caffeine constricts blood vessels, easing headaches caused by enlarged vessels. But coffee addicts develop tolerance to constricted vessels; when they reduce caffeine intake, they suffer headache as vessels enlarge.

ing the swollen vessels back toward their normal, pain-free size. More important, people who are prone to toxic headaches can prevent them by avoiding the toxin that serves as a trigger—provided that the toxin can be identified. This task is not always a simple one, for the possible triggers are numerous and astonishingly varied.

The aches in wines and spirits

Among the foods and drinks that poison the system to initiate head pain, alcoholic drinks are probably the best-known villains. How many drinks are too many is hard to predict—not only among the population at large but even on an individual basis—for the cause of the hangover is not alcohol alone. Other ingredients in the drink may exert more influence, as may the personality of the drinker and the circumstances of the drinking.

The alcohol itself is certainly one factor. It is consumed primarily for its effects on the nervous system, which include the relaxation of muscles such as those around blood vessels. The relaxation seems to be caused not by alcohol as such but by one of the by-products of its processing in the body, acetaldehyde. When the muscles are made to relax, the blood vessels expand.

This effect can help relieve a tension headache—a small drink of liquor is, indeed, a common and effective treatment for such head pains. But large amounts of alcohol seem to carry the expansion of blood vessels too far; eventually, the head hurts from the stretching of the nerve endings in the enlarged vessels.

Compounding the effects of alcohol are various nonalcoholic substances called congeners, which contribute the color, aroma and taste of particular wines and spirits. Congeners may have an even more powerful effect than alcohol on the cranial blood vessels, and they are largely responsible for the aftereffects of drinking.

These facts have emerged from a number of experiments conducted in England and the United States since the 1950s. One researcher, Dr. Gaston Pawan of the Middlesex Hospital Medical School in London, attempted to confirm the suspected role of congeners by offering them in pure form to groups of volunteers. His subjects refused to take them—the taste was too bad. But when the volunteers drank liquors from which all the congeners (but not the alcohol) had been filtered, they reported aftereffects milder than those noted with unfiltered drinks.

Tests by several other researchers have demonstrated that the congener content depends partly on the raw material that is fermented to make an alcoholic beverage, so that some congeners appear in certain spirits and not in others. Furthermore, some congeners are introduced during the aging process, so that older and more expensive liquors tend to cause worse hangovers than less expensive ones bottled shortly after manufacture. Bourbon and brandy, both beverages that are aged for some time in wooden barrels, absorb from the wood large amounts of congeners that make them notorious for their hangover potential; the older and costlier the liquors are, the greater the quantity of hangover-producing congeners they contain.

A ranking of alcoholic beverages in order of congener content would begin with aged bourbon and brandy at the top of the list; these would be followed by the rest of the bourbons and brandies and then, more or less in order, dark rum, rye, aged scotches, blended whiskeys, light scotches, gin and vodka. Vodka is the hard liquor that is lowest in congeners. A colorless, almost odorless and tasteless, unaged distillate from grain such as rye or barley or from potatoes, vodka is little more than unflavored ethyl alcohol and water. Theoretically, then, drinking excessive amounts of vodka is less likely to bring on a hangover than consuming otherwise equal quantities of other alcoholic beverages.

Wines have only small amounts of congeners and are less likely than other drinks to cause a headache. But some wines bring more risk than others.

Many red wines are richly endowed with a chemical naturally manufactured by the body, histamine, that enlarges blood vessels (an excess of histamine is responsible for the stuffiness of allergies). Vintage French red wines from Burgundy may have 10 times as much histamine as other reds and 15 times as much as white wines, and thus may cause nasal congestion. But Dr. Pawan found in his research that, histamine content notwithstanding, expensive red wines are less likely to cause headaches than cheap ones. The reason again seems to be their lower congener content. (Dr. Pawan's recipe for getting the headache out of inexpensive red wine: Open the bottle several hours before you plan to serve the wine and allow it to "breathe"—the congeners evaporate faster than the alcohol.)

Hangover headaches sometimes depend less on what is drunk than on how it is drunk. Psychological effects seem to be as important as physical ones. If the alcohol and congeners were the only cause, the headache would be expected to appear before the drinking ended, while their concentration in the bloodstream was high. But the hangover comes much later, at a time when the chemical levels may have subsided in the bloodstream.

In search of other triggers, Dr. Harold Wolff of New York Hospital conducted repeated experiments with a group of people who often suffered headaches. He found that when these individuals were given two to three ounces of 95 per cent ethyl alcohol, roughly equivalent to four to six ounces of 90-proof vodka, in the laboratory, they never experienced hangover headaches. Dr. Wolff reasoned that "the taking of alcohol under laboratory conditions is quite different from social drinking. The discipline imposed by experimental sit-

Rating drinks for hangover

Which drinks lead to the worst headaches and nausea was determined by some rather jolly research conducted in London by Dr. Gaston Pawan of the Middlesex Hospital Medical School. In experiments over a decade, Dr. Pawan invited groups of men to weekly drinking sessions in a friend's apartment. After an ordinary meal was served, drinking began. Each week the men drank effectively equal amounts of alcohol—the equivalent of almost a pint of 70-proof whisky—but from different liquors. Most subjects left the sessions "inebriated but not drunk," said Dr. Pawan.

The next day the men reported their hangovers, and from their accounts Dr. Pawan derived numerical ratings indicating the severity of the headaches and other symptoms caused by various drinks. The results of one test are graphed below. Brandy produced the worst hangovers and gained the highest rating, with red wine a close second. Vodka and gin won the lowest ratings. The reason, Dr. Pawan and many other doctors believe, is the drinks' different concentrations of chemicals called congeners—by-products of fermentation and distillation that give each liquor its characteristic taste and aroma. The amounts are very tiny. Brandy, for instance, contains about .0036 ounce of congeners in a jiggerful, vodka only .0000428 ounce. The British experiment did not test the popular American drink bourbon, which is notorious as a headache source; its congener content *(overleaf)* is comparable to that of brandy.

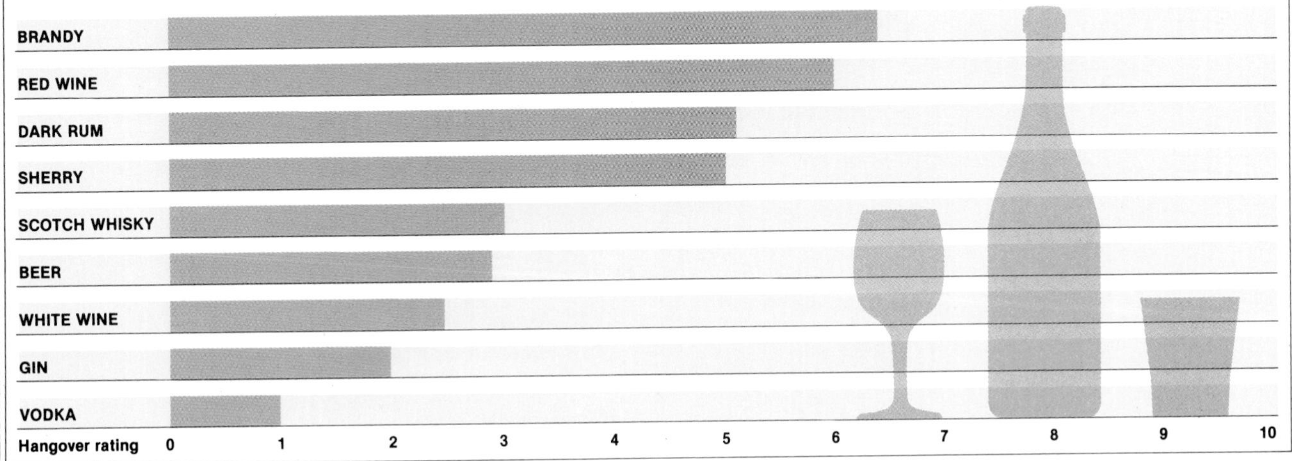

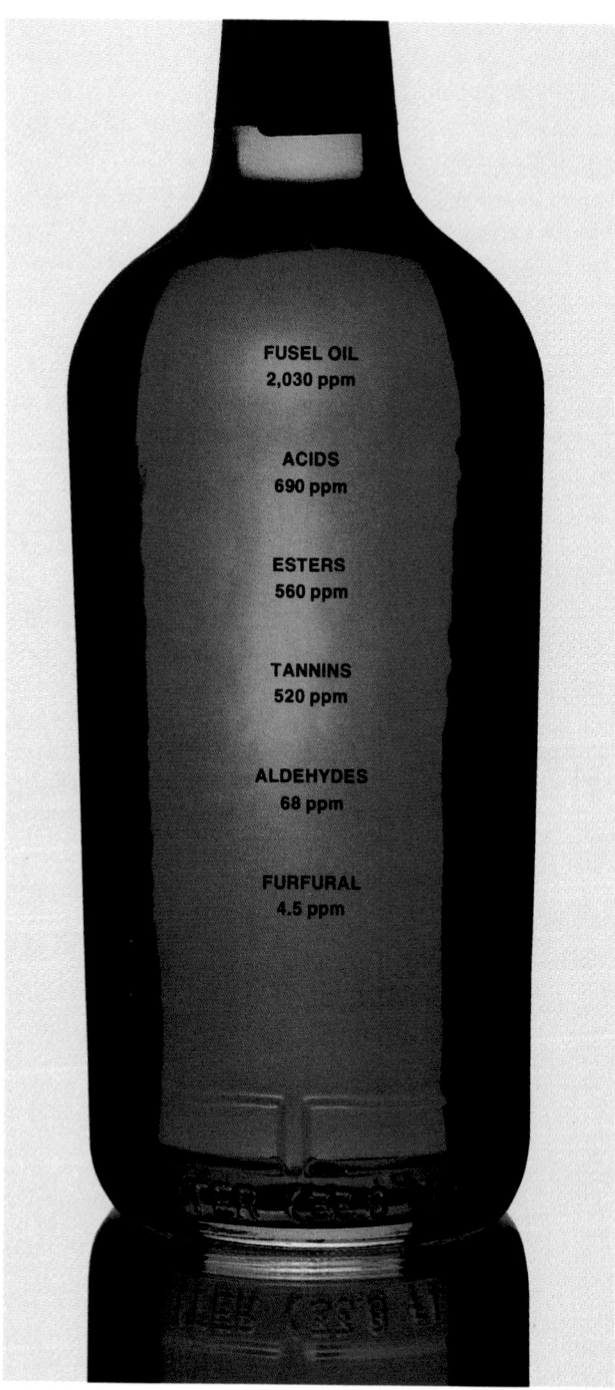

The amounts of hangover-causing chemicals, or congeners, in bourbon whiskey—second only to brandy as a hangover-inducer—are listed above; "ppm" stands for parts (of chemicals) per million parts of bourbon. Although fusel oil, from fermentation, is most plentiful, tannins and other substances that arise during aging may contribute as much to hangover headache.

uations precludes the excitement that accompanies its use in a party setting."

Although Dr. Wolff's research was carried out before the effects of congeners were demonstrated experimentally, most authorities agree with his basic conclusion: The hangover headache results not only from the action of alcohol and impurities on cranial vessels, but also from the cumulative effect, on those who drink, of late hours, the excitement of talking, singing and laughing, loss of self-restraint, "and perhaps some remorse."

If remorse stimulates restraint in eating and drinking, it can, of course, prove to be an effective preventive against future hangovers. For a hangover headache that is already in residence, many of the traditional morning-after remedies are indeed effective. Aspirin, a cold compress and rest will bring relief for this or any other vascular headache. So will drinking black coffee or tea—the caffeine they contain forces blood vessels to constrict, counteracting the dilation that is the cause of the headache.

An antidote not to try is another drink, folklore to the contrary notwithstanding. "The hair of the dog that bit you" will only bring on another bite. Also, you can cross off the raw eggs and Worcestershire sauce that your black-sheep uncle swore by. To anyone who felt queasy to begin with, such gustatory assaults on the stomach might tip the scales toward total gastrointestinal upset. They will do nothing at all for the headache.

The standard remedies may relieve the pain of a hangover headache, but recovery is speeded if the chemical toxins are eliminated from the body as rapidly as possible. One method of ridding the system of remaining alcohol is to eat and drink foods high in fructose, one of the common sugars. Fructose increases by 15 to 30 per cent the rate at which the body can break alcohol down into innocent chemicals. Foods high in fructose include that old stand-by, tomato juice, but also honey, apples and grapes in juice or solid form. The sugar in table sugar and in cakes and candies will not help, however; it is chemically different and lacks fructose's metabolic effect on alcohol.

Dehydration also plays a significant role in the discomfort

experienced during a hangover headache, and attending to that effect also helps cure the pain. Alcohol is a diuretic; that is, it stimulates urine production, in part by interfering with the hormone ADH, which serves to maintain a steady rate of water retention by the body. Hangover victims will recognize systemic dehydration as a furry tongue, a bad taste in the mouth, a dryness in the mouth and throat. The body is laboring additionally under some chemical deficits because the diuretic action of the alcohol has flushed certain needed nutritive materials through the body at an uncommon speed; food that was eaten has not been properly absorbed.

The antidote to dehydration is the measured restoration of the missing fluids and chemicals, not so fast as to further irritate the stomach, but just fast enough to be comfortably absorbed—perhaps 12 ounces of liquid every one to two hours. Any of the packaged broths are an excellent choice because they not only contain salt, one of the missing chemicals, but counteract the bad taste accompanying hangover, provide nourishment, and are relatively bland. Acidic drinks such as orange juice are not recommended; they can cause problems in digestion.

Eat, drink and be wary

Better than any cure are the methods for avoiding hangovers in the first place. Obviously, anyone who is particularly susceptible to hangovers ought to drink something other than alcohol. If that seems too puritanical a solution, there are reasonably effective alternatives that work for most people some of the time.

You can, for example, prepare for an evening of partying by eating properly beforehand. Remember that foods high in fructose will help the body process alcohol; in addition, foods high in protein, such as meat, milk and cheese, are excellent for "lining the stomach" to help it resist irritation. Try to be well rested, too, even if it means taking time out beforehand for a relaxing nap.

If it is possible to do so, avoid partying altogether if you are angry, tense or emotionally exhausted: Alcohol in combination with emotional tension tends to be exceptionally potent, and the tendency to drink more than usual under such pressures adds to the risk of over-indulgence and the likelihood of a hangover.

For self-protection while drinking, avoid beverages high in congeners and histamine. Take what you do drink with a mixer, such as one of the fructose-high juices or a carbonated base such as soda or quinine water. The mixers will attend to the thirst aspect of drinking, possibly reducing total alcohol consumption, and most certainly speeding its processing and elimination by body metabolism.

Take advantage of bland cocktail snacks, such as the ones with cheese, but avoid the salty tempters such as nuts, which only induce more drinking. If you are doing your drinking with smokers, find the best-ventilated spot you can and then go outside for extra doses of fresh air as often as you can. Many headaches are not so much reactions to alcohol as they are reactions to the toxic air of smoke-filled rooms. And lastly, when you go home, have a bedtime snack of honey on crackers. Full of fructose, the snack will be working on your behalf while you, presumably, sleep the rest of the night away in comfort.

That drinking alcoholic beverages can bring on headaches has been known for millennia. But only recently have scientists been able to link head pains to a number of other substances that are routinely ingested; in most cases a single chemical has been identified as the culprit. Among the most common offenders singled out are the caffeine in coffee and other beverages, the seasoning MSG (monosodium glutamate) and the nitrate and nitrite compounds commonly employed as preservatives.

Caffeine—a cause and a cure

The coffee headache—which many doctors suspect is more common than generally thought—is a paradoxical result of the physiological effect of caffeine. Caffeine does not cause enlargement of cerebral blood vessels, the vascular action that raises pressure inside the head and makes it hurt. Rather, caffeine constricts the vessels—that is why coffee is a useful antidote for hangover headache. In fact, caffeine is an ingredient in many common headache remedies.

But as with alcoholic drinks, what can be helpful in rea-

A PANTRY PACKED WITH ACHY AMINES

Foods as diverse as chocolate, cheese and citrus fruits share a common headache trigger: They contain natural compounds of nitrogen called amines. Amines are useful in many bodily functions, but in concentrated amounts they can change the size of blood vessels and thus provoke headaches.

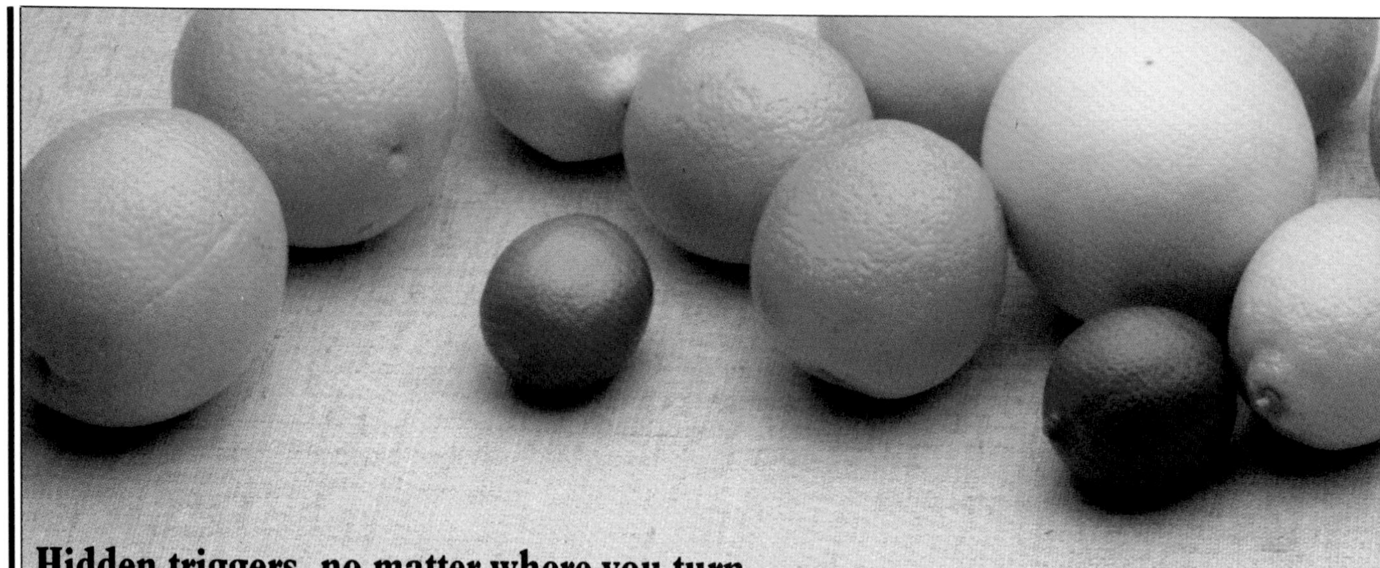

Hidden triggers, no matter where you turn

A Chinese-restaurant patron sipping won-ton soup, a house painter working in a closed room, a farmer eating oranges as he picks them—all are potential headache victims because substances they breathe or consume can trigger headaches. Some 2,000 years ago Hippocrates linked this ill to certain foods, warning against the possible effects of milk and "heavy wine." Modern researchers have added to the list many additional foods, along with a number of chemicals widespread in the environment; all can make cranial blood vessels either shrink or swell, provoking the vascular type of headache.

Some people can develop a tolerance to such headache triggers but lose this protection when the trigger is absent for a time. Workers in explosives plants, for example, find their nitrate-caused headaches recur when they come back to the job after a vacation. To maintain their tolerance for nitrates, some of them keep tiny packets of dynamite in their hatbands.

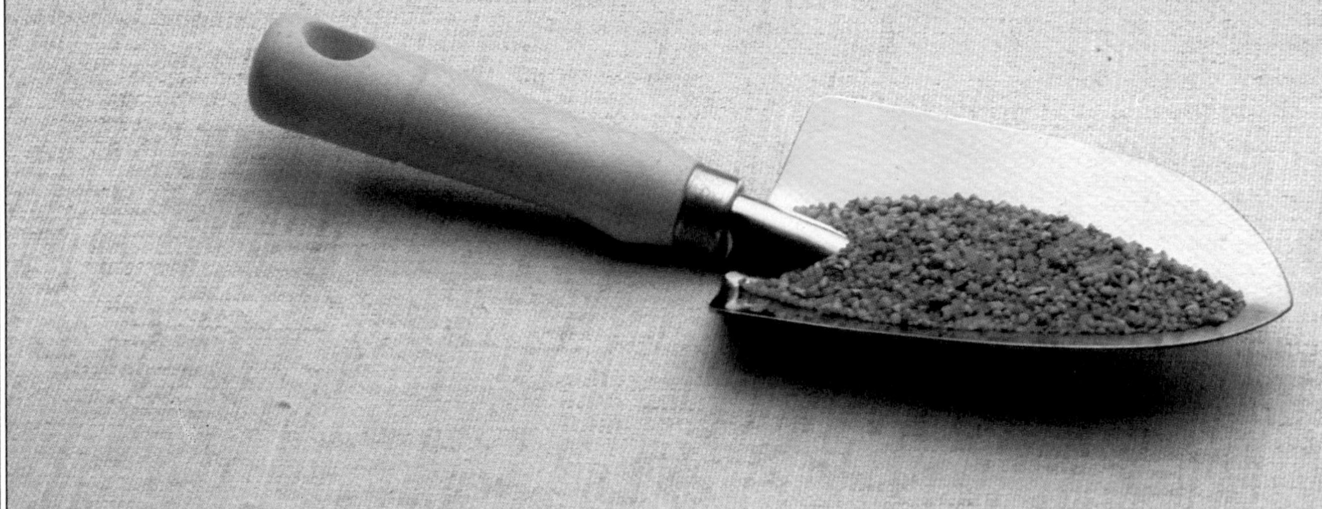

PAIN FROM NITRATES AND NITRITES

It has been nicknamed the hot-dog headache but it can also afflict the gardener inhaling fertilizer fumes. The triggers in either case are, like those in oranges, nitrogen compounds, but in the form of nitrates or nitrites. Nitrites preserve meats; nitrates make fertilizer, explosives and nitroglycerin heart medicine.

THE CHINESE-RESTAURANT SYNDROME

Within half an hour after eating at a Chinese restaurant, some diners suffer a reaction no fortune cookie ever foretold: pounding headache, dizziness and tightness across the chest and face. The culprit is monosodium glutamate—MSG—a flavor-enhancer used in Oriental cooking and in many processed foods.

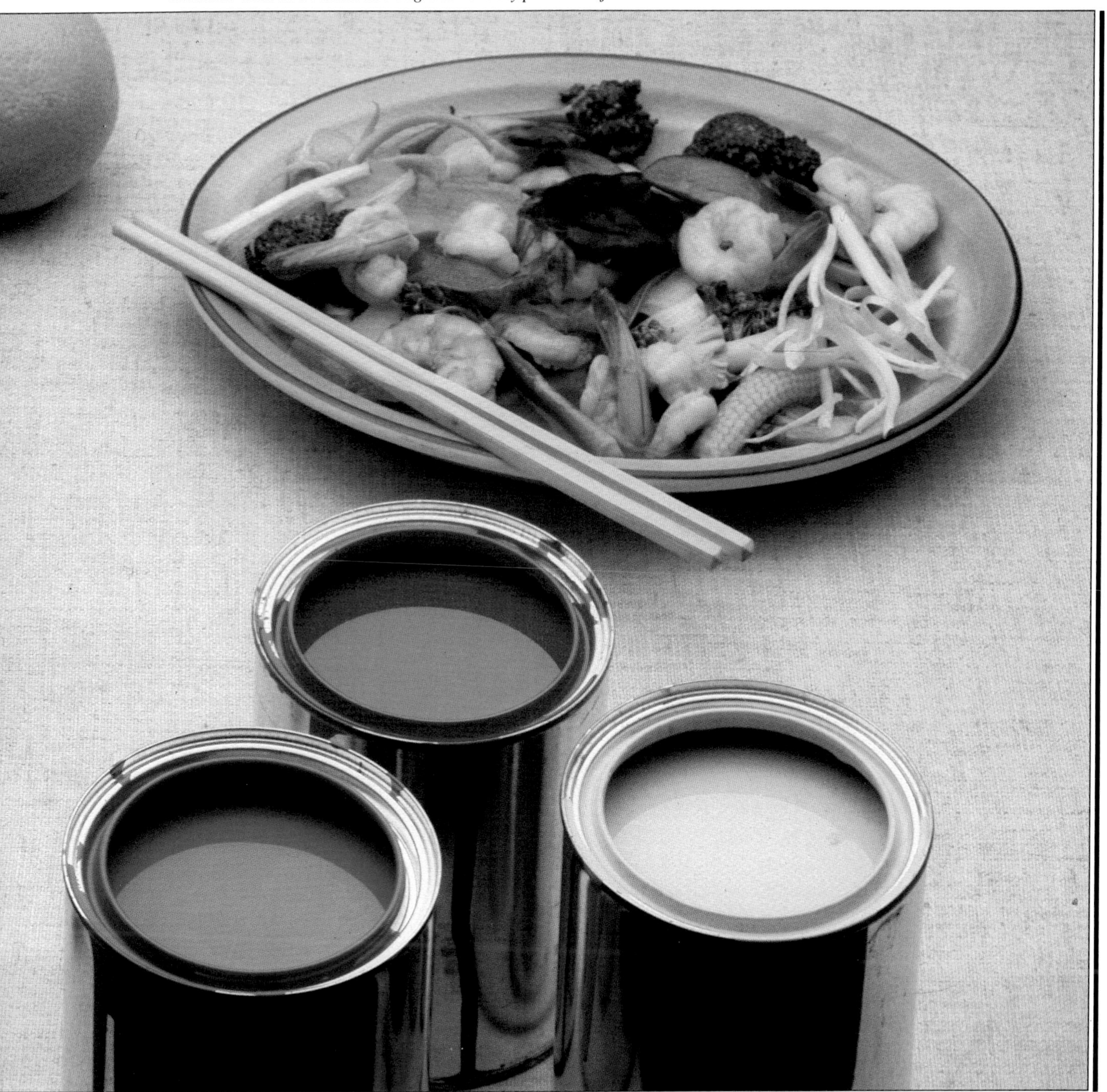

SICKENING FUMES FROM SOLVENTS

Spring cleaning can bring on headaches in more ways than one. Fumes from organic solvents—turpentine, brush cleaners, benzine in gasoline and benzene in paints, dyes, glues and linoleum—are a source of vascular headaches. Formaldehyde, present in some foam insulation, is another trigger.

sonably small quantities can be the trigger of trouble in larger quantities. A coffee addict may consume 10 or 15 cups per day, ingesting so much caffeine that his blood vessels are continuously subjected to its constricting effect; they adapt to it. So long as he gets his customary coffee fixes, he feels no head pain (although the excessive intake of this stimulant has been blamed for digestive troubles and irregular heartbeat). However, when the coffee drinker does not get his usual heavy dosage of caffeine, he gets a withdrawal headache. His arteries, uncustomarily released from the grip of the constricting drug, rebound and dilate excessively: The result is a toxic vascular headache.

Withdrawal headaches, which are seldom recognized for what they are, often strike coffee drinkers on weekends—the regularly refilled cup on the corner of the workday desk is not at hand on the tennis court. When a withdrawal headache develops, short-term relief can be obtained by stopping for coffee or by taking antisleep tablets charged with caffeine. However, the habitual coffee drinker would be wise to wean himself from his caffeine dependency; for most people this means establishing a limit of two to four cups a day. As tolerance to caffeine declines accordingly, coffee will again become a practical emergency antidote to the occasional vascular headache.

Although coffee has been described as the primary offender in this category of toxic vascular headaches, other popular beverages, such as tea, cocoa and cola drinks, can also bring on caffeine dependency and its subsequent withdrawal symptoms when they are consumed to excess. However, coffee is much more potent, containing up to four times as much caffeine per ounce as any of the other beverages. In addition, certain caffeine-boosted medicines *(Chapter 5),* if heavily used and then dropped abruptly, will bring on the same kind of rebound headache.

The Chinese-restaurant syndrome

Unlike caffeine, monosodium glutamate, or MSG, is believed to cause headaches (as well as other, more frightening symptoms, such as chest pain) directly by enlarging blood vessels. A seasoning that has no taste of its own but enhances the flavor of other ingredients, it has long been used in the Orient and now is commonly added in small quantities to such prepared foods as TV dinners, frozen and canned meat, and powdered soups.

MSG is used with a rather heavy hand in Chinese cooking, and the reaction to it has become known as the Chinese-restaurant syndrome. Avoidance of the headache is relatively simple once an individual has identified the cause and determined his personal level of sensitization to the additive. If his system's intolerance is very great, then he should read carefully the labels on packaged foods before sampling their contents. If on the other hand the threshold of tolerance is fairly high, then only certain Oriental foods are potential trouble-makers (the Japanese, who have an extremely high threshold, are believed to eat about three times as much MSG as Americans). Mild-flavored soups such as won ton and egg drop, which tend to be heavily enhanced, should be avoided. And in most Oriental restaurants, chefs respond solicitously to a request that dishes be prepared without MSG.

Far more common than MSG are a number of chemically related headache triggers that are not only eaten but also may be inhaled. These are the nitrates and nitrites, compounds characterized by the presence of a group of nitrogen and oxygen atoms (the difference between the two compounds is that nitrates contain a group made up of one nitrogen atom and three oxygen atoms, nitrites a group of one nitrogen and two oxygen atoms).

Both types of compounds have been employed for thousands of years as food preservatives, particularly in meats—before the days of refrigeration, nitrites and nitrates enabled hams and sausages to be stored over a winter without spoiling. Almost coincidentally, they color the meat that they preserve an appetizing pink (without the preservative, hams and hot dogs would be a dull gray or dark brown). Despite their long history of useful and seemingly danger-free service, both nitrates and nitrites have now come under suspicion as possible cancer-inducers (although the risk of cancer seems to be outweighed by the risks from tainted meat), and there is no doubt that these compounds can cause headaches.

Both nitrates and nitrites relax involuntary muscles, including those that control the size of arteries. The arteries may stretch enough to bring on a headache. Most people are likely to suffer a nitrate or nitrite headache only if they consume unusually large amounts of preserved meats. However, large amounts of these compounds may enter the bodies of some persons in other ways, for nitrates and nitrites are components of many substances other than foods and they do not have to be eaten to cause trouble.

The nitrate group, for example, is part of the nitroglycerin molecule, and nitroglycerin is not only the explosive ingredient in dynamite but a medicinal ingredient widely used to treat the cardiovascular ailment angina. As a medicine, nitroglycerin is seldom swallowed as a pill but is absorbed through the skin. As the resilience of arteries tends to diminish with age, and as circulatory problems that might be treated with nitroglycerin tend to increase with the years, the possibility grows that the blood-vessel enlargement nitroglycerin causes may be enough to bring on a headache.

The same effect can trouble workers who handle nitrate explosives in munitions factories or on construction jobs; they may develop headaches from skin contact and from breathing contaminated air. Even home gardeners with a tendency toward vascular sensitivity sometimes develop a headache as a result of spreading fertilizer, which contains nitrate compounds.

Nitrate headaches generally have a dull, aching quality and are accompanied by a flushed face. Other symptoms are a rapid pulse and a feeling of lightheadedness. In many instances regular exposure to modest quantities of nitrates, as in taking a daily prescription, will eventually lead to a tolerance for the toxin, and assuming the dosage remains constant, discomfort and other side effects will gradually lessen. In the case of hot dogs, children who cannot handle them comfortably when young may very well develop greater tolerance later on.

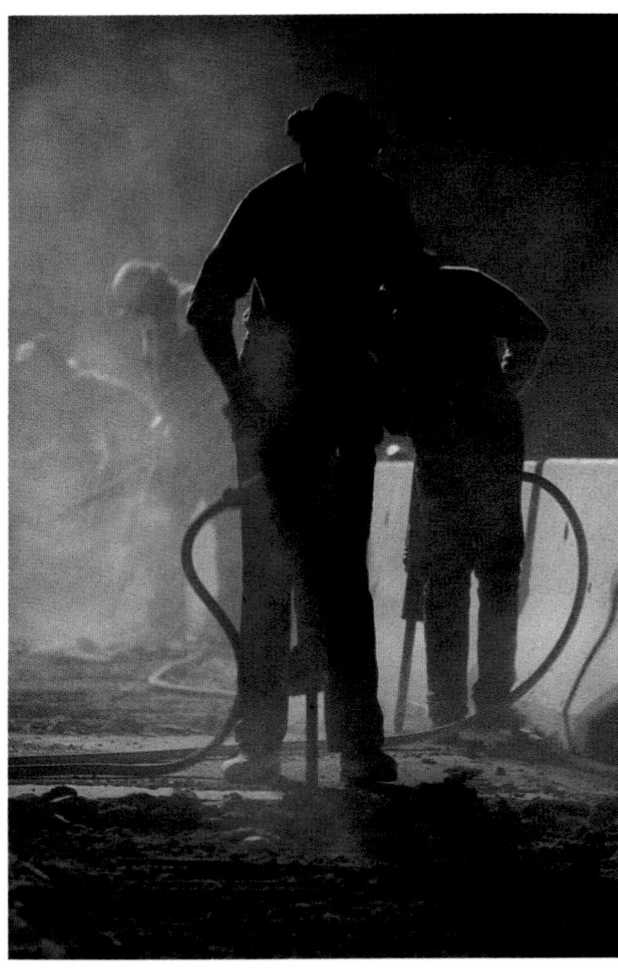

A jackhammer operator laboring amid dust and din risks two headaches at once: a toxic vascular headache from airborne debris and the muscle-tension variety from the vibration and clamor produced by the tool. This man guards against one with a breathing mask but seems to disregard the other— his ear shields are pushed above his ears.

Aches in the air you breathe

Among the other headache-causing toxins that may be inhaled are chemicals in polluted air. Some are, for most people, only occasional problems, such as the vapors that are given off by paints and dyes. But at least one of these toxins is almost ubiquitous in the urban environment: carbon monoxide. Carbon monoxide is a colorless, odorless and exceedingly poisonous gas yielded as a by-product of numerous chemical reactions. It is found chiefly in the exhaust fumes of automobiles and in the combustion fumes of improperly operating gas stoves, space heaters and oil furnaces. When low levels of carbon monoxide build up in the atmosphere of a poorly vented room, or even out of doors in an area that is subject to heavy automobile traffic, a headache is one of the first signs of danger.

The head pain and other symptoms, including tightness across the forehead, rapid heartbeat and dizziness, are linked to carbon monoxide's extraordinary affinity for hemoglobin, the compound in the blood responsible for carrying oxygen from the lungs to all body tissues, including the brain. Carbon monoxide's ability to latch on to hemoglobin is 200 to 300 times greater than that of oxygen, and thus it, not hemoglobin, gets most of the oxygen that is breathed in, preventing the delivery to tissues of this essential element. The body reacts, enlarging the arteries in the head in an effort to compensate for lack of oxygen by bringing in more carriers in the blood. A headache soon develops. (When the carbon monoxide content of air reaches .2 per cent, the hemoglobin transport system is fully saturated and the headache gives way to unconsciousness and death.)

Living and breathing on a street where traffic stalls is not likely to kill anyone, but carbon monoxide is so dangerous that anyone who suffers frequent vascular headaches and suspects that this chemical may be the cause should take immediate steps to check out the suspicion. If carbon monoxide is to blame, there is but one remedy: Eliminate it entirely from the air supply.

Not quite so deadly but generally quick to cause headaches are a variety of volatile solvents in paints, paint removers, brush cleaners, spot removers, gasoline, glue and certain types of foamed insulation. These solvents are so volatile that they quickly fill the atmosphere, and many are rapidly absorbed through the skin. Most of them are carbon compounds, generally derived from petroleum, that can cause damage to nerve cells or the heart muscle. In many cases they provoke headaches because their molecules are constructed like those of the chemicals that transmit nerve signals, including the transmitters of dilation signals. The solvent compounds are such close imitations that they substitute for the real thing, and the nerves, fooled by the mimicry, order blood vessels to expand.

Not only can these solvents trigger headaches, but in sufficient doses they can do permanent damage to the nervous system. They can be used safely if cautions are taken. Some can be used only if protective gloves are worn. All require adequate ventilation. Rod Wolford, health and safety director of the International Brotherhood of Painters and Allied Trades, suggested the use of two portable fans when these materials are used indoors. One should be located so that it evacuates polluted air from the room, preferably out a window. The second fan should be set higher up to pull in fresh air from another room or from an opposite window and direct it at chest height to the working area.

Such safeguards are not practical in all cases. The solvent used in some insulation—particularly the type that is forced as a foaming liquid into the space inside house walls—poses special problems. Its vapors, from formaldehyde, may continue to spread in the air for a considerable period of time after the insulation is installed.

Aches of altitude

The atmosphere can set off toxic headaches even when it is free of man-made pollution. Natural variations in the concentration of oxygen in the air, which depend on altitude, are a common cause of head pain. The headaches associated with altitude sickness are like those caused by carbon monoxide in that they arise from an insufficiency of oxygen, but the mechanism is different. Most people have bodies adapted to air that has the density normal near sea level. At higher elevations, the oxygen content of the air decreases sharply, falling to 83 per cent of its sea-level value at 5,000 feet and to 69 per cent at 10,000 feet.

People accustomed to living in such thin air adapt to it, developing increased proportions of red corpuscles in their blood, the better to transport the oxygen needed. But those coming from lower elevations are likely to experience symptoms of oxygen deficiency periodically between six and 96 hours after arrival. These symptoms include a throbbing headache, usually distributed over the head, a sensation of fullness in the head (related to an accumulation of fluids there), hot flushes of the face, and an extreme sensitivity to light. The pain is often aggravated by sudden motions or coughing, or by lying down.

Most lowlanders are soon able to acclimate themselves to the new atmospheric conditions so that high-altitude headaches are rarely more than a temporary problem. And the adverse reaction to sudden altitude change may diminish with repeated visits, indicating that, for reasons not yet understood, some kind of carry-over effect is conferred with each successive exposure.

High-altitude headaches are usually a problem at elevations above 8,000 feet and are best known to mountain climbers, though tourists and skiers who fly up to mountain resorts from coastal starting points suffer them too. The pains can develop even at elevations as moderate as 5,000 to 7,000 feet—the altitudes of a number of cities popular among tourists—if a newly arrived lowlander exacerbates his oxygen deficiency by exercising strenuously.

Short-term help for mild high-altitude headaches is available from aspirin or acetaminophen, or in more severe cases from the ergotamine prescribed for migraine. For the mildest cases a slightly increased intake of coffee may turn the trick; cold nonalcoholic drinks also help. In any case, anyone traveling to the high mountains will do himself and his head a great favor by keeping his schedule of activities relatively light and by avoiding active sports for a few days. A stopover of a day or two at some intermediate altitude, if that can be arranged, will also ease the transition and reduce the likelihood of headache.

Bright sun—often intense at high altitudes—also can

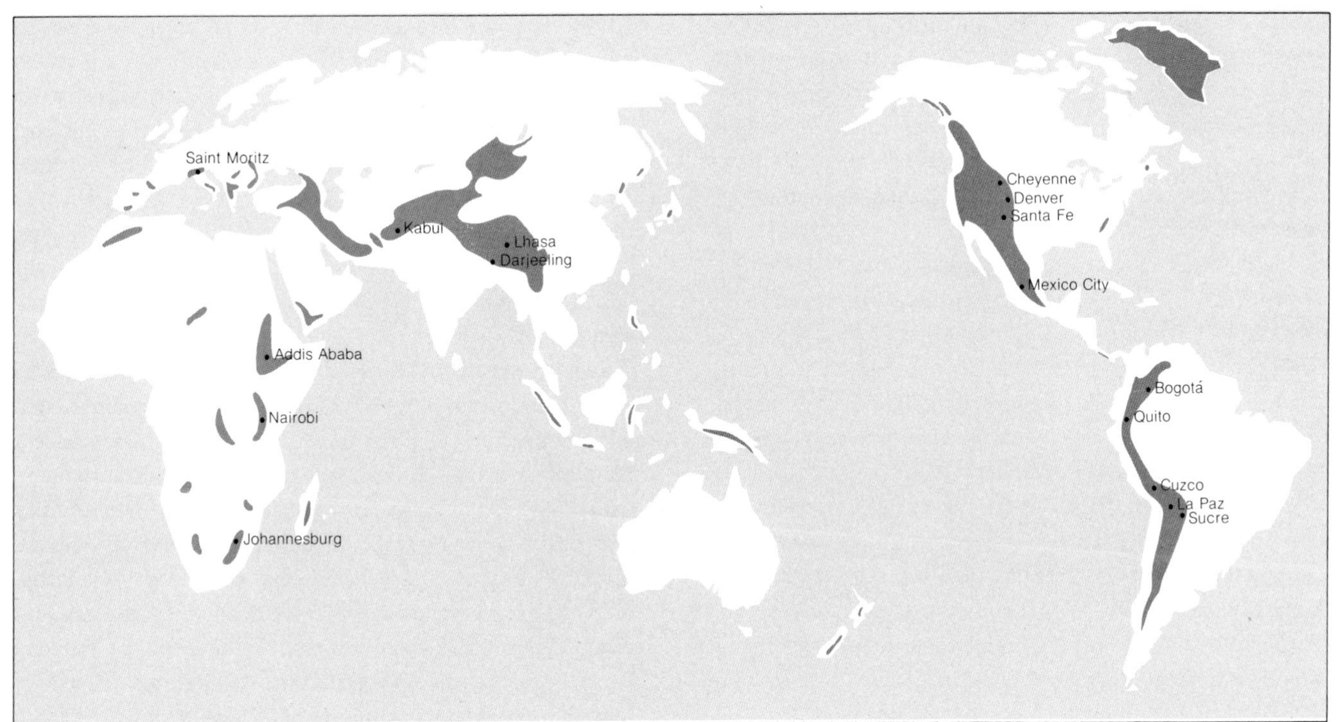

Visitors to cities within these red-shaded regions—all more than 5,000 feet above sea level—may suffer altitude headaches, caused partly by reduced oxygen. The risk increases with height: At Denver, 5,280 feet high, such headaches may occur only after exertion, but at Bogota, 8,659 feet, some visitors suffer even at rest. At La Paz, 12,795 feet, head pain strikes most visitors.

bring on acute headache. Headache researchers regard this as typically a combination of muscular and vascular responses. The muscular reactions are caused by prolonged squinting, usually in glaring light at the beach or in snow. The squinting provokes a tension headache *(Chapter 2)* and can be prevented by shielding the eyes with sunglasses. A hat helps and also may prevent the vascular part of the headache. The vascular response is brought on by the sun's heat, which dilates blood vessels; the sun also bakes body moisture and salts out of the skin, causing subtle chemical and electrical disturbances in body fluids. As arteries swell, blood pressure falls, bringing on dizziness along with headache. This portion of a sun-caused headache can be prevented or alleviated by limiting exertion and drinking plenty of fluids, especially bland ones such as fruit drinks, iced tea or plain water. Do not drink alcoholic beverages, which not only dilate blood vessels but also stimulate the elimination of body fluids and thereby aggravate the dehydration.

Most toxic headaches are set off by a trigger that originates outside the body, such as air pollution or food, but others arise because substances normally present inside the body set them off. Such headaches develop in response to periodic changes in the body's internal chemistry—changes brought about by hunger, by the intermittent release of hormones or by an intensive physical effort. In each case the pain sensations arise when cerebral blood vessels swell beyond their normal limits.

The right foods for hunger headache

Hunger headache is a broad term for an assortment of head pains that, some experts say, may be brought on by changes in the level of sugar in the bloodstream. Blood sugar—a type of sugar compound called glucose—is, along with fats, one of the body's chief sources of heat and energy. It enters the body, some hours before becoming fuel, as a food carbohydrate (either a sugar or a starch compound), goes through a series of digestive processes, and is absorbed into the blood. The bloodstream transports blood sugar to hungry tissues where, with the help of the hormone insulin, it is utilized for body operations and finally broken down into wastes.

At any given time the blood of an average adult may contain about one quarter of an ounce of blood sugar, less than half an hour's supply for the needs of the entire body. Much more is stored in the muscles and liver as glucose reserves, some actively being converted to blood sugar, the rest held in temporary storage; the total amount in the body may come to around three quarters of a pound. When blood-sugar levels fall below the system's basic requirements, particularly if the drop is relatively large or very sudden, many people experience a headache.

The causes of such a sharp sugar-level fluctuation can be as straightforward for some people as postponing a meal, dieting or fasting, particularly if this underconsumption alternates with overconsumption. Exertion is another cause, using up more glucose than the unconditioned body is accustomed to replenishing. Less predictable are sugar-level variations brought on in reaction to eating excessive amounts of sugar compounds—a binge of birthday cake and ice cream, to take a common example.

The antidote for a hunger headache is marvelously easy in most cases: Eat something—preferably protein, which rebuilds the glucose supply slowly. A glass of milk should bring about temporary restoration of the body's chemical equilibrium. Sugary foods such as candy are the wrong remedy for a hunger headache; they encourage the rapid sugar fluctuations that cause such a headache in the first place. If hunger headaches come on with regularity, they could indicate an imbalance in sugar metabolism, and a doctor should be consulted.

A different kind of internal fluctuation triggers the headaches that afflict many women during their menstrual periods. In a number of cases these pains are migraine attacks, but similar vascular headaches are experienced by women who do not ordinarily suffer from migraine. These head pains are triggered by the cyclical production of the female sex hormone estrogen, which regenerates the uterus each month.

Women typically experience two declines in estrogen levels during each menstrual cycle, the first around the 14th day (ovulation), the second approaching the 28th day or just before onset of the next cycle. Dr. B. W. Somerville of Prince

Henry Hospital in Sydney, Australia, noted that vascular migraine headaches coincided with those episodes of estrogen depletion. Such headaches may occur only in some months; the reason apparently is the additive feature in vascular headaches: It often takes more than one factor or influence to get a headache going.

Similar vascular headaches can be brought on by almost anything that stirs up the body's operation physically or emotionally: anger, extreme exertion, even sexual orgasm. The pains always follow close upon the heels of the triggering event and they generally subside within a few minutes as the enlarged blood vessels return to normal. Increasing heart rate leads to increasing blood pressure; simultaneously the blood vessels in the head expand.

Orgasmic headache is of particular interest to researchers because it is frequently preceded by muscle tension, which might be expected to constrict blood vessels rather than enlarge them. Men suffer from this ailment much more than women. Except in a small percentage of cases, orgasmic headaches seem to have no serious long-term consequences, and most sufferers can eliminate them by taking one of the blood-pressure medicines or, more simply, by changing their position during intercourse. According to some of those affected, a fully reclining position, combined with somewhat slower arousal, helps.

Keeping fever pains out of your head

There is one kind of toxic vascular headache that almost everyone experiences from time to time: the fever headache. Fever is most often brought about through a process that begins with infection by bacteria or viruses. The invaders make white blood cells release a fever-producing substance known as endogenous pyrogen. In a complex series of events these chemical mediators enter the bloodstream; when they reach the brain, they stimulate production of yet another class of chemicals, the prostaglandins. The prostaglandins inform the hypothalamus, the brain's tiny thermostat, that an attack is under way; the hypothalamus initiates responses in the rest of the body that are designed to send internal temperatures upward—a reaction that usually is uncomfortable and sometimes can be dangerous, but may, some experts believe, help repel the invasion.

In the final stages of this fever-producing process, the body's metabolic rate accelerates, the heart beats faster, and arteries near the skin, which normally dissipate a considerable amount of heat, are constricted so as to slow down blood flow. Slowing of the blood flow reduces heat loss through the skin, thus increasing internal heat.

When the new, higher, body temperature is reached, the body's use of oxygen and food increases, requiring in turn an increase in the rate of blood supply. Now all arteries—including those that supply the brain and are the starting points for vascular headaches—must expand. At this point of arterial dilation, fever headache sets in. The particular symptoms of fever headache are much like those that mark other toxic headaches; the sensations experienced are typically dull, deep, aching and generalized, though there may also be a more intense area of hurt localized at the back of the head.

For temporary relief from a fever headache, try pressing with your thumbs against the common carotid arteries, which rise on either side of the windpipe in the neck; the pressure restrains the surging flow of blood in the overstretched and tender arterial branches long enough for them to shrink briefly. (Caution: Do not press hard or long, or you may shut off blood flow and faint.)

While a fever headache rages, rest with your head elevated, avoiding any jolting movement, which only serves to intensify the pain. Apply cold compresses to the forehead, and take aspirin or acetaminophen to lower the fever and reduce the headache simultaneously. Because fever-induced vascular headaches are secondary symptoms of systemic illnesses such as mumps, influenza and measles, they are likely to remain or recur until the primary disorder goes away. At that point, the headache should go away, too, permanently.

Go away it almost certainly will. For almost all toxic headaches, unlike the much more severe migraine and cluster pains described in Chapter 4, are transient complaints. Seldom are they related to important underlying disorders. And the discomfort they bring can usually be relieved by simple, safe self-treatment. ✱

Solving the mysteries of migraine

Strange sights of a classic attack
Key causes in heredity and hormones
Evil winds of pain
The migraine personality
Drugs to prevent or end the misery
A catastrophe for men: cluster headaches

"It started with the wallpaper, which I suddenly observed to be shimmering like the surface of water when agitated. A few minutes later, this was accompanied by a vibration in the right hand, as if it were resting on the sounding board of a piano. Then dots, flashing, moving slowly across the field of vision. Patterns, as of Turkish carpets, suddenly changing. Images of flowers continuously raying and opening out. Everything faceted and multiplied: bubbles rising towards me, apertures opening and closing, honeycombs. These images were dazzling when I closed my eyes, but still visible, more faintly, when the eyes were opened. They lasted 20 or 30 minutes, and were succeeded by a splitting headache."

To some readers the imagery of this account, the events and the sudden, painful climax are familiar companions. The anonymous patient who, in 1970, recorded the sequence of symptoms for the British physician Oliver Sacks, was a victim of the chronic, agonizing headache called migraine. This disorder and its relative, the cluster headache, are both vascular, involving expansion of blood vessels. Migraine and cluster headaches, however, are graver and more complex than the immense variety of vascular headaches that are linked to chemicals of one kind or another and are generally lumped under the heading "toxic" *(Chapter 3)*.

Migraine and cluster headaches differ from the toxic type in several distinctive ways. In addition to the sheer intensity of pain, both are chronic; they afflict the sufferer over a period of years, and sometimes for a lifetime. Unlike the occasional attacks of toxic headaches, they are congenital disorders, rooted in the unique physical constitution of the victim. And while toxic headaches are marked by no more than a simple dilation of blood vessels, both migraine and cluster headaches consist of complex series of events, with far-reaching consequences.

A migraine attack is a two-stage affair. In the first stage, corresponding to the spell of visions and hallucinations reported by Dr. Sacks's informant, blood vessels that carry blood to the brain are drastically constricted. In the second, vessels near the surface of the scalp dilate as drastically, to produce an excruciating headache. The extreme constriction and dilation not only affect circulation, but bring other symptoms in their wake: Almost 90 per cent of migraine sufferers are racked by nausea, and more than 50 per cent by vomiting; almost three quarters of them have disturbing feelings of lightheadedness, and about four out of five are pained by even ordinary daylight.

Whereas attacks of migraine headache are largely unpredictable, cluster headaches come—as the name implies—in daily or weekly groups, and between groups the victim may be free of pain for months or years at a time. The explosive pain of a cluster headache is its single, unvariable symptom; by contrast, migraine, although it follows some unfortunates from the cradle to the grave, may take different forms at different ages. In small children, for example, the full array of migraine symptoms is rare, but certain other symptoms, such as colic, chronic motion sickness and periodic vomiting

The bizarre sensory disturbances typical of migraine headache—perceptions of bright-colored lights and distorted shapes, coupled with a throbbing nucleus of pain—are suggested by a photograph originally created to advertise a headache remedy.

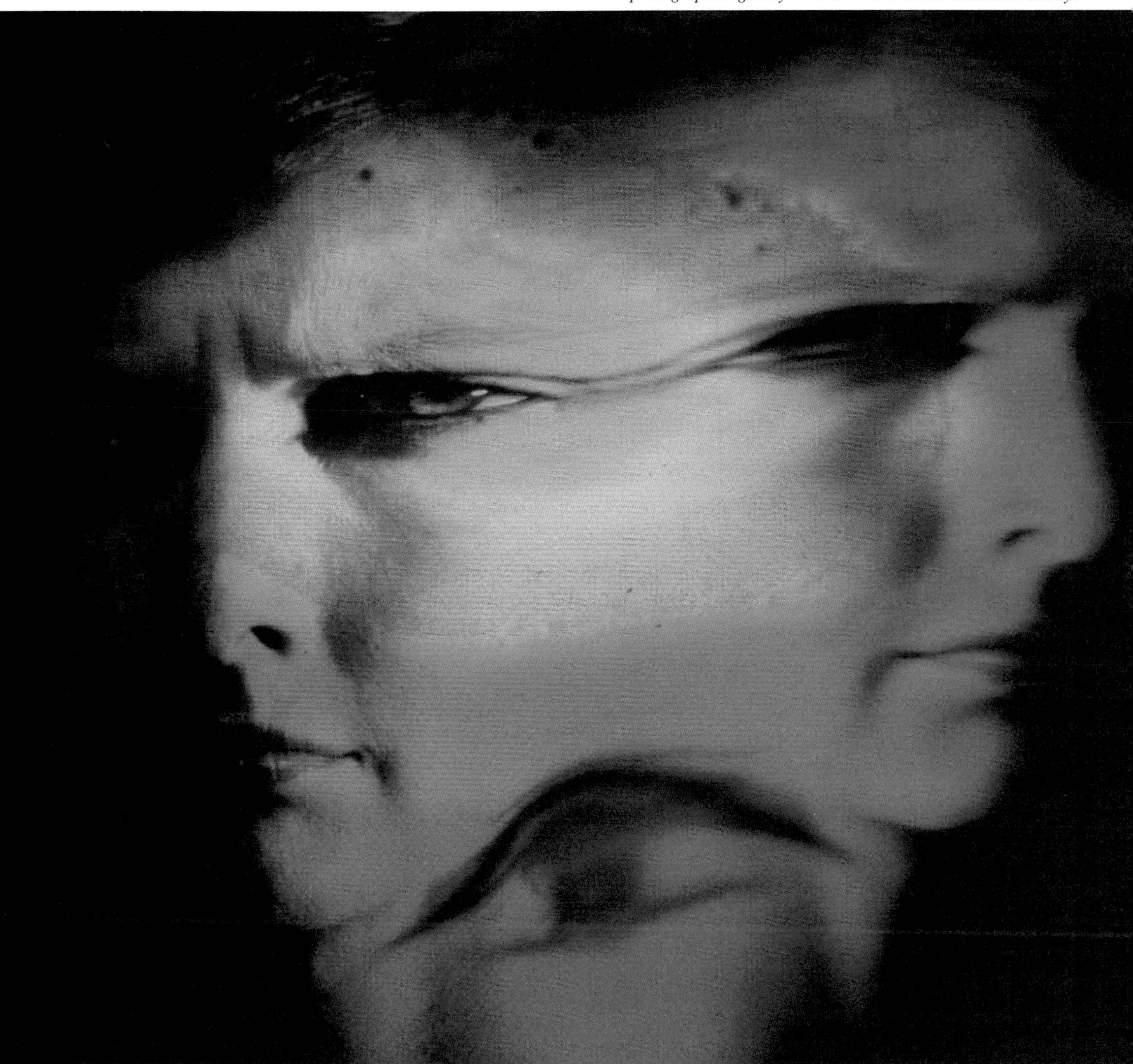

unrelated to intestinal infections, are now recognized as so-called migraine equivalents, which indicate a disposition to develop migraine later on.

Another difference between the two disorders lies in the pattern of attacks with respect to gender. Among juvenile migraine sufferers, boys slightly outnumber girls, but with the onset of puberty the distribution changes markedly; by adulthood, women victims outnumber men by about three to one. Cluster headache reverses the ratio: Four out of five sufferers are men. And though the two related disorders may attack the same victim, migraine is far more common. For every victim of cluster headache, there are 10 or more—according to some estimates, as many as 50—victims of migraine, which is thought to afflict one in every five men, women and children.

After centuries of anguish, effective control

Although cluster headache was first recognized as a distinct ailment only a century ago (it was not fully described in clinical terms until the 1950s), migraine has been studied as well as suffered for as long as humanity has had words to apply to it. Doctors have sought for its causes and mechanisms as far back as written medical history can be traced. References to its ravages turn up in the Sumerian writings of 6,000 years ago, and Egyptian scribes in the time of Pharaoh Akhenaton, about 1400 B.C., set down medicinal formulas for its treatment, including a scalp ointment to be prepared from hippopotamus hide and poppy seeds. Aside from any comfort that the patient might receive from the laying on of hands, however, there was little that could be done to ease an attack or prevent the next one.

Three thousand years later, treatment of migraine had improved little, but understanding of some of its distinctive features was clear. In a description that is echoed in many modern reports on the disease, Dr. Thomas Willis, physician to England's King Charles II and a specialist in nervous disorders, told in the 1660s of the suffering of Lady Anne Finch Conway. He first saw her when she was in her thirties and suffering from migraine almost constantly. "She was of great wit, so that she was skilled in the Liberal Arts, and in all sorts of Literature, beyond the conditions of her sex; and as if it were thought too much by Nature, for her to enjoy so great endowments, without some detriments, she was extremely punished with this Disease."

He went on to describe the course of her attacks, which "troubled her sometimes on one side, sometimes on the other, and often through the whole compass of the Head. During the fit (which rarely ended under a day and a night's space, and often held for two, three, or four days) she was impatient of light, speaking, noise, or of any motion; sitting upright in Bed, with the chamber made dark, she would talk to no body, nor take any sleep or sustenance."

At the heart of Dr. Willis' account was the story of Lady Conway's desperate resort to "very many Remedies by the most skilful Physicians, both of our own Nation and the prescriptions of others beyond the Seas, without any success or ease." One of these remedies was quicksilver, or mercury, a poison that was commonly administered as an intestinal irritant and purgative (it also induced continuous copious drooling). "Some years before, she had endured an oyntment of Quicksilver so that she ran the hazard of her life. Afterwards twice a Cure was attempted (though in vain) from a Mercurial Powder, which the noted Empirick Charles Hues ordinarily gave: with the like success.

"She tryed the Baths, and Spa-waters of almost every kind and nature; she admitted of frequent Blood-letting, and also once the opening of an Artery; she had also made about her several Issues of blood, sometimes in the hinder part of her Head, and sometimes in the forepart, and in other parts. She also took the Air of several Countries, besides her own native Air, she went into Ireland and into France. There was no kind of Medicines, both Cephalicks, Antiscorbuticks, Hystericals, all famous Specificks, which she took not, both from the Learned and the unlearned, from Quacks, and old Women; and yet notwithstanding, the contumacious and rebellious Disease refused to be tamed, being deaf to the charms of every Medicine."

In a notable early step toward better treatment, Dr. Willis proposed a few "evident causes" of Lady Conway's headaches. He observed that the onset of her attacks seemed to be linked with changes of season, weather conditions, certain phases of the sun and moon, violent passions and errors in diet. Doctors have been tracking evident causes, or triggers, and finding increasingly more effective treatments ever since.

The disorder that proved to be wholly inescapable for the beleaguered Lady Conway is no longer so. Through medical treatment and the individual's attention to his own set of triggers, migraine has become subject to significant control and moderation. A number of drugs are now available to relieve the pain and the dreadful sick feeling. In some cases, particularly where the immediate causes of migraine attacks are identified as specific features of diet or behavior, the victim can avoid migraine headaches altogether. And though

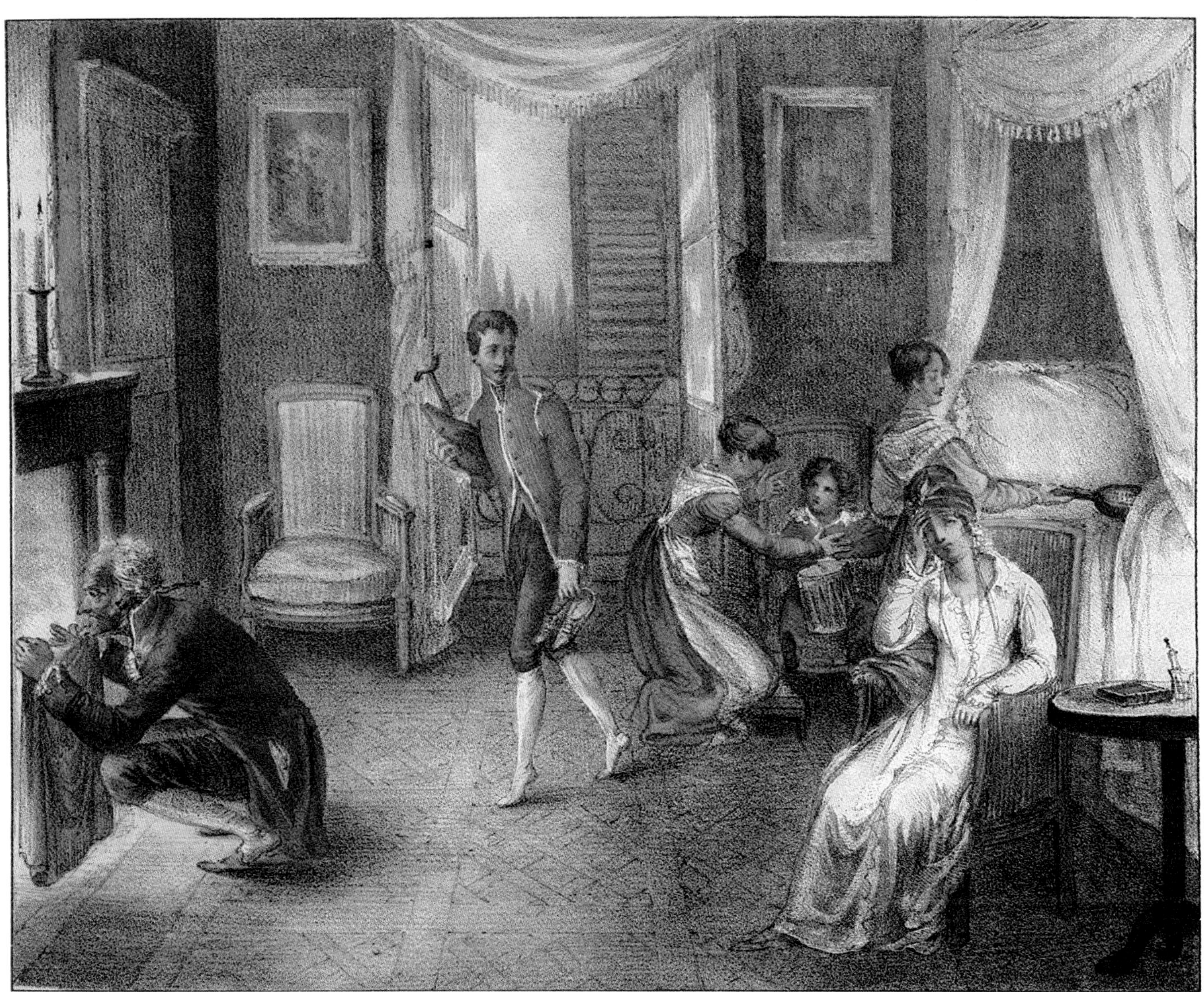

A migraine victim's need for quiet, darkness and soothing warmth is dramatized in this 19th Century French lithograph, "La Migraine," which depicts a family's efforts to ease the mother's suffering. While a servant shields her from firelight, her husband tiptoes shoeless across the floor, the child is made to cease his drumming, and another servant warms the bed with a heated pan.

avoiding migraines is not the same as eliminating the predisposition to them, it does constitute the most effective kind of management of the ailment.

Strange sights of a classic attack

The first step in the management of migraine is an accurate diagnosis. It is not so simple as might be expected, for no tidy set of events fits all migraine experiences. Some of the variations are surprising. An attack can take place without head pain, for example: Headache is only one symptom, albeit the best known, of a system-wide process. But, allowing for the myriad exceptions, certain useful guidelines for identifying most migraines are now recognized.

The vast majority of migraines fall into two classifications—classic migraine, on the one hand, and common migraine, also known as sick headache or simple migraine, on the other. Classic and common migraines differ partly in their prevalence—nine out of 10 migraines are the common variety—and partly in the manner of their onset.

Classic migraines have what doctors call a prodrome or aura—a set of harbinger symptoms that precede a headache. An aura, which may last from 15 minutes to a half hour or more, consists in painless but often distracting or even incapacitating disturbances of sight, hearing, touch, smell and speech. Often, the aura is accompanied by a temporary "high" or a sense of generalized excitement. Less often, it produces transient alterations in judgment, memory and behavior rather similar to those that are exhibited during intoxication. More disconcerting heralds of a classic migraine attack may include numbness, weakness and even temporary paralysis in one or more limbs.

Though the aura is almost always followed by a bout of head pain and other disorders, and is thus anything but welcome, it can be in itself a rather rich experience. Saint Hildegard of Bingen, a 12th Century abbess of Rupertsberg, Germany, was given to rapturous visions *(pages 81-83)* that have since been diagnosed as migraine prodromes.

Describing what she called "The Fall of the Angels," in her manuscript *Scivias,* or *Know the Ways,* Hildegard tells of seeing "a great star most splendid and beautiful and with it exceeding multitude of falling stars." Modern medical interpretation defines this display of visual fireworks as a scintillating scotoma. In other prodromes, Hildegard knew moments in which all visible objects went dark, "all annihilated, being turned into black coals and cast into an abyss so that I could see them no more," a phenomenon known to present-day migraine specialists as negative scotoma; her visions also sometimes included images of zigzag lines, which she interpreted as the "edifices of the City of God," but which investigators now describe, less reverently, as fortification phenomena.

Lewis Carroll, another migraine sufferer, was subject to distortions in his perception of size and scale—and these distortions became grist for his whimsical literary imagination when he wrote *Alice in Wonderland.* In the modern medical literature of migraines, Carroll's visual experiences are termed Lilliputian (for diminished size) and Brobdingnagian (enlarged size)—terms taken from still another literary creation, Jonathan Swift's *Gulliver's Travels.* Other distortions of perception that may occur in a classic migraine aura are mosaic vision, in which images are fractured into irregular facets or dots, and cinematographic vision, in which movement is seen as if in a rapidly running slide show—one still picture after another.

Common migraine, the garden variety that accounts for most migraines, was once thought to have no prodrome or aura—to come on, in effect, with no warning at all. Extensive investigation and interviews with sufferers have revealed, to the contrary, that a sick headache is occasionally preceded by a spell of abnormal moodiness or excitement, beginning as much as a day before the headache. By comparison with the classic aura, it is vague, untheatrical and gradual in its onset; indeed, for many people, it is too subtle to merit notice ordinarily.

Many ills from a one-sided ache

The next stage in migraine is essentially the same in both the classic and common varieties. The dominant symptom is a painful headache, often throbbing to the rhythm of the pulse—a sure sign of vascular origin. Typically, the pain

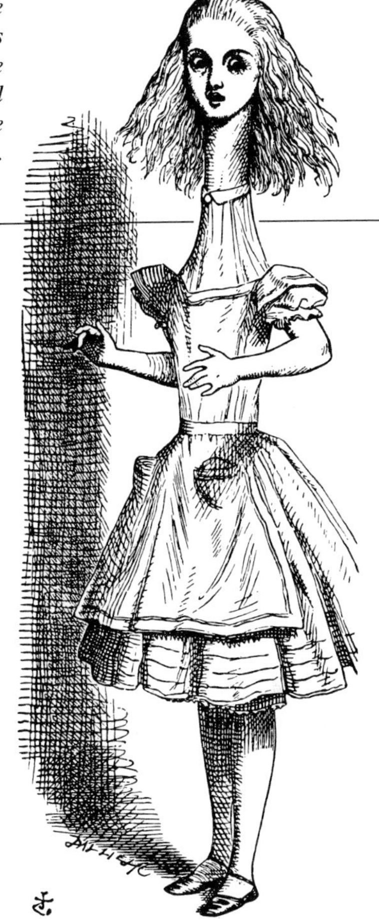

In John Tenniel's illustration for Alice in Wonderland, the heroine's neck grows so long that her feet "seemed to be almost out of sight" —a sensation typical of migraine headaches such as those suffered by Alice's creator, Lewis Carroll.

strikes one side of the head at its onset: Its very name, in fact, derives from the Greek word *hemikranios,* or "half head," first bestowed upon the mysterious disorder by the Greek physician Galen in the Second Century A.D. In medieval Latin the term survived in a corrupted form as *hemigrania;* an early English version, now almost obsolete, was *megrim,* while the French adopted the word that has gained general acceptance, *migraine.*

As Dr. Willis carefully noted more than 300 years ago, the pain may shift to the opposite side of the head as the episode continues, or may become generalized. Wherever the pain occurs, it can be frightful. The author Joan Didion, a nearly lifelong victim of classic migraine, became, according to her own description, "almost unconscious with pain, with a debility that seems to stretch the limits of endurance."

In contrast to ordinary vascular or tension headaches, which usually set in fairly late in the day as pressures build, migraine attacks often disrupt sleep or appear within minutes after awakening. Classic migraine may last from one to six hours, with pain at full intensity for most of the period; common migraine often takes several hours to reach its full strength, but may last from one to three days.

The headache is usually accompanied by other symptoms, including nausea, vomiting, loss of appetite, diarrhea, dizziness, tremors and spells of sweating and chills. Fingertips may turn bluish and hands are icy. For many sufferers, sensitivity to daylight and ordinary household sounds becomes so intense that nothing short of a solitary retreat in a dark room can get them through an episode. Tears well up in the eye closer to the pain area or in both eyes, and the sufferer's face often becomes pallid. One or both of the arteries in the temples may become so distended that their pulsations are visible to an observer several feet away. The nose feels and sounds blocked, though it is free of discharge.

The body tends to retain an excessive amount of salt and water, so that hands and feet become visibly and painfully swollen; for 95 per cent of migraine sufferers, a temporary weight gain of two to five pounds occurs, and in some extraordinary cases gains of as much as 17 pounds have been recorded. Feelings of apathy and an overriding sense of psy-

The Alice-in-Wonderland syndrome

"I'm very brave, generally, only to-day I happen to have a headache," bemoaned one of the fantastic characters dreamed up for *Alice in Wonderland* and *Through the Looking-Glass* by mathematician Charles Lutwidge Dodgson, who used the pen name Lewis Carroll. He himself suffered classic migraines, with physical sensations now known as "the Alice-in-Wonderland syndrome."

Carroll's miseries helped him devise adventures for his heroine. *Alice in Wonderland* begins with the girl dozing, then feeling herself falling through space—a vivid description of the dizziness common to migraine. Elsewhere Alice feels herself growing tall *(above)* or shrinking—"shutting up like a telescope," as she puts it. Carroll also gave a fanciful account of the migraine "blind spot," or blank area that appears to blot out vision directly ahead, when he described Alice in a shop in *Through the Looking-Glass:* "Whenever she looked hard at any shelf," he wrote, "that particular shelf was always quite empty, though the others round it were crowded as full as they could hold."

chological prostration may match the body's physical debility. Less often, the psychological response takes the form of irritability and hostile feeling.

Any or all of these symptoms can arise from both classic and common migraines, which account for the vast majority of severe vascular headaches. Several rare near-relatives, collectively known as complicated migraines, carry disquieting symptoms of their own. Though the division of these other ailments into categories varies from specialist to specialist, the most widely accepted variants are hemiplegic, ophthalmoplegic and basilar migraines.

Hemiplegic migraine is a moderate to severe headache lasting as long as five days. Its distinguishing feature—once termed, for lack of better information, an "apoplectic seizure"—is some form of temporary numbness or paralysis. The condition, called hemiplegia (for "half stroke"), is usually limited to one side of the head and body. It usually affects speech in much the way a stroke does (in some cases, actual strokes have occurred). The symptoms are alarming, but the paralysis and speech disorder typically disappear within 48 hours.

Ophthalmoplegic migraine, too, is marked by a moderate headache and a temporary paralysis. In this case the paralysis strikes the eye on the same side as the headache, producing double vision, a drooping eyelid and an enlarged pupil. The immediate cause is well understood: Under extreme pressure from swollen blood vessels directly behind the eye, an oculomotor nerve, which controls the muscles of an eye, produces the eye-related symptoms.

In basilar migraine, pain is typically localized at the back of the head around the branches of the basilar artery, which supply blood to the base of the brain and the back of the cerebral cortex. Once again, the secondary characteristics are extraordinary: Spasms in the artery produce giddiness, fainting, loss of equilibrium, dizziness and slurred speech—symptoms that might well be mistaken for those of drunkenness. Only recently identified and studied, basilar migraine is still a maze of unanswered questions. The disorder seems to be peculiar to young people, especially young women. In the first detailed analysis of a group of victims, conducted in 1961 by Dr. Edwin R. Bickerstaff of the University of Birmingham in Great Britain, almost 95 per cent were less than 23 years of age, and in this youthful group 76 per cent were adolescent girls, in whom the onset of migraine was closely timed to the menarche, the first occurrence of the menstrual cycle.

Every attack of migraine, whether simple or complex in origin, eventually ends; the migraine pain and other symptoms subside, and characteristic postheadache symptoms follow. Like other aspects of the illness, they vary from patient to patient. Some frequent signs are little more than consequences of the trying experience the patient has just endured—a feeling of profound fatigue, an extremely tender scalp and soreness in the muscles of the head and neck, perhaps a remnant of a muscle-tension headache induced by hours of clenched resistance to the migraine itself.

Other effects are more dramatic. For some people, the resolution of pain comes with extreme suddenness and even violence—in a climactic siege of vomiting or sneezing, for example. A more gradual recovery may be marked by unusual amounts of perspiration, the need to urinate copiously, or a period of weeping, as though the body's entire system were undergoing a physical and emotional catharsis. Any of these events may be followed by a deep, exhausted sleep, from which the victim awakes with normal energy restored and even a feeling of euphoria.

Why migraine hurts so much

When the pain finally goes away, the sufferer is in one sense simply rejoicing in a return to normal health. But the euphoria, like the depression and other symptoms that precede it, has physical as well as mental roots. Each is a part of nature's programing for migraine. Researchers now feel reasonably certain that all of these events arise in the arterial system and in the system of nerves that instruct the arteries to constrict or dilate. In migraine sufferers, these systems are inherently unstable. When confronted with a wide range of internal and external challenges, which the normal individual can handle with equanimity, they overreact. Among the factors in this overreaction are certain blood components; arterial

A warning of an attack in bizarre visions

For one migraine victim in 10, the staggering pain of an attack is preceded by a warning: Bizarre images flash and flicker across the field of vision. These "migraine auras," usually made up of zigzag lines, bright pinwheels or starlike pinpoints, are so distinctive that some have acquired special names. For example, the zigzags, which may resemble the crenelated top of a castle, are called the fortification phenomenon. The visions are so striking that many victims have recorded them in drawings and paintings.

The most famous pictures of migraine auras are those created in the 12th Century under the direction of Saint Hildegard of Bingen, abbess of Rupertsberg convent *(right)*. Hildegard, who left behind not only pictures but writings indicating she suffered from classical migraine, considered her visions to be divinely inspired allegorical symbols. To record the images and her interpretation of them, she supervised the preparation of two illustrated manuscripts, portions of which are reproduced overleaf.

Modern victims of migraine also have recorded their auras in paintings and drawings. Leslie Crespin, an artist of Taos, New Mexico, often has used her visions in her work *(page 84)*. Their form has changed since her doctor prescribed drugs to control the attacks—she no longer sees human figures—but they remain bizarre, including in one vision "a fly's eye made of millions of light-blue Mickey Mouses."

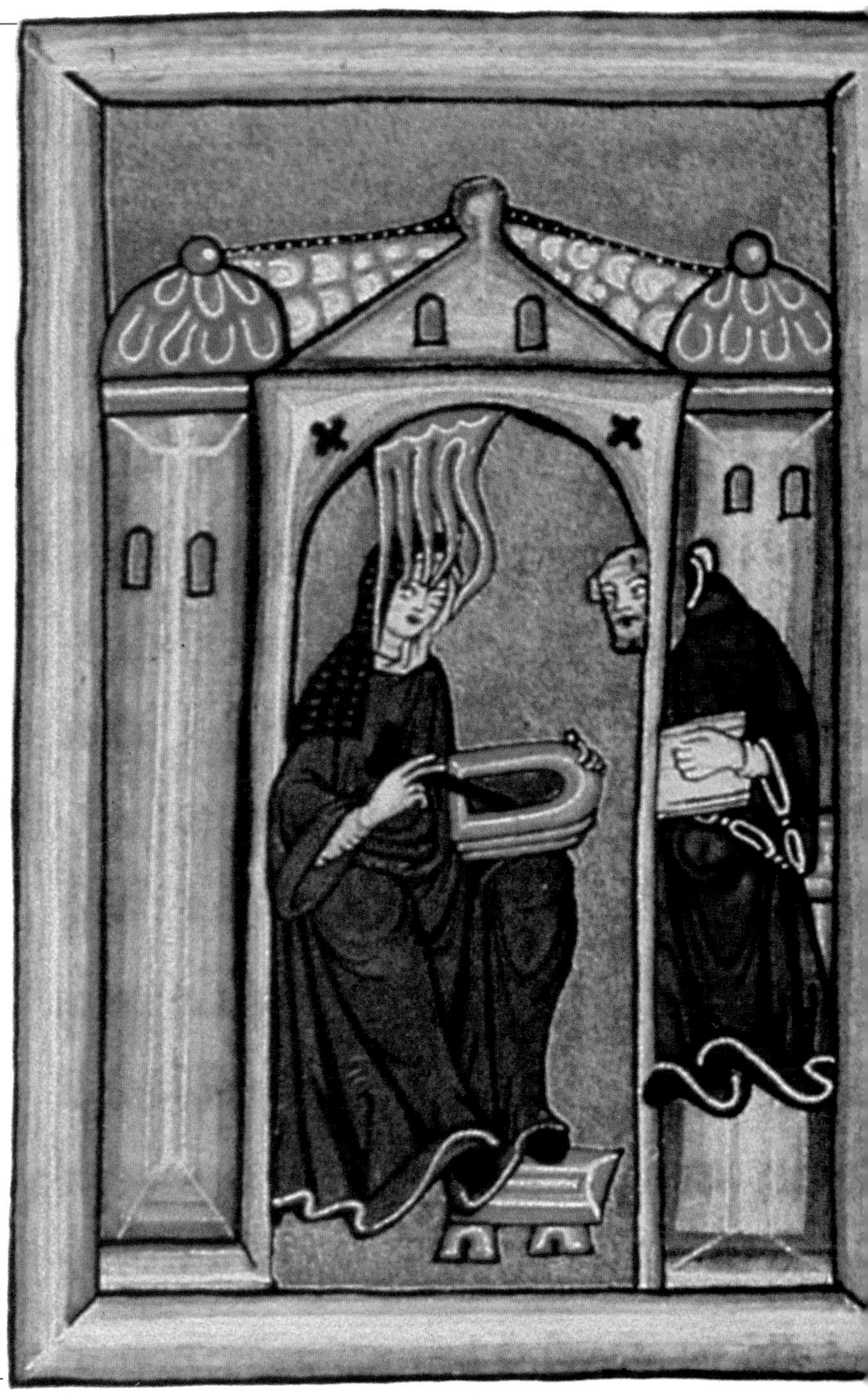

A 12th Century manuscript illustration portrays migraine sufferer Saint Hildegard as she records a vision, represented as flames above her head, while a monk observes. Hildegard derived religious meaning from the images she saw, typical of those preceding a migraine attack.

Lines resembling the walls of a fortress—a so-called fortification phenomenon—trail from a three-winged head in a 12th Century artist's representation of one of Saint Hildegard's visions. The scintillating lines, a common feature of migraine auras, signified to Hildegard the walls of the City of God.

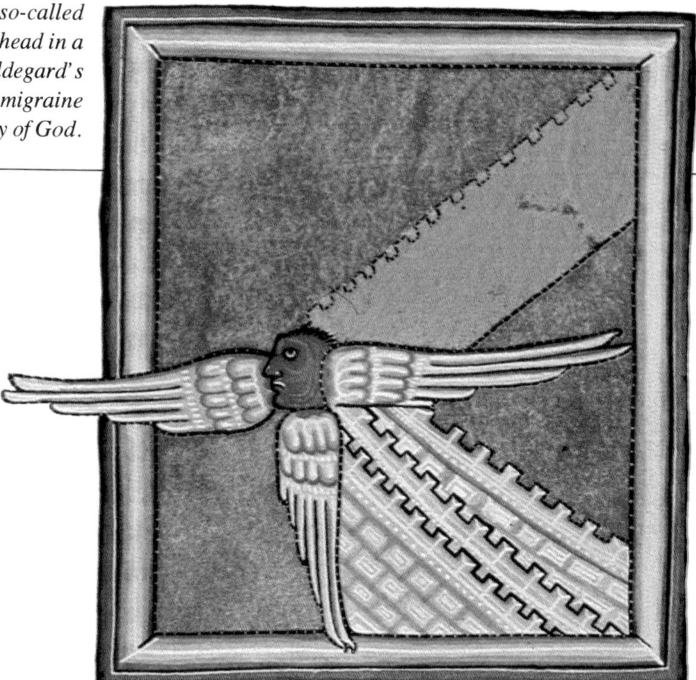

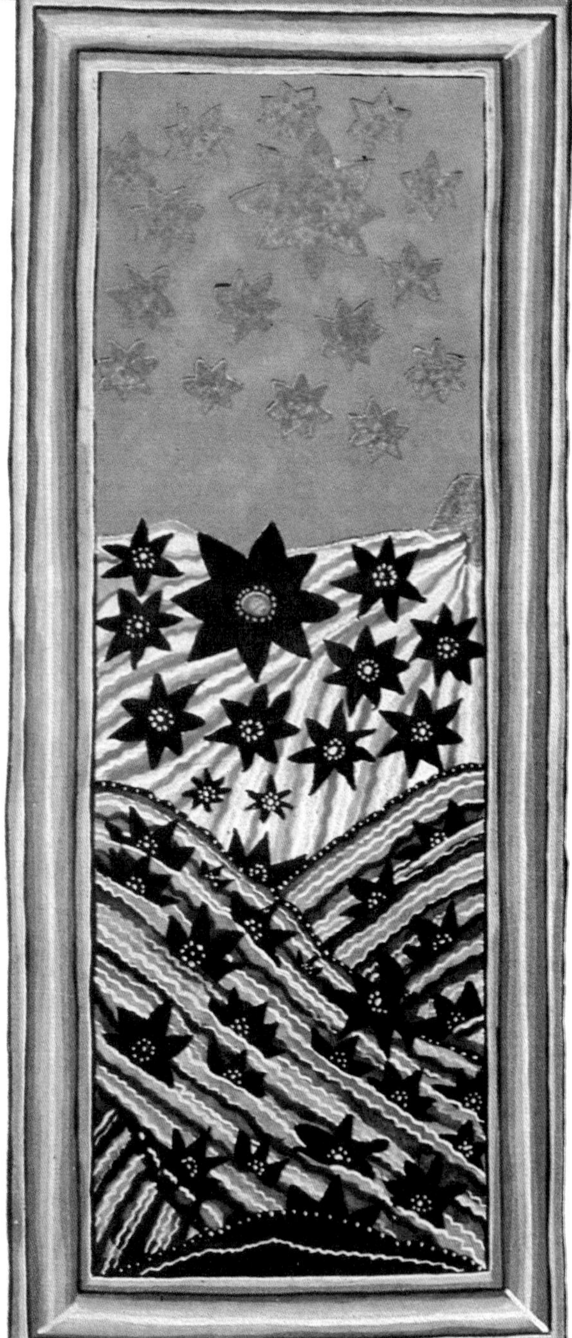

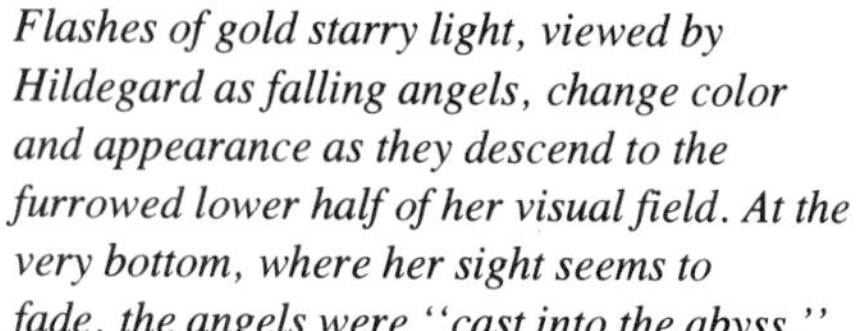

Flashes of gold starry light, viewed by Hildegard as falling angels, change color and appearance as they descend to the furrowed lower half of her visual field. At the very bottom, where her sight seems to fade, the angels were "cast into the abyss."

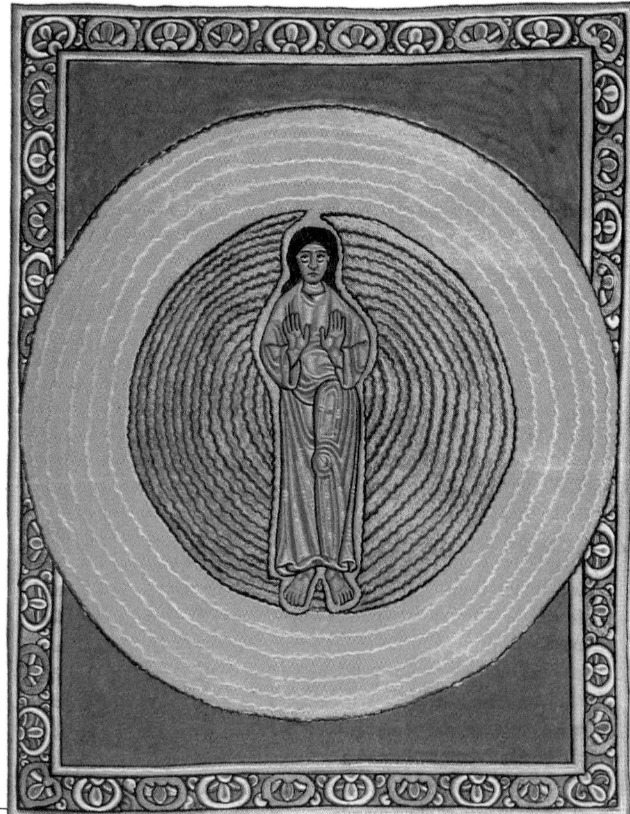

A brilliant, shimmering pinwheel shape, one of the most common images of a migraine aura, surrounds a radiant human figure identified by Hildegard as Christ. She described the pinwheel as "a most shining light" and interpreted it as God. It contained, she said, "a human form of a sapphire color which glittered with a gentle but sparkling glow."

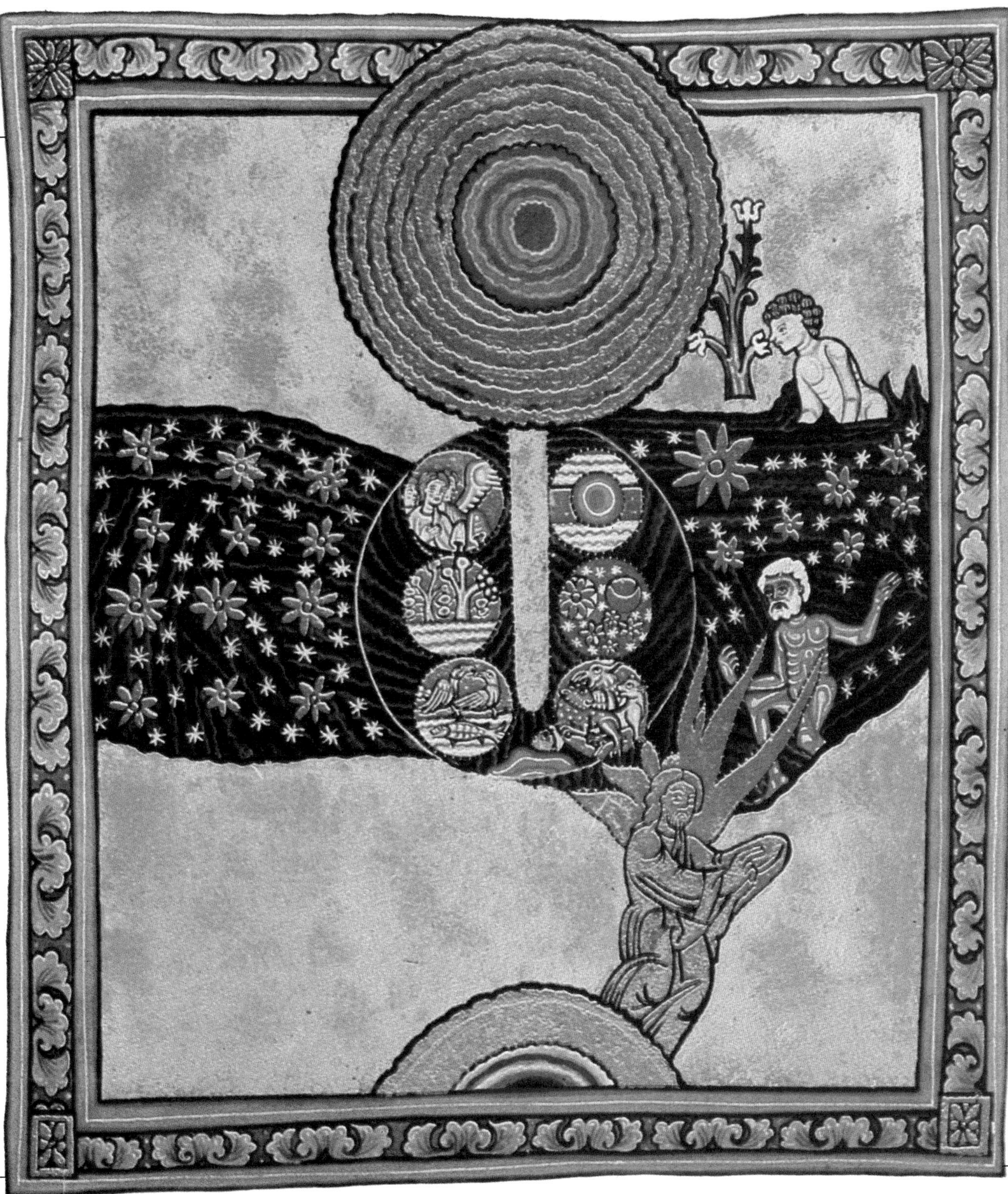

In one of the most elaborate depictions of Hildegard's visions, migraine symbols portray Biblical history: The top pinwheel represents God. At center six small circles illustrate the six days of Creation. Adam, young and innocent at top right, sniffs the flower of obedience; at center right, sinful and aged, he falls into darkness, to be uplifted by Christ rising out of the dawn.

A modern artist's eerie images

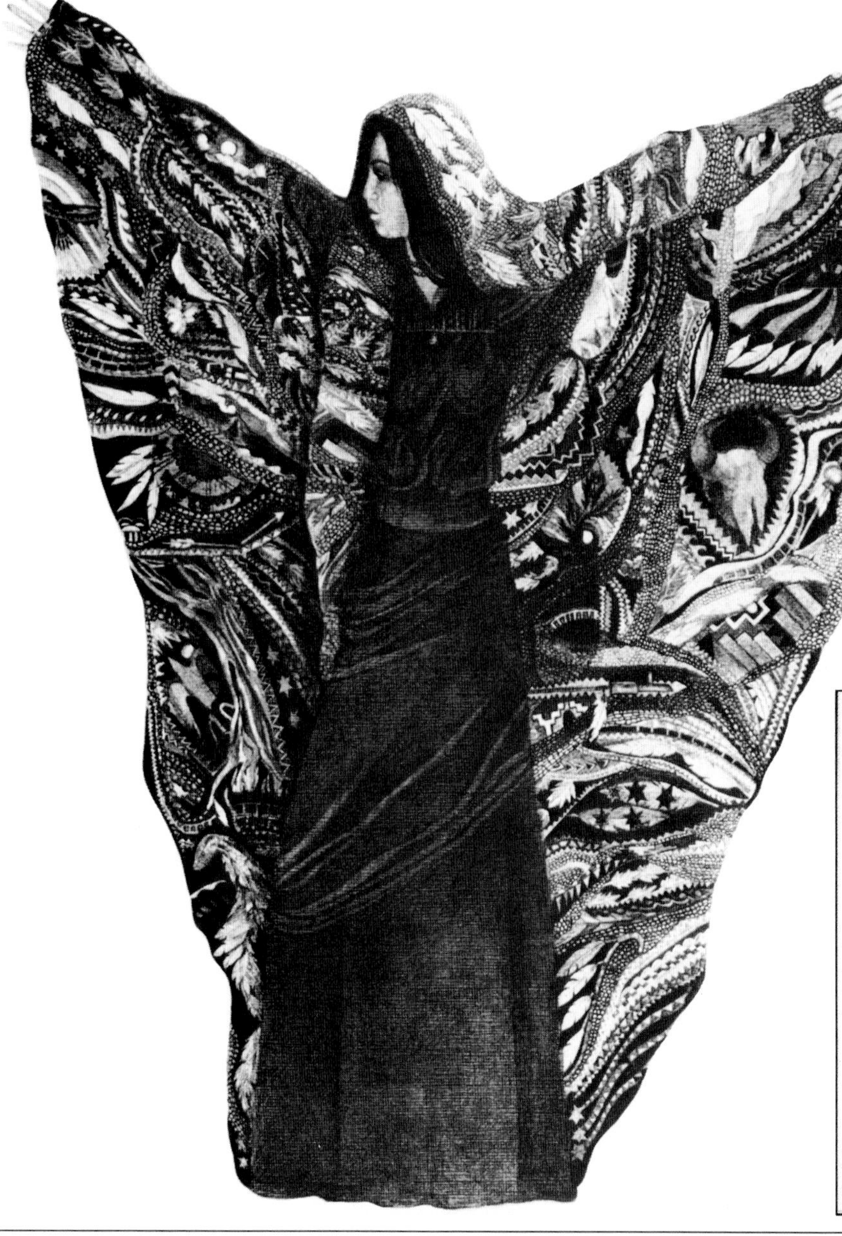

Shimmering zigzag lines and stars of migraine visions are emblazoned on the robe of an Apache woman in New Mexico artist Leslie Crespin's sketch of an apparition that appeared in her room before the painful throbbing of a migraine headache began. She saw such apparitions for as long as an hour at a time.

Drawn in the throes of an actual migraine attack, the slashing ink strokes of a work that Leslie Crespin entitled "Death with Long Hair" express the artist's anger at her intense pain.

responses to the substances called hormones, which induce constriction and dilation in blood vessels; other chemicals, called neurotransmitters, that convey signals along nerves; and individual responses to stress. These factors act on the blood vessels in sequence.

According to Dr. John Graham, director of the Headache Research Foundation at Faulkner Hospital in Boston, Massachusetts, an attack begins when small arteries near the center of the brain constrict; the volume of blood flowing through the narrowed vessels is correspondingly reduced. This is not in itself an uncommon event—in a normal individual, blood flow varies in response to the stresses of everyday life, and slight constrictions are commonplace. In those with migraine, however, the constriction is extreme. In one test, conducted at Baylor University in Houston, Texas, in 1977, migraine patients inhaled a harmless radioactive gas before and during an attack, and the rates of blood flow in their brains were measured by a counter. Among the victims of classic migraine, blood flow in some areas was down an average of 50 per cent.

A deficiency of blood to the face soon produces the pallor associated with the warning disturbances of the aura. Similarly, the disruptions in the senses can be traced to specialized parts of the brain that are deprived of blood. For example, anomalies in vision indicate a constriction of small vessels in the occipital lobes of the brain, where visual impulses are interpreted, while hearing disturbances suggest arterial constrictions and reduced blood supply in the temporal lobe, where the acoustic center is located.

Any widespread constriction of cerebral vessels, however, is dangerous as well as disturbing. A drastic insufficiency of blood, with its load of oxygen and nutrients, could threaten the very life of the brain. To protect itself, the body quickly mounts a defense. Larger arteries near the surface of the brain suddenly dilate. Such compensatory dilation is a routine reaction whenever arteries constrict, but in migraine the rebound, like the original constriction, goes to excess. Vessels swell to diameters half again as large as normal, stretching their walls and the nerve endings embedded in the walls. This stretching alters the electrical voltage in the nerves, resulting in a pain impulse. The characteristic throbbing migraine begins, each throb corresponding to a pulse of blood coursing through the arteries and stretching them.

It was long assumed that arterial dilation alone accounted for all the pain of migraine. As tools of investigation became more sophisticated, however, other causes were identified. According to the most widely held theory, migraine pain arises not only from the stretching of dilated arteries but also from chemical irritation caused by substances in the blood or around the swollen area.

Some of these substances normally link the nerves and muscles that regulate the circulatory system. For example, chemicals called neurotransmitters are released from the nerve ends and stimulate muscle fibers to take a specific, limited action. But if neurotransmitters such as norepinephrine, epinephrine and acetylcholine are released in excessive amounts, or if certain countervailing substances that normally neutralize or inhibit them after their release fail to function, then it seems reasonable to suppose that stimulation becomes irritation, leading to local inflammation and additional pain.

Furthermore, the chemicals called hormones, which normally travel through the bloodstream to stimulate distant organs, may make their own contribution to pain. Among their many chemical properties, certain hormones have powerful irritant effects. Carried along in the blood, they may seep into the areas around dilated blood vessels through the stretched and consequently more permeable vessel walls. As they collect there, they may increase the pain that is caused by the stretching itself.

Key causes in heredity and hormones

Although the chemistry of migraine is still largely a matter for speculation, other aspects of the disease now are known in detail. Scientists can report who gets migraine, when they get it and, perhaps most interesting of all, what sort of people they are—information that suggests clues to causes.

Migraine clearly seems to run in families. More than 70 per cent of the victims, when asked to go back over their family history, find a near blood relation who has also suffered from it or from a related type of vascular headache. Naturally enough, most researchers now argue that migraine is inherited—a result of a nervous system that cannot provide close, steady control over artery contractions. But the matter is not settled. To some extent, the high incidence of migraine in some families may be mere coincidence; there is also a possibility, argued by some researchers, that the ailment is not inherited but rather is a reaction subconsciously selected as a family pattern for coping with stress.

More intriguing—and more firmly established—is a connection between migraine and hormones over the course of a lifetime. Migraine attacks most often begin at or soon after adolescence, when the pattern and amounts of hormones in the bloodstream change radically. At middle age, another time of hormonal change, many migraine sufferers find to their relief that their attacks diminish in frequency and severity, though certain migraine equivalents, such as periodic nausea and vomiting, may continue. Some women regularly suffer migraine attacks just before or at the start of a menstrual period—a time of changing hormone levels—but find that their disorder subsides after menopause, when female sex hormones diminish.

Pregnancy, another time of increased hormonal activity, has a markedly favorable effect, particularly on common

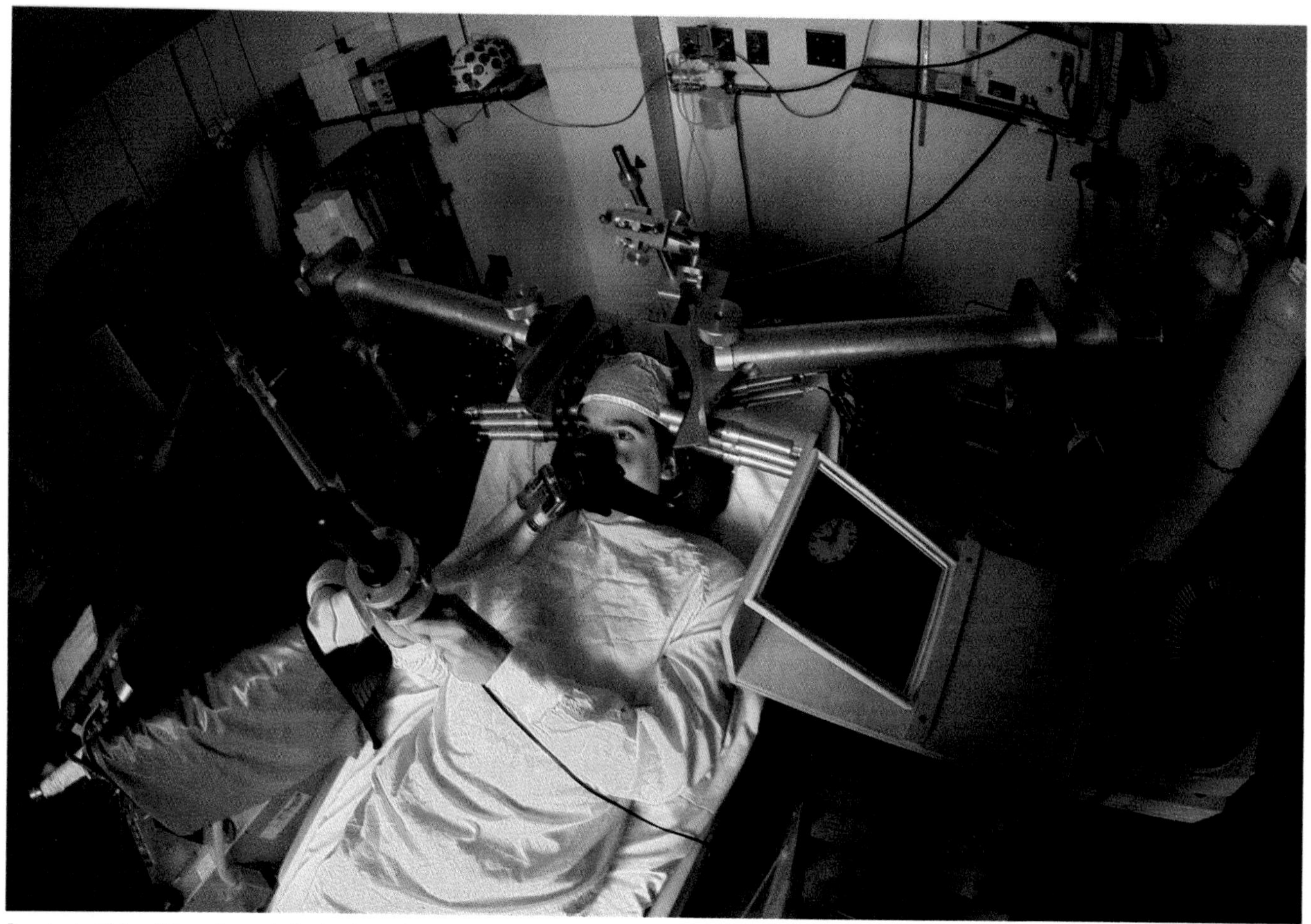

In a test of blood flow through the brain—the data help evaluate headache remedies—a volunteer inhales radioactive gas while detectors around his head track its progress in the blood. To show how mental activity affects the flow, he uses a flashlight rod to answer questions projected onto the ceiling with an angled mirror (right), which also picks up a wall-clock reflection.

migraine. In a 1972 study of pregnant women at the Prince Henry Hospital in Sydney, Australia, 77 per cent of the subjects who had previously suffered migraines reported that their attacks disappeared completely, occurred less often, or were milder in the second and third trimesters. (Among the remaining migraine victims, some women reported worsening pain. A few women who had never had migraine before suffered their first attack while carrying a child.)

It is not surprising, then, that the deliberate administration of hormones has an equally strong effect. Oral contraceptives, which are a mixture of the hormones estrogen and progestin, influence some women's susceptibility to migraine, as does the administration of estrogen to relieve symptoms of menopause. The additional hormones, particularly in the contraceptives, can bring on a migraine attack, exacerbate an existing condition or introduce a complication of migraine, such as stroke—but not always. Sometimes they do just the opposite, and they have been known to interrupt a long history of migraine susceptibility.

Evil winds of pain

Such quirky, often contradictory, effects are not unique to hormones. As in the ordinary run of vascular headaches, dozens of potential triggers have been implicated in repeated attacks of migraine. Not all the triggers are chemical, and to the layman they often appear to have no rhyme or reason. One typical attempt to unravel their mysteries has been the long hunt for a link between migraine and weather.

Bone and muscle pains, of course, have long been attributed to the decrease in barometric pressure that precedes a storm, and many a rheumatic grandparent serves as a family weather forecaster. In 1877, the noted American neurologist Weir Mitchell published a report on this phenomenon, describing "a belt which may be called the neuralgic margin of the storm," in which "the stir and perturbation of the elements" was sensed. Dr. Mitchell correctly blamed lessened barometric pressure for much of the effect, but he also included as causes temperature, humidity, winds and possibly "some as yet unknown agency productive of evil. Such an agency may be either electricity or magnetism." Electricity may indeed be a factor in migraine, particularly associated with the "witches' " winds that strike various parts of the world at certain seasons.

"Hot winds of ill repute in all parts of the world affect mental and physical well-being and may constitute a factor in provoking headaches in weather-sensitive patients," wrote Dr. Felix Gad Sulman of Hebrew University, Jerusalem, in an article on his migraine research in *Hemicrania,* the journal of the British-based Migraine Trust. "Such winds are known by various terms, e.g., the Santa Ana of Southern California; the desert winds of Arizona; the Argentine Zonda; the Sirocco and Tramontana of the Mediterranean littoral; the Meltemia of Greece; the Xlokk of Malta; the Chamsin or Sharkiye of the Arab countries; the Sharav of the Old Testament, which still scourges Israel; the Foehn of Switzerland, Southern Germany and Austria; the Autun of France; the North winds of Melbourne; the Thar winds of India, the Chinook of Canada; the Gonding and Koembang of Java and the Bohoroh of Sumatra."

These brooding winds, Dr. Sulman said, are notorious for their association with headaches, depression, discomfort and irritability. That association, he thought, might well relate to another phenomenon—the abnormally high concentrations of positive ions intrinsic to such winds.

In the atmosphere, a molecule of air is normally electrically neutral. An ion is a molecule that has either lost or gained an atomic component bearing a negative electrical charge; as a result an ion has either a positive or a negative electrical charge. In ordinary weather, the air is fairly well balanced, with mostly neutral molecules and about 2,000 ions, roughly evenly divided between positive and negative, in each cubic centimeter of air. But in weather that creates a high state of atmospheric friction—thunderstorms and "ill winds" being prime examples—the number of ions and their proportions are drastically altered: Many more molecules are ionized. In a spell of Israel's Sharav weather, for example, the number of ions may rise to 8,500 per cubic centimeter, and 4,500 of these ions are positive.

Dr. Sulman and his colleagues studied migraine patients selected for their susceptibility to the Sharav. They isolated particular characteristics of the wind that were consistently present when attacks were reported by their subjects: Relative humidity dropped below 30 per cent; temperature rose as much as 27 degrees (Fahrenheit) above the average for the time of year; and the winds blew from the east, roaring in from the desert. The researchers also analyzed the biochemistry of the sufferers and found that their production of a neurotransmitter known as serotonin was increased as the ratio of positive ions rose. Serotonin is a blood-vessel constrictor. It is, in fact, exactly the kind of substance that could be responsible for the extreme vessel constriction of the first stage of a migraine episode.

By his own admission, Dr. Sulman was still a long way from cracking the mystery of wind and migraine, and research by other investigators failed to confirm his findings. But he noted that human beings breathe some 2,500 gallons of air every 24 hours; given the fact that electricity is a critical element in biological processes at the cellular level, it seems only reasonable that it play a role on a larger scale in various states of health and illness, migraine among them. Some inconclusive experiments with negative-ion machines, small room-sized generators of negative ions, suggest that changing the ratio of positive to negative ions may indeed alleviate migraine symptoms.

Winds, of course, represent only one possible trigger for migraine. A partial list of agents *(page 90)* drawn up in 1980 by two American headache authorities, Drs. Neil Raskin of the University of California and Otto Appenzeller of the University of New Mexico, indicates their extraordinary range; the list includes fatigue, glaring light, excessive sleep, cold foods and perfume.

Some researchers say, ruefully, that almost anything can be found to spark an attack in some migraine tinderbox somewhere. And though minor triggers may be almost indiscernible, they are cumulative in their effects. Like the straw that broke the camel's back, each of these various influences by

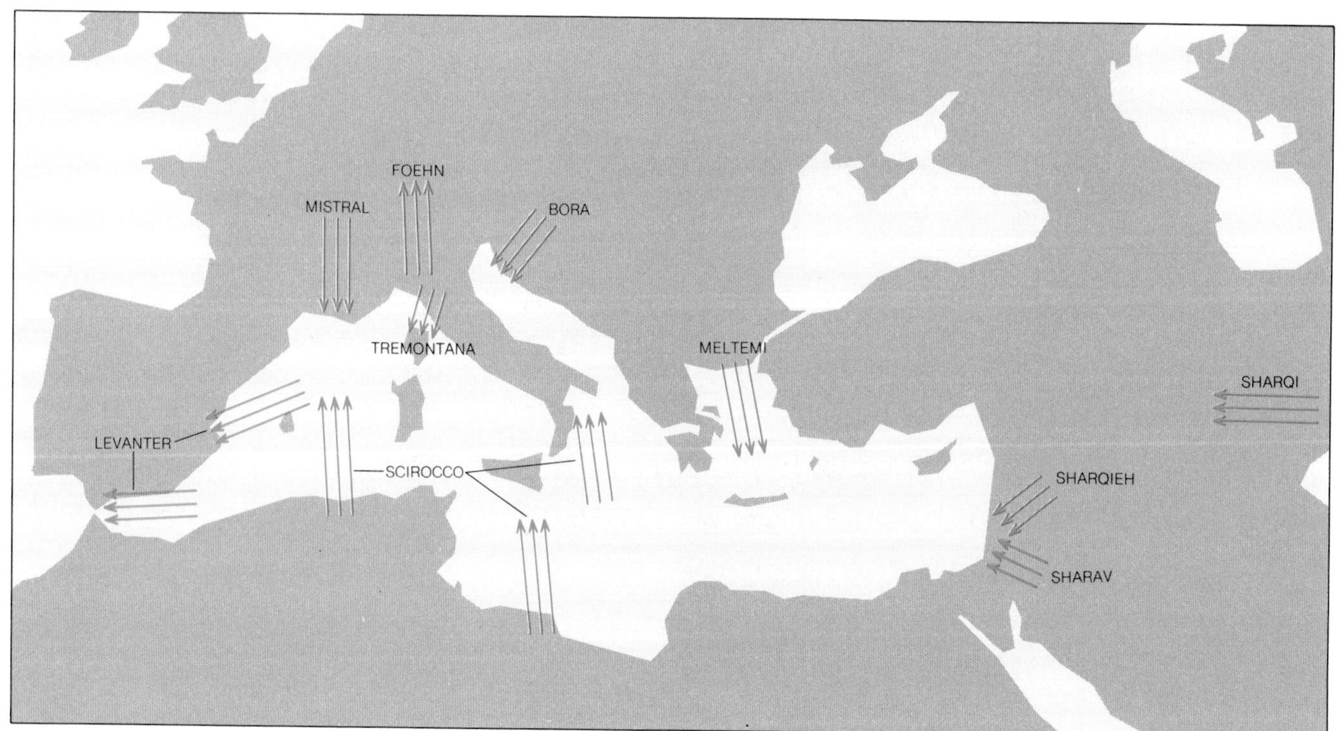

Long blamed for headaches, hot, dry "witches' " winds are common around the Mediterranean—this map locates 10 listed by Dr. Felix G. Sulman, who studied such phenomena in Israel and laid their effect to electrified air molecules. Similar winds in California and elsewhere have equally sinister reputations.

itself may have no visible impact on the system, but when the body is burdened successively by numerous triggers, they strain it beyond its limits.

The migraine personality

Triggers alone, however numerous, complex and subtle they may be, do not account for all attacks of migraine. The Australian headache authority Dr. James Lance of the University of New South Wales observed that even after a specialist had catalogued every trigger and potential trigger for a group of victims, "many patients go on having their attacks without relation" to any or all of them.

One such case was documented by a specialist of particularly wide experience, Dr. Arnold Friedman, Professor of Neurology at Columbia University's College of Physicians and Surgeons, and President of the American Association for the Study of Headaches. Dr. Friedman had followed the patient through every conceivable variation of situation and event that could bring on an attack. The patient's experience was indeed diverse: He had, as Dr. Friedman noted, "an occupation that takes him through the world from the Himalayas in Tibet to Somaliland, indeed from the highest altitudes to the lowest, from the wettest to the driest—experiencing climatic, food and culture changes. But his migraine remains, for he carries his personal environment with him."

That personal environment was, in large part, the patient's distinctive and inescapable psychological make-up, and it is not surprising that, in addition to trigger phenomena, certain common personality features among migraine victims have long been under investigation. In the 1930s Dr. Harold G. Wolff, a pioneer in many aspects of headache research, used detailed life histories of 46 sufferers to develop a profile of the typical migraine personality. Dr. Wolff found that, as children, more than half his subjects had been delicate in health and shy and withdrawn in personality. He described them as "extremely obedient to the desires of their parents, sober, conscientious," but noted that in some situations their docility was replaced by "unusual stubbornness or inflexibility." In general the migraine sufferers took good to obsessive care of their possessions as children, and were uncommonly preoccupied with moral and ethical problems as adolescents.

In their adult years, Dr. Wolff found, 90 per cent of the subjects were "unusually ambitious and preoccupied with achievement and success." Almost all of them "were conscientious, persistent, and exacting, attempting to arrange or bring order wherever possible. They were meticulous, the surroundings in which they placed themselves reflecting their neatness and fastidiousness." Because of such qualities, Dr. Wolff's subjects tended to be put in positions of considerable responsibility. If they had a shortcoming in these posts, it was in not delegating tasks to others, for fear that the jobs would not be done satisfactorily. In their own work, they typically exhibited tireless persistence and a willingness to work long, irregular hours to get things finished. Interruptions in work, for the weekend or even for a few minutes to take care of other pressing business, brought anxiety and tension. Despite the praise and admiration of others, few felt the satisfactions of achievement.

In their personal pleasures and habits, Dr. Wolff's subjects tended to be equally orderly and meticulous. Few were able to relax successfully. Weekends and social engagements were highly structured, hobbies tended to involve carefully organized collections of things, and home projects began with detailed lists and inventories. Dr. Wolff even discovered certain consistencies in creative and esthetic pursuits. "Most cultivated persons were fond of contrapuntal music and were particularly partial to Bach, Haydn and Mozart. They were unsympathetic to less formal and more voluptuous expression. In the plastic arts, notably painting, lithography, and etching, the same enthusiasm for the formal or architectural was observed." In personal relations, behavior was cool, combining courteousness with detachment. Inflexible in their standards for themselves, they were unforgiving of others, frequently harboring deep, unexpressed resentments toward workmates and family members.

Migraine attacks in Dr. Wolff's group were almost as likely to be precipitated by success as by failure, or by the letdown after exertion as by the exertion itself; in effect, any change in activity was stressful. Dr. Wolff reported an incident in the life of a perfectionist scientist who had submitted a

The myriad triggers of migraine headaches

A migraine headache, like a leaking gas main, can be touched off by almost any spark. One migraine victim reported headaches only on the days after haircuts; others have blamed yellow-colored medicines and tap water. Surveys of regular sufferers, however, have shown more predictable patterns of physical, psychological and environmental factors *(below)* that trigger headaches. They seem unrelated except in one respect: Many represent extremes. Too little sleep, for example, is a trigger. So is too much sleep.

Once identified, many triggers can be avoided. Glaring light, for example, can be reduced by tinted or polarizing eyeglasses; suspect foods can be eliminated—or extra meals added if hunger is a trigger. Many women using oral contraceptives avoid headaches by using pills with less estrogen.

Climatic changes and emotional tension, two common triggers, are not so readily avoided. A more escapable trigger is the period of letdown after stress: Teachers commonly report migraines at the start of school holidays, and many accountants suffer migraines the day after the deadline for income taxes. People in such high-pressure jobs often find relief if they avoid relaxing too much too soon—for example, by not sleeping late on the weekend after a hectic week.

TWENTY-TWO WAYS TO START A MIGRAINE ATTACK

Common triggers	Occasional triggers
Emotional tension	Relaxation after stress
Lack of sleep	Excessive sleep
Weather changes preceding hot, dry winds and thunderstorms	High humidity
Intense light and glare	Flickering light
Physical exertion and fatigue	High altitude
Head injury	Visual problems such as myopia and astigmatism
Menstruation and menopause	Pregnancy
Oral contraceptives	Drugs containing nitroglycerin, histamine and reserpine
Hunger	Excessive vitamin A
Alcohol	Pungent odors from perfumes, solvents or smoke
Certain cheeses, chocolate and red wines	Cold foods

paper to a professional journal. "Several weeks later he was confronted by an envelope containing his returned and supposedly rejected article. He was deeply humiliated and disappointed. An hour passed before he opened the envelope, and during this period a severe headache developed." When the anxious scientist finally did open the envelope, he found good news: Not only had the manuscript been accepted, the journal's editor had written a special letter of commendation. Nevertheless, the headache mechanism, once in gear, was not to be thwarted by good news; his migraine ran its full and all-too-familiar course.

Dr. Wolff's group was small and possibly unrepresentative. Many migraine sufferers are not meticulous, ambitious or cool, and thus do not fit his personality profile; they suffer their chronic vascular headaches simply because they are physically predisposed to migraine and expose themselves to environmental triggers. As one especially articulate migraine victim, Joan Didion, put it: "Not all perfectionists have migraine, and not all migrainous people have migraine personalities. I have tried in most of the available ways to escape my own migrainous heredity . . . but I still have migraine."

Nevertheless, Dr. Wolff's description works often enough to be useful in making a preliminary diagnosis of migraine for persons who have chronic headaches and who exhibit the appropriate personality pattern. Migraine is known to be strongly related to stress and to the method by which stress is resolved. Clearly, the meticulous, ambitious, controlled and cool individual is more vulnerable than the person who is free and easy, and given to expressing feelings openly.

The psychological pattern shared by so many migraine sufferers has strongly influenced methods of treatment. Although a number of drugs are available to relieve the ailment's pains and even to prevent attacks, much emphasis today is placed on helping a patient to manage his daily life in ways that minimize the impact of migraine.

Drugs to prevent or end the misery

The drugs most commonly used to relieve migraine pain are modern versions of an old one: ergotamine *(pages 94-103)*. Given at the right time, by the right method and in the right dosage, it can, according to Dr. Egilius Speirings of the University Hospital at Rotterdam, relieve up to 90 per cent of migraine headaches. Yet, curiously, ergotamine is not, strictly speaking, a painkiller. Over-the-counter painkillers, such as aspirin, are generally too mild to help migraine sufferers much, even in the maximum allowable dosages. Painkillers available only by prescription, though more potent, are dangerous to migraine sufferers: Because migraine is a chronic condition requiring constant medication, these drugs carry the possibility, even the likelihood, of addiction. What is needed is a drug that will attack the physical cause of a migraine headache. Ergotamine fills the bill: It is a powerful constrictor of blood vessels, counteracting the dilation of vessels that brings on the pain of migraine.

Knowledge of the action and correct use of ergotamine was long in coming; for centuries, in fact, the drug's original source, a fungus called ergot that attacks the rye plant, was a terror rather than a boon. Ergot is the cause of a dreaded, often fatal disease called ergotism, marked in its course by delusions and hallucinations; a close chemical relative of the substance is lysergic acid, or LSD, perhaps the best-known hallucination-producer of modern times. As a disease, ergotism was identified in an Assyrian tablet dating back to 600 B.C., and it has erupted in sporadic outbreaks throughout recorded history.

But in the 1880s, physicians in Germany, England and the United States began to use ergot on a trial-and-error basis as a drug to relieve the pain of migraine. From then on, progress was comparatively rapid. In 1918, ergotamine was isolated as the active ingredient of the drug; this substance can now be produced synthetically. And in the late 1930s, when the first modern descriptions of a migraine attack were made, physicians finally were able to clarify the action of ergotamine. They could, for example, explain that, since this drug is a powerful constrictor, it has little or no effect during the aura stage of classic migraine, when blood vessels in the head are naturally constricted, but goes to work during the headache phase, when they are dilated.

While ergotamine remains the drug of choice for migraine, it is rarely given in its simple form nowadays. To enhance its action, it is often compounded with other blood-vessel constrictors, such as caffeine. Other additions are designed to reduce its side effects. Ergotamine causes nausea, one of the characteristic symptoms of migraine itself; to ease the cumulative nauseas produced by the drug and the disease—which, in combination, could make it impossible for the patient to keep the medicine down—an antinausea drug such as belladonna is often added to the mix.

Beyond ergotamine lies a still-unattainable goal—a medicine that would prevent a migraine attack rather than merely relieve its symptoms. On the one hand, researchers are experimenting with drugs called beta blockers, most notably propranolol, which may relax the system of muscles that, in a migraine sufferer, causes the chronic pattern of arterial constriction and dilation. Though effective as a means of lowering blood pressure and preventing heart attacks, propranolol has yet to be proven as a migraine preventive. More promising, but also more mysterious, is the action of a drug called methysergide, basically a blood-vessel constrictor, but one that can sometimes restore the basic chemical balance that is missing in a migraine victim.

Such drugs are only part of the treatment that helps control migraine. The physician also attempts to identify the triggers that set off each patient's attacks—some triggers may simply be certain foods—in the hope that once isolated, they can be avoided. In addition, personality characteristics may be investigated to seek inner frustrations or feelings of insecurity that can provoke or intensify migraine responses. This "whole-person" approach to migraine has achieved gratifying—and sometimes breath-taking—results. At The New England Center for Headache, in Cos Cob, Connecticut, for example, 98 per cent of a sample of 150 patients treated in 1981 showed dramatic improvements.

A catastrophe for men: cluster headaches

Some of the medical advances in the treatment of migraine have been extended to its variant, the cluster headache, which is beginning to yield to some of the same drugs and in much the same way.

Cluster headaches are unique in the intensity of pain they

These angiograms—X-rays of blood vessels that have been injected with dye to make them stand out—were taken during the onset of a cluster headache, a severe type that occurs in batches. The pictures reveal an unfelt symptom: The internal carotid artery deep in the head, shown at normal size in the circle at left below, begins to constrict (right) as the headache begins.

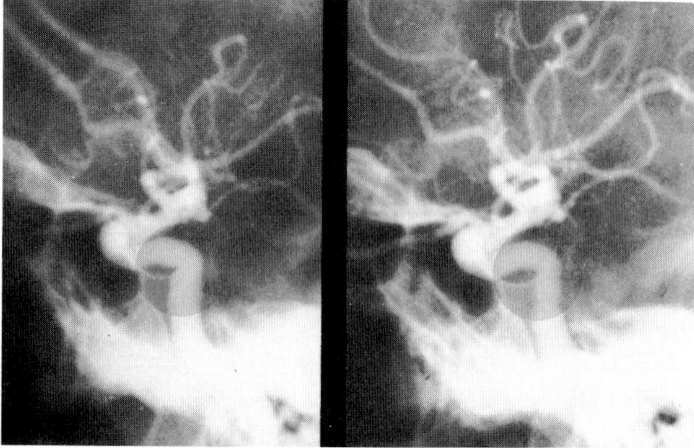

deliver. Sufferers have long since exhausted the lexicon of pain-related words in trying to describe the excruciating sensations that come over them when an attack is in full flood. Unlike migraine victims, cluster sufferers do not—indeed, they cannot—sit still during an attack. They cry out, writhe and pace the floor in their agony, frequently so losing control that they pound their fists through walls, break furniture and risk inflicting serious injury upon themselves and others. The notion of suicide as the only possible escape from this pain is frequently voiced and the threat has, on occasion, been carried out.

Cluster headaches are also unusual in their predictability. Victims know with a certainty not only that an attack will end—but that it will be renewed soon. Often they can even predict the very hour. One of the mot provocative—and still inexplicable—features of the disorder is its cyclic nature; it recurs at certain fixed hours of the day and at certain seasons of the year. This regular recurrence suggests some relationship between the onset of attacks and the biological rhythms within the individual—that is, his biological clock. The pattern of attacks may be one of headaches 45 minutes long recurring two or three times each day (usually at the same specific hours) for six to twelve weeks, or headaches two hours long once a week for a year, and so on. Then, almost as unexpectedly as the first episode in the cluster series began, the disorder abruptly vanishes, not to be revived for months or years, perhaps never again. (In rare instances the headache persists without remission; this is termed chronic cluster and is uniquely debilitating.)

Cluster headache is the only primary headache disorder in which afflicted males outnumber females. Further, many of the victims of cluster headache seem to have a number of physical characteristics in common.

Dr. John Graham, who laid out the commonly accepted description of a migraine attack, was also the first to compile data on cluster headache systematically. He found that male sufferers from this disorder have what he described as a "leonine appearance," with a ruddy complexion, thick facial skin (which he termed "orange-peel"), visibly dilated blood vessels, particularly across the bridge of the nose, a deeply furrowed forehead, and a broad chin and skull. Dr. Graham also found a high correspondence between cluster headache and a tall, trim, rugged body type. On the average, his cluster-headache subjects were about two and a half inches taller than the adult male population at large. Of course, none of these physical characteristics—including the fact that one in three subjects had hazel-colored eyes as compared with one in 11 among healthy individuals—sheds any light on the physical origins of cluster headaches.

Later studies by Dr. Lee Kudrow and his associates at the California Medical Clinic for Headache, in Encino, essentially confirmed Dr. Graham's observations, and added another piece to the physical jigsaw puzzle. Along with the abnormally high proportion of hazel-eyed persons, there was an abnormally low proportion of blue-eyed persons. Dr. Kudrow suggested that cluster-headache patients might also have in common some defect in the regulation of melanin, a pigment associated with eye and skin color. Whether this defect plays a role in causing the headaches or is merely an additional symptom of some deeper chemical disorder, he was not able to determine.

Attempts to draw a personality profile of a typical victim, comparable to that of migraine sufferers, have left cluster specialists in disagreement. Dr. Graham characterized his male patients as "mice living inside lions," men with aggressive behavior masking feelings of dependency and inadequacy; other studies, based on larger samples and using more extensive personality probes, put this assessment in question. But as with most migraine sufferers, difficulty in handling stressful situations is now regarded as a critical personality factor in predisposing an individual to cluster headaches. And two forms of social behavior indirectly related to personality were noted: Male cluster sufferers tend to smoke substantially more and to drink more coffee and alcoholic beverages than men of ordinary good health. (However, they almost always abstain from alcohol during cluster episodes, since even a small quantity will precipitate another attack.)

Cluster susceptibility seems to have nothing to do with a familial or inheritable trait (despite the connection to eye color, which is genetic). The possibilities that the release of histamine in the blood or some hormonal instability is at fault have been intensively studied, with little success.

Harm from a macho life style

In an attempt to find a link between cluster headache's cyclic nature and the life styles peculiar to some people, especially young men, Dr. Kudrow, for one, revived the debate over the existence of a distinctive cluster personality. Working on a series of hypotheses that linked life style to brain injury, he proposed that in cluster victims certain bodily rhythms, such as the daily ebb and flow of hormones, are distorted as the result of injury to the brain centers controlling them—and that the injury, in turn, is caused by a distinctive way of life.

"The male psyche at an age between the teens and late twenties," he wrote, "is one mixed with bravado and uncertainty, responsibility and self-indulgence, and deliberation and impulsiveness." In this psychological setting, Dr. Kudrow argued, "periods of excessive drinking, sleep deprivation, drug use, and other potentially damaging experiences may cause toxic or metabolic injury."

Cluster headaches are so painful that radical measures are sometimes employed to treat them. In extreme cases, surgery has been used experimentally, but surgical procedures are risky at best, and as often as not they are ultimately unsatisfactory. In one typical operation, the surgeon cuts the nerves that control the constriction and dilation of cranial blood vessels; according to a 1970 report by Dr. Averill Stowell of the Hillcrest Medical Center at Tulsa, Oklahoma, 32 in a sample of 36 cluster patients were relieved of pain by the operation—but 15 of the 32 relapsed into the cluster pattern after a period ranging from one to three years. An even more drastic procedure is cryosurgery, in which liquid nitrogen is used to freeze and destroy tissue, including the distended arteries that cause cluster-headache pain. Roughly a third of the patients reported some relief of their pain, but about the same number suffered permanent facial numbness.

Most treatment is based on drugs that constrict blood vessels, such as methysergide, taken several times a day throughout a cluster period; and the migraine remedy ergotamine, taken at the first sign of each attack. Techniques of behavior modification, helpful in many headaches, have proved less useful. Dr. Kudrow, for example, drawing on his experience with patients at the California Medical Clinic for Headache, stated that "biofeedback training, psychiatry, hypnosis, physical therapy and manipulation techniques appear to be of little value" in preventing or moderating attacks of cluster headache.

For one special type of cluster headache, however, a drug has been found that provides a wonderfully effective treatment. The ailment, chronic paroxysmal hemicrania, is fortunately rare—it is described as the worst-of-the-worst headaches. It was identified as a separate disorder only as recently as 1974 and traced to some 25 individuals by 1980. Among the first patients to be studied, attacks struck 10 to 18 times a day, year in and year out for as many as 20 years, rendering the victims virtually incapable of participating in life. Then, in 1976, physicians discovered that regular and continued doses of indomethacin, an anti-inflammation drug, made the headaches virtually disappear; for some patients the relief was permanent.

The victory over chronic paroxysmal hemicrania is not only heartening in itself, but strengthens the hopes of every variety of headache sufferer. Drugs can indeed perform near-miracles in alleviating some head pains and warding off others—in most cases by mechanisms that only now are beginning to be understood. ❋

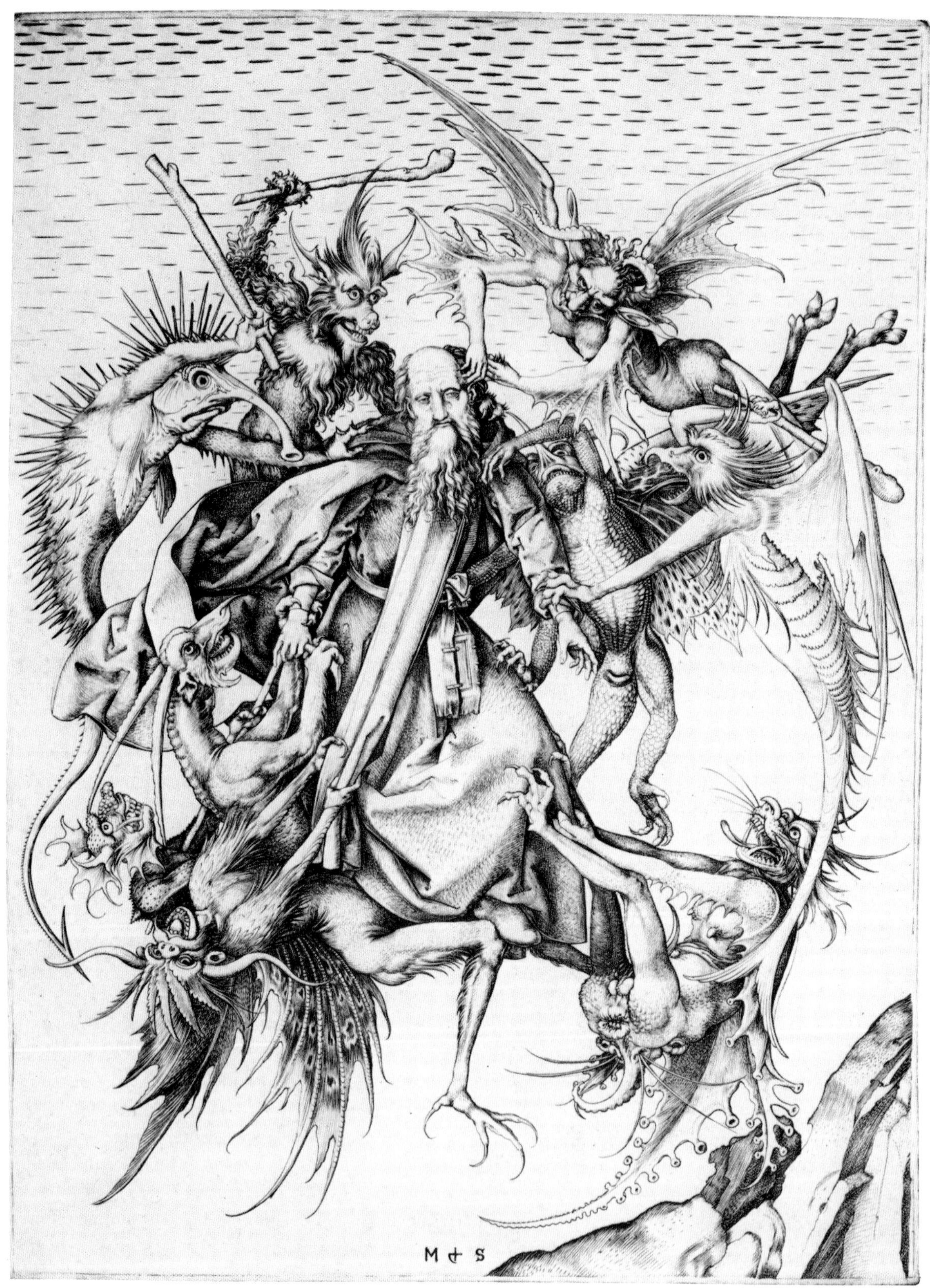

Saint Anthony Tormented by Demons, a 15th Century German engraving, depicts the monk assailed by unearthly creatures like those described in his writings. The monk's terrifying visions were similar to the hallucinations of ergotism, and during the Middle Ages, ergotism was called St. Anthony's fire. Victims prayed at his shrine for relief from the burning pains.

From a curse of the past, a present blessing

The grain parasite ergot is one of medicine's notorious Jekyll-and-Hyde characters: Dreaded through history as an insidious killer, it emerged in modern times as a magical treatment for migraine.

As early as 600 B.C., an Assyrian tablet named ergot as a poison, and in the Middle Ages ergot-induced mass poisonings ravaged Western Europe. A fungus that grows on rye and other grains, ergot ferments in certain kinds of weather and yields a form of LSD, the powerful hallucinogen that can cause psychotic "trips" or even death. Mysterious outbreaks of convulsions, delusions and painful burning sensations—blamed on devils and witches in more superstitious eras—were probably due to this ergot derivative. The recurring struggles of the Third Century monk Saint Anthony with what he called spectral demons *(left)* have been blamed on ergotism. So has the odd behavior of adolescent girls that led to the 17th Century Salem witch trials *(below)*. Modern grain-processing methods have all but eliminated the threat of ergotism—although 1951 saw a terrifying outbreak of the condition in a small town in France *(overleaf)*.

The other side of ergot's personality—that of healing agent—has also been long known. It constricts muscles and has been used to speed uterine contractions during childbirth and reduce bleeding afterward. Ergot's active ingredient, ergotamine, was isolated by Swiss chemist Arthur Stoll in 1918, and in 1925 a colleague noted the drug's migraine-healing properties—it constricts the enlarged blood vessels that cause the pain. In large doses, however, ergot remains a poison, and demands caution in use.

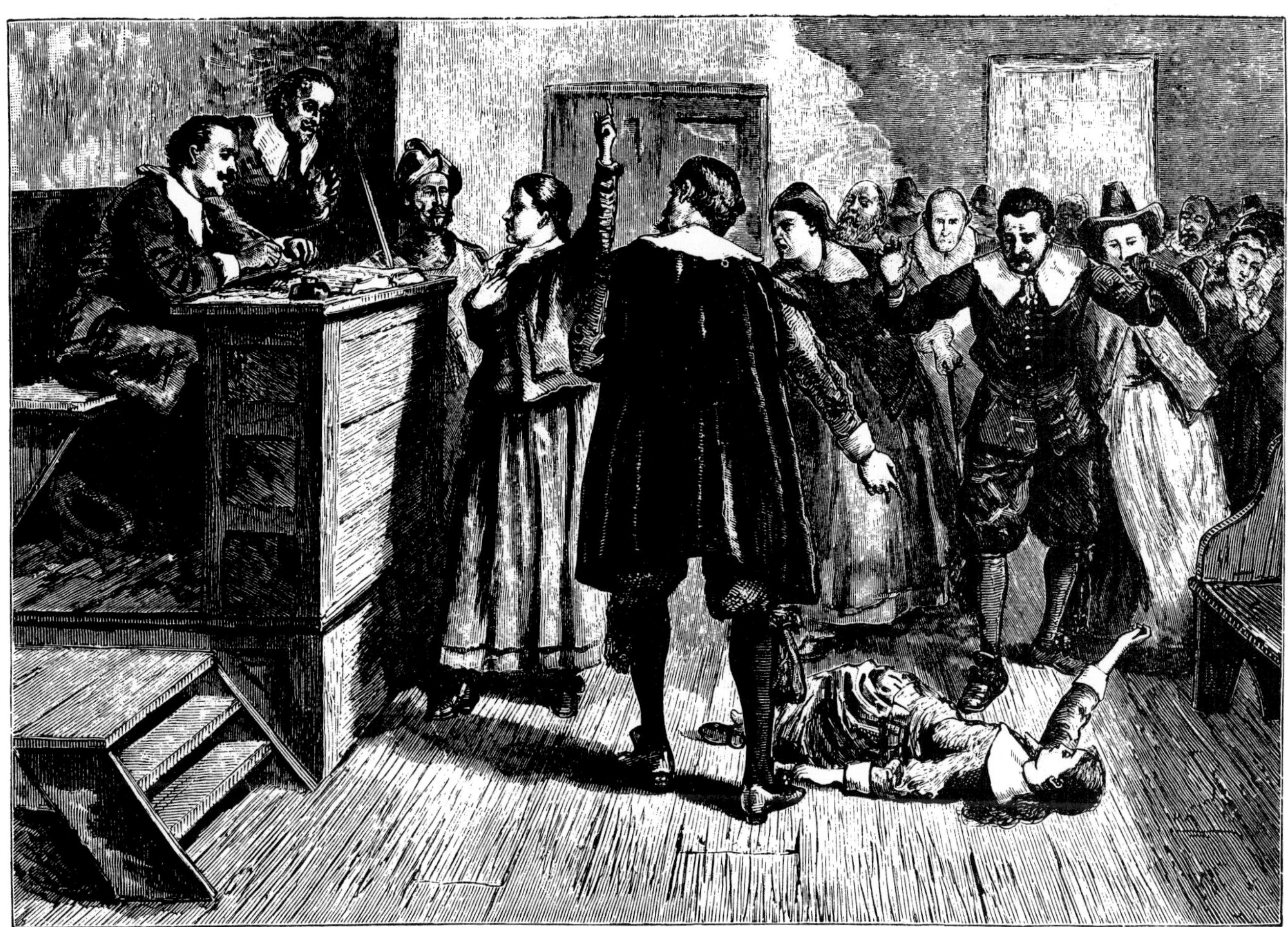

A girl seized by fits sprawls on a courtroom floor in this picture of the Salem witch trials in colonial Massachusetts. Puritan leaders, calling such symptoms proof of a soul taken over by the devil, executed 20 people during a witch-hunt in 1692. But ergot may have caused the fits. The preceding summer was very damp and may have stimulated ergot infestation of rye.

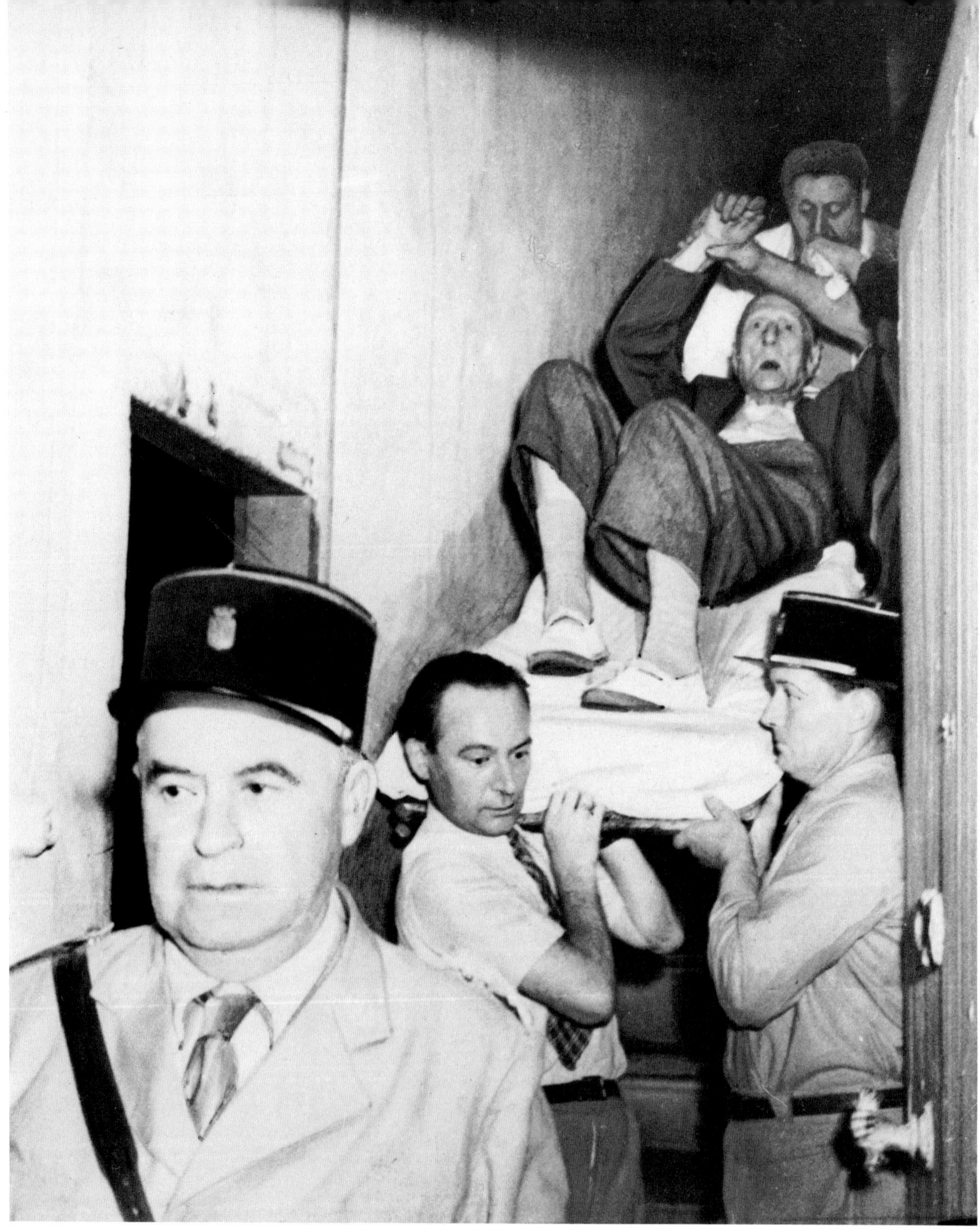

Screaming in terror at visions that only he can see, a 75-year-old man is carried from his home by police and hospital attendants. Local hospitals were quickly filled with hysterical, pain-racked patients. Doctors could only use straitjackets and leather straps to keep the most violent victims from injuring themselves while waiting for the poison to wear off.

Death in the staff of life

In the summer of 1951, a quaint village in southern France, Pont-St.-Esprit, was struck by a malady that terrified and mystified inhabitants. What seemed to be food poisoning appeared in epidemic proportions. Sufferers experienced violent stomach pains, chills, insomnia and strange burning sensations. Dogs, cats and ducks died in agonizing convulsions after eating table scraps.

French authorities soon traced the mystery to ergot-infested flour shipped from a mill 300 miles away and innocently baked into bread by a village baker. But nothing could stop the poison's snowballing effects. Once in the bloodstream, ergot's hallucinogenic component starts a chain reaction that builds momentum before exhausting itself days or weeks later. No cure was known.

The epidemic reached a peak on the night of August 24—called in Pont-St.-Esprit the Night of the Apocalypse. Victims ran through the streets gripped by fearful delusions or odd compulsions. Some screamed that wild beasts pursued them, others leaped from windows to escape imaginary flames. All told, more than 200 were stricken and seven died from *le pain qui rend fou*—"the bread that causes madness."

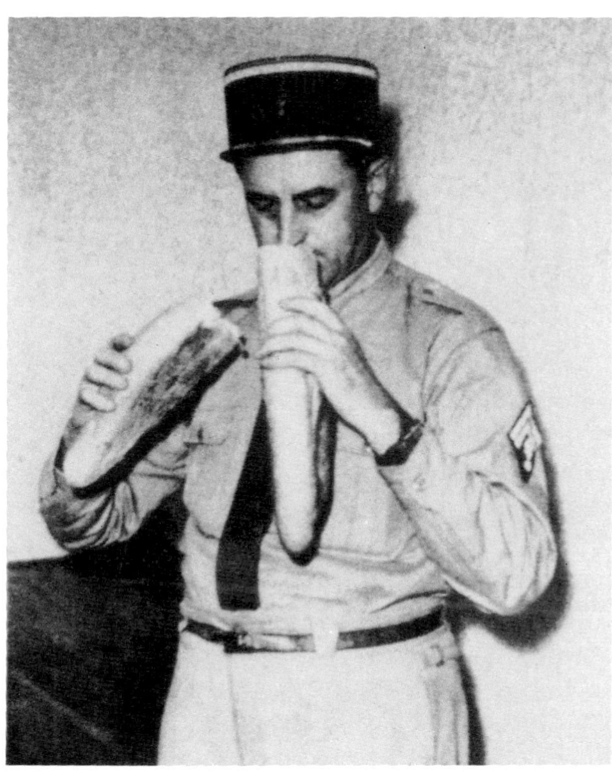

A village gendarme sniffs a loaf of suspect bread, searching for a telltale oily odor produced by the fungus in infested flour. Authorities arrested a baker and a miller who were suspected of having shipped the bad flour from a neighboring province even though they were aware that something was wrong with it. The two were later released for lack of evidence.

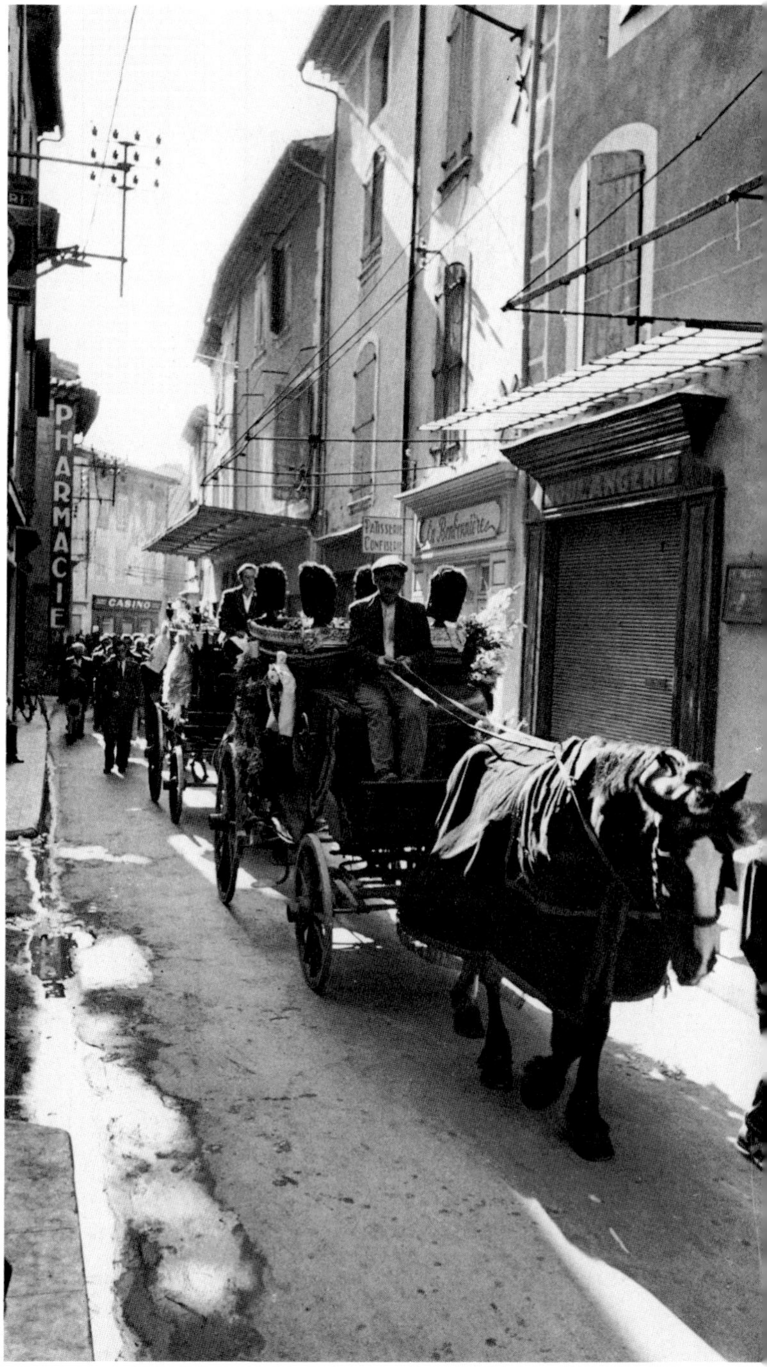

Bearing the bodies of an elderly couple who died from ergot poisoning, horse-drawn hearses lead a funeral procession past the closed shutters of the bakery ("Boulangerie") where the victims had bought the bread that killed them.

Good medicine from bad grain

The ergot fungus begins its life cycle as a cluster of spore sacs *(below)*. Ergot is scattered by wind or insects in the spring to infest the flowers of rye and other grains; it produces a spore-filled mucus called honeydew that quickly spreads to other plants. The spores from the mucus feed on the plants for several weeks, consuming the kernels while transforming themselves into black, purple or brown pods that resemble grain kernels.

Since 1925, when Swiss chemist Ernst Rothlin discovered that the fungus could alleviate migraine, ergot has been harvested from infested rye fields. When ergot supplies were cut off during World War II, the Swiss pharmaceutical company Sandoz began artificially cultivating it, using machines to inject spores directly into the grain ears *(opposite)*. In the 1960s, Swiss scientists learned to synthesize ergot's active ingredient; today, laboratory cultivation *(overleaf)* provides most of the ergot used to make drugs.

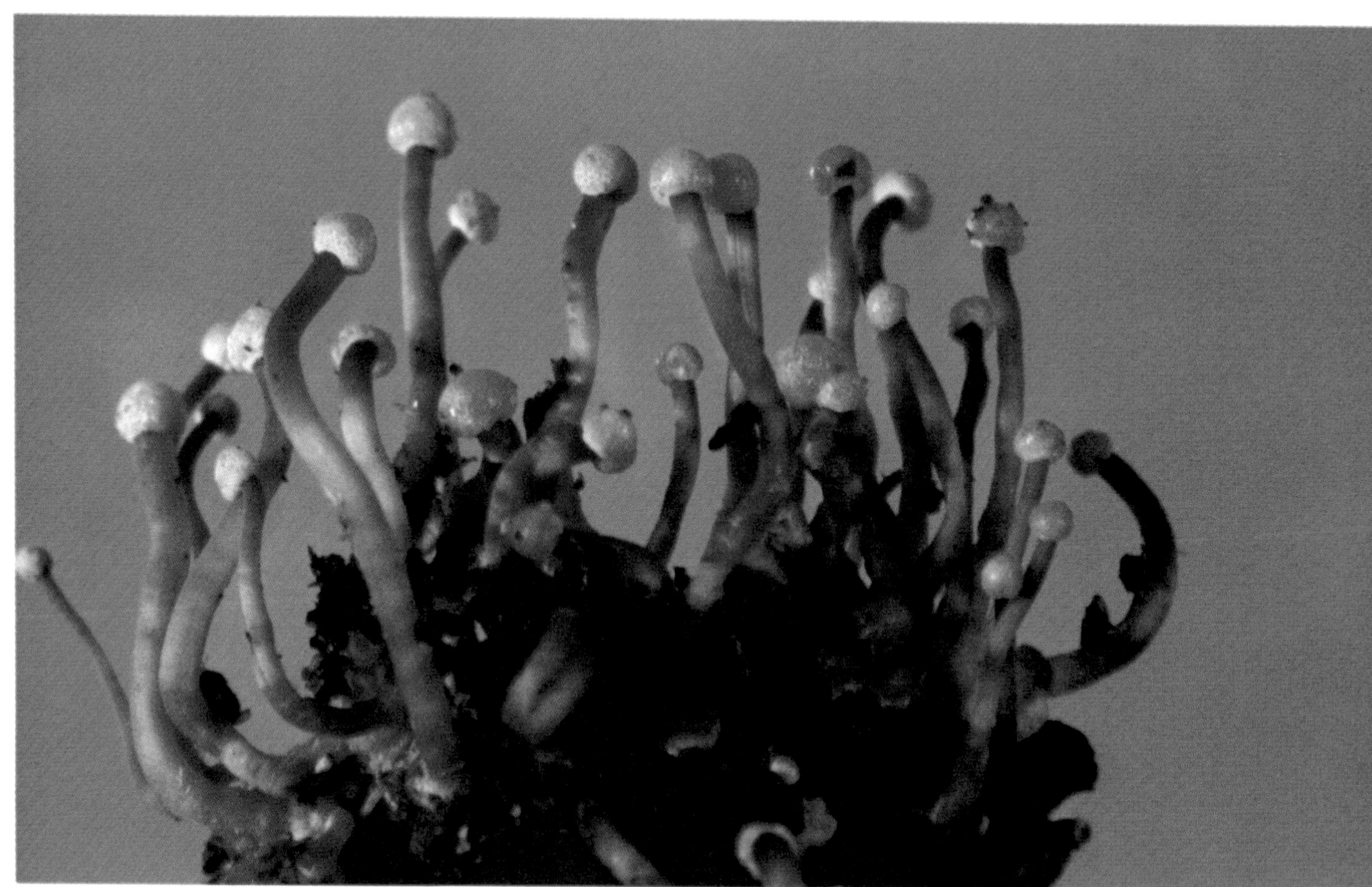

Resembling a forest of tiny antennae, the bulbous projections above are naturally growing ergot—or Claviceps purpurea, a relative of the common mushroom—at the reproductive stage. These fruiting bodies, magnified about five times, sprout in grain fields in the spring from ergot pods that fell the previous season. The spores inside will spread to infect the new generation of grain.

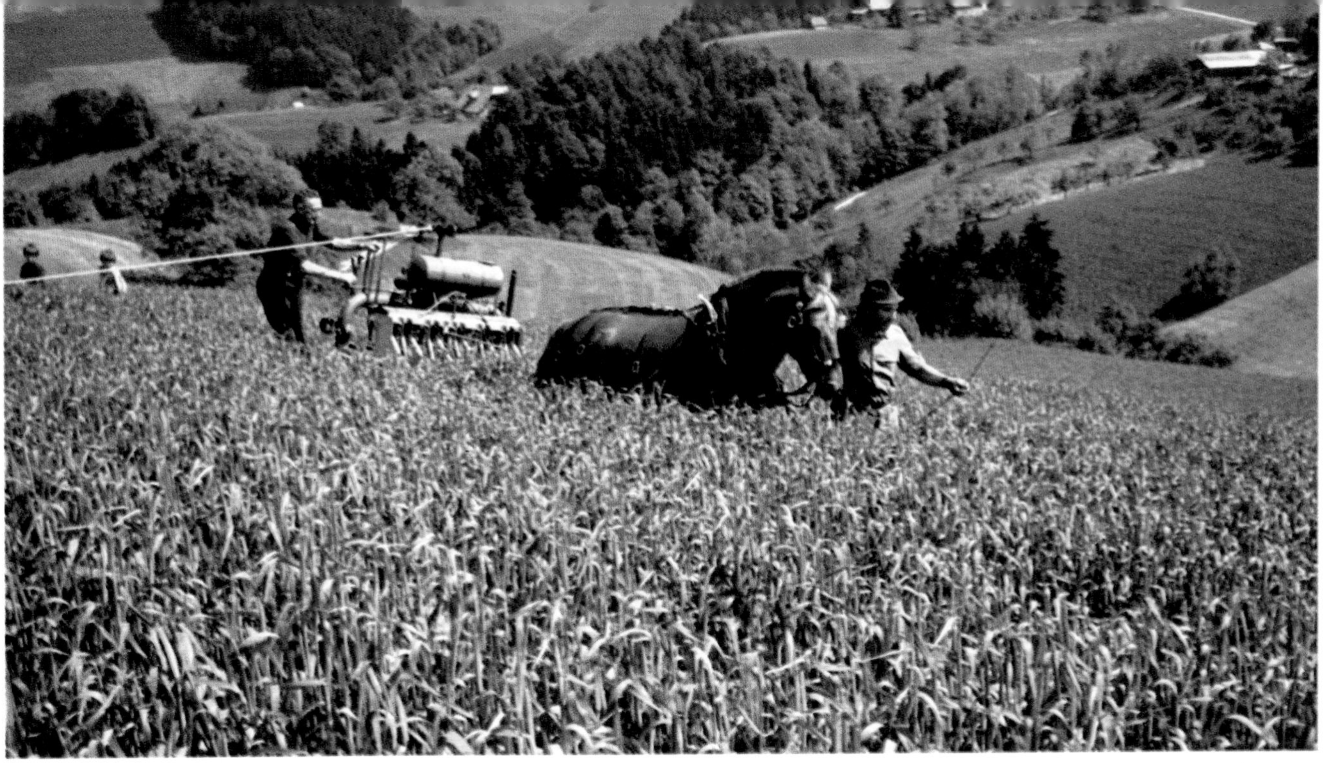

Horse-drawn inoculating machines, used in fields too steep or rocky for tractors, spread ergot spores on a rye crop for medicine production.

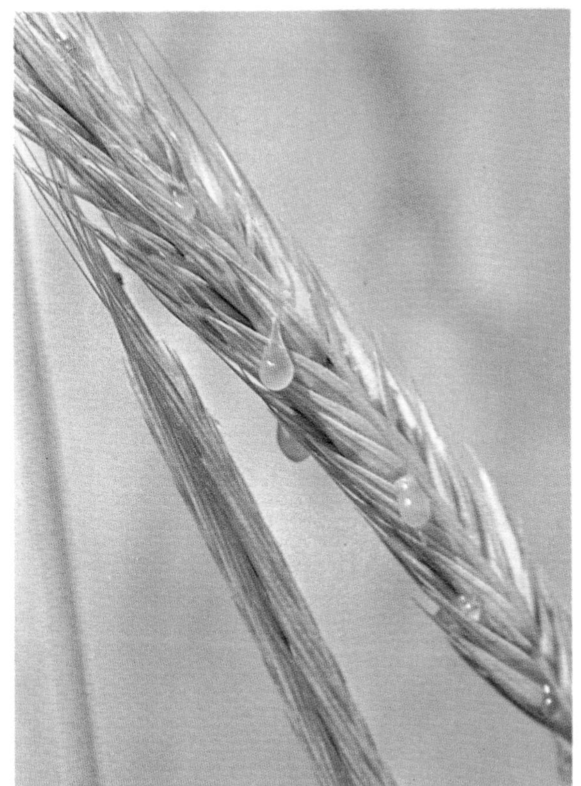

Within a week, the parasitic spores begin to feed off the rye kernels, excreting a sticky fluid called honeydew. Laden with spores, the honeydew drips onto other grain ears, where the spores grow and harden into pods that replace rye grains.

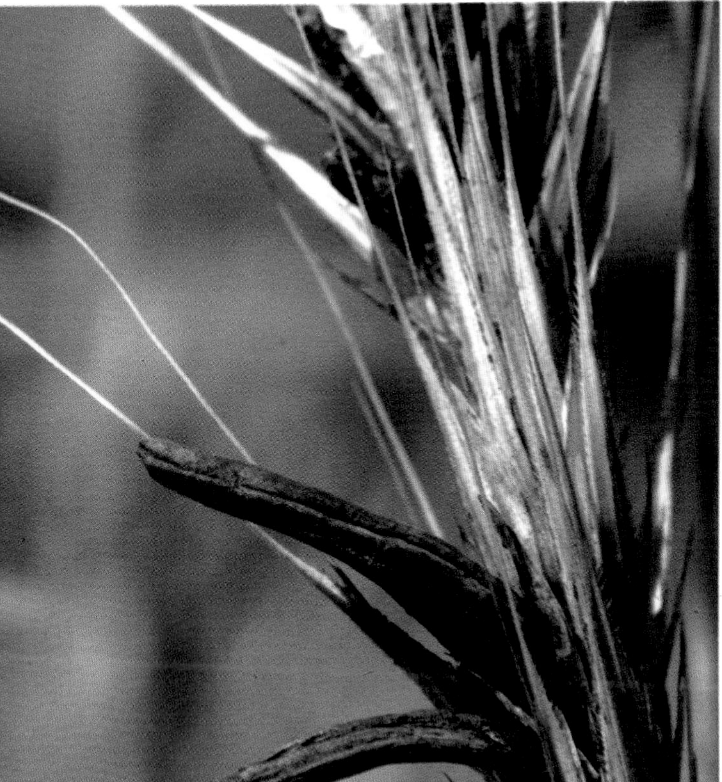

Mature ergot pods growing on rye (above) are ready for harvesting six to eight weeks after inoculation. During harvesting, some of the inch-long pods drop to the ground to hibernate through the winter and sprout again, beginning a new life cycle.

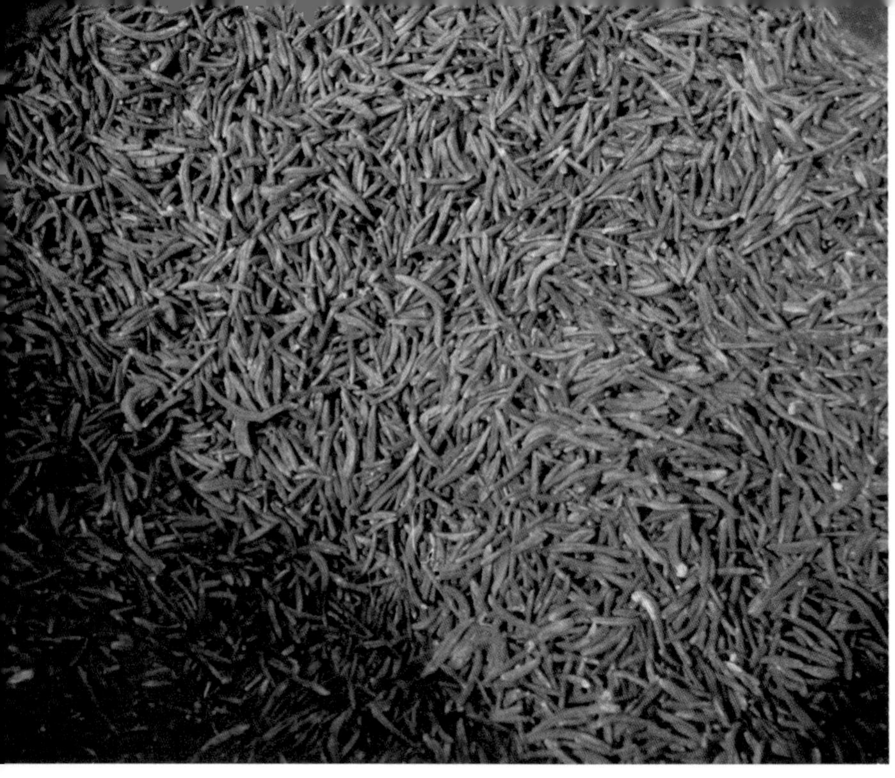

A barrel full of ergot pods harvested from a specially cultivated rye field awaits shipment to a drug processing plant, where active chemicals will be extracted. Most modern firms now bypass the rye-field and harvesting stages, and instead grow fungus from spores in laboratory flasks and tanks (below and right).

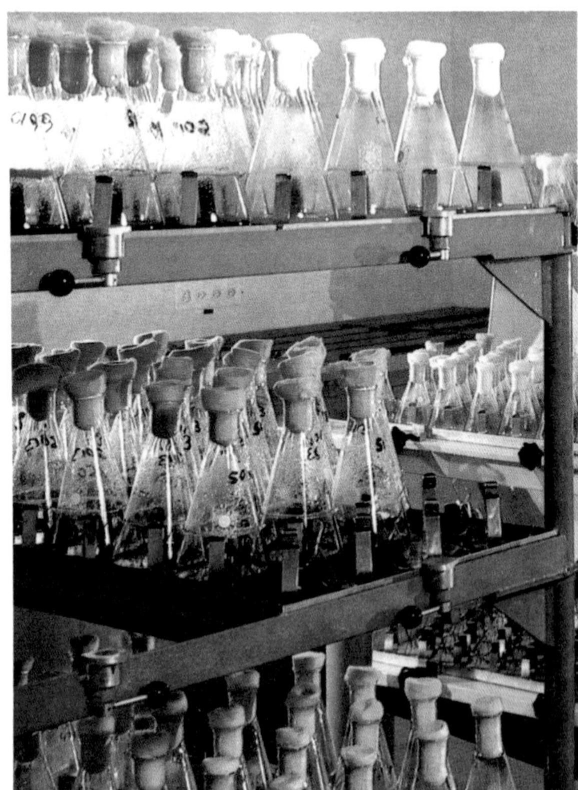

In a laboratory, ergot fungus grows in flasks plugged with colored cotton wads to indicate the different cultures used to produce various strains. The strongest batches are selected for fermentation (right).

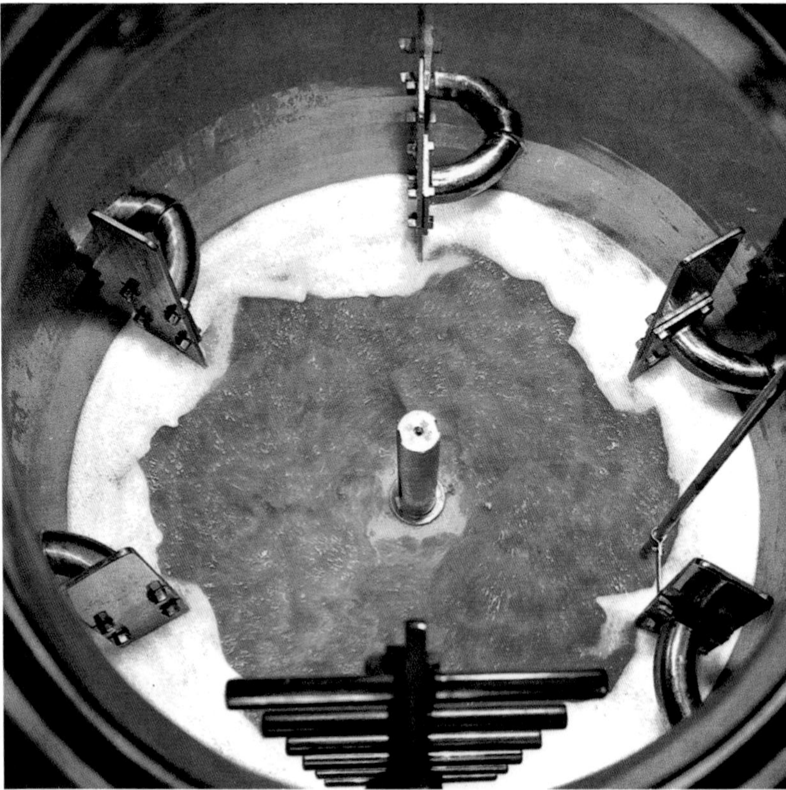

Ergot culture bubbles in an 800-gallon fermentation drum at the Sandoz plant in Switzerland. This process produces a chemical called paspalic acid, which is later converted to the lysergic acid used as the base for drugs containing ergot. A variation of this base—lysergic acid diethylamide—is the hallucinogen LSD.

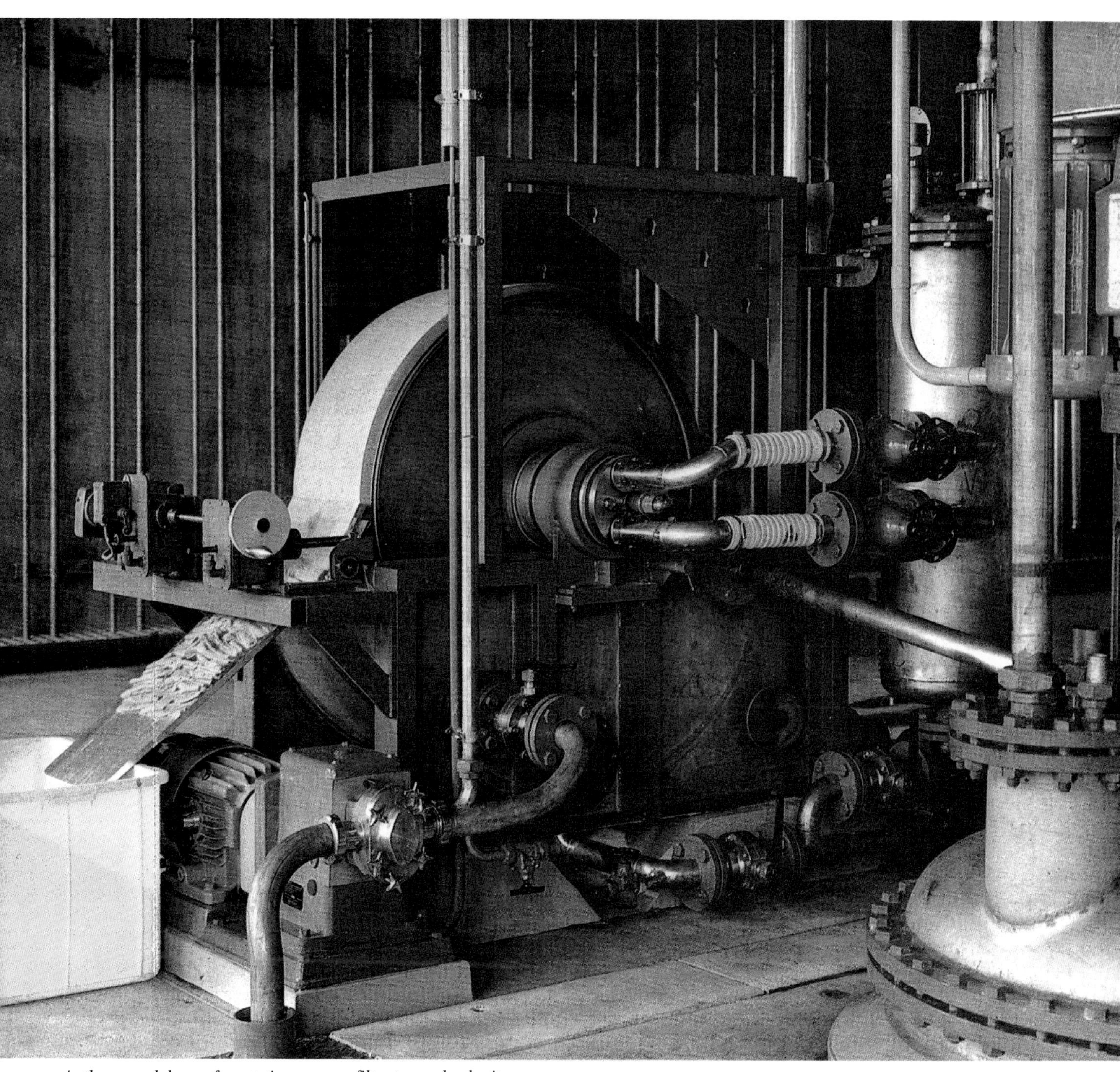

As the curved drum of a rotating vacuum filter turns slowly, its lower portion dips into the foaming fermentation vat beneath to skim off paspalic acid. The acid is dried and in a series of reactions is converted to ergotamine, which is shipped abroad in the form of a crystalline salt, ergotamine tartrate.

Ergotamine in many guises

Few medicines come packaged in as many ways as ergotamine, a drug that, while it is very effective for migraine relief, is often hard to stomach. Because nausea is one of the side effects of ergotamine—as well as a migraine symptom—some patients must take forms of the drug that bypass the digestive system and enter the bloodstream directly through injections, inhaled sprays, rectal suppositories or tablets that dissolve under the tongue and are absorbed there.

The active ingredients, which may include drugs other than ergotamine, are carried by the blood to overexpanded blood vessels in the head. Some forms of the medicine reach the pain site faster than others—an important factor in treating acute migraine attacks: The sooner ergotamine is used after symptoms appear, the better it works to stop the headache.

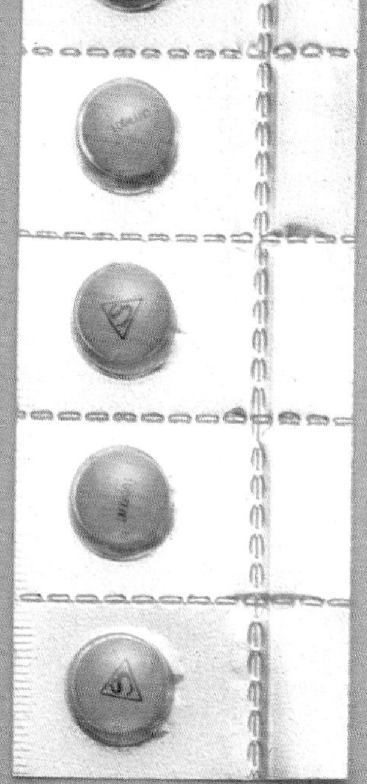

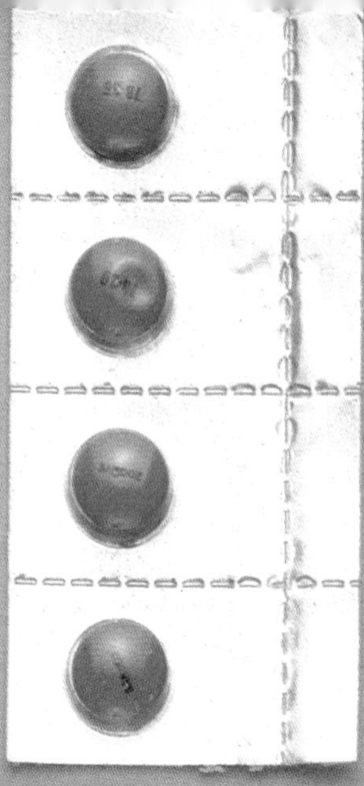

TABLETS WITH BOOSTERS AND BUFFERS ADDED
Two types of oral Cafergot tablets, above, combine ergotamine with caffeine—which also shrinks blood vessels, thus allowing a smaller dose of the powerful ergotamine. The pills on the right contain belladonna as well to relax stomach muscles, and pentobarbital to reduce tension. Simple to use but slower to act than other forms, tablets start working within half an hour.

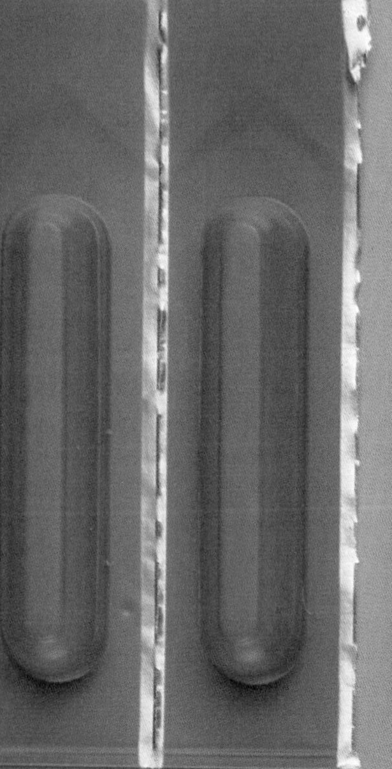

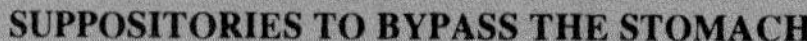

SUPPOSITORIES TO BYPASS THE STOMACH
When nausea is a problem, Cafergot may be taken in suppositories (below). It enters the bloodstream through the large intestine and begins to take effect within 15 minutes.

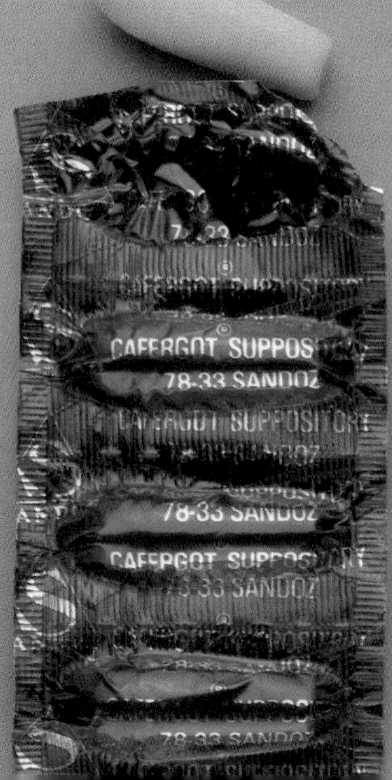

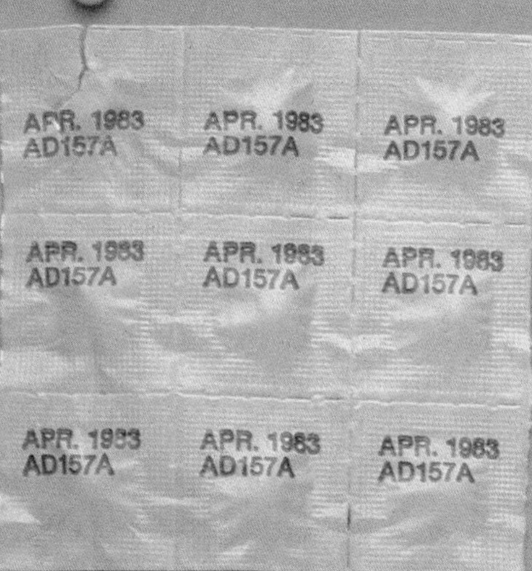

INJECTIONS FOR SWIFT RELIEF
The ergotamine solution in these vials—two still packaged and one unwrapped—is injected by needle directly into a patient's bloodstream. Acting in five to 10 minutes, injections are the speediest and surest remedy but also the most cumbersome.

PILLS THAT TUCK UNDER THE TONGUE
The tiny tablet of ergotamine above is another form that bypasses a troubled stomach. Uncoated for fast absorption, the tablets are placed under the tongue, where they dissolve and enter the bloodstream, taking effect within 15 minutes.

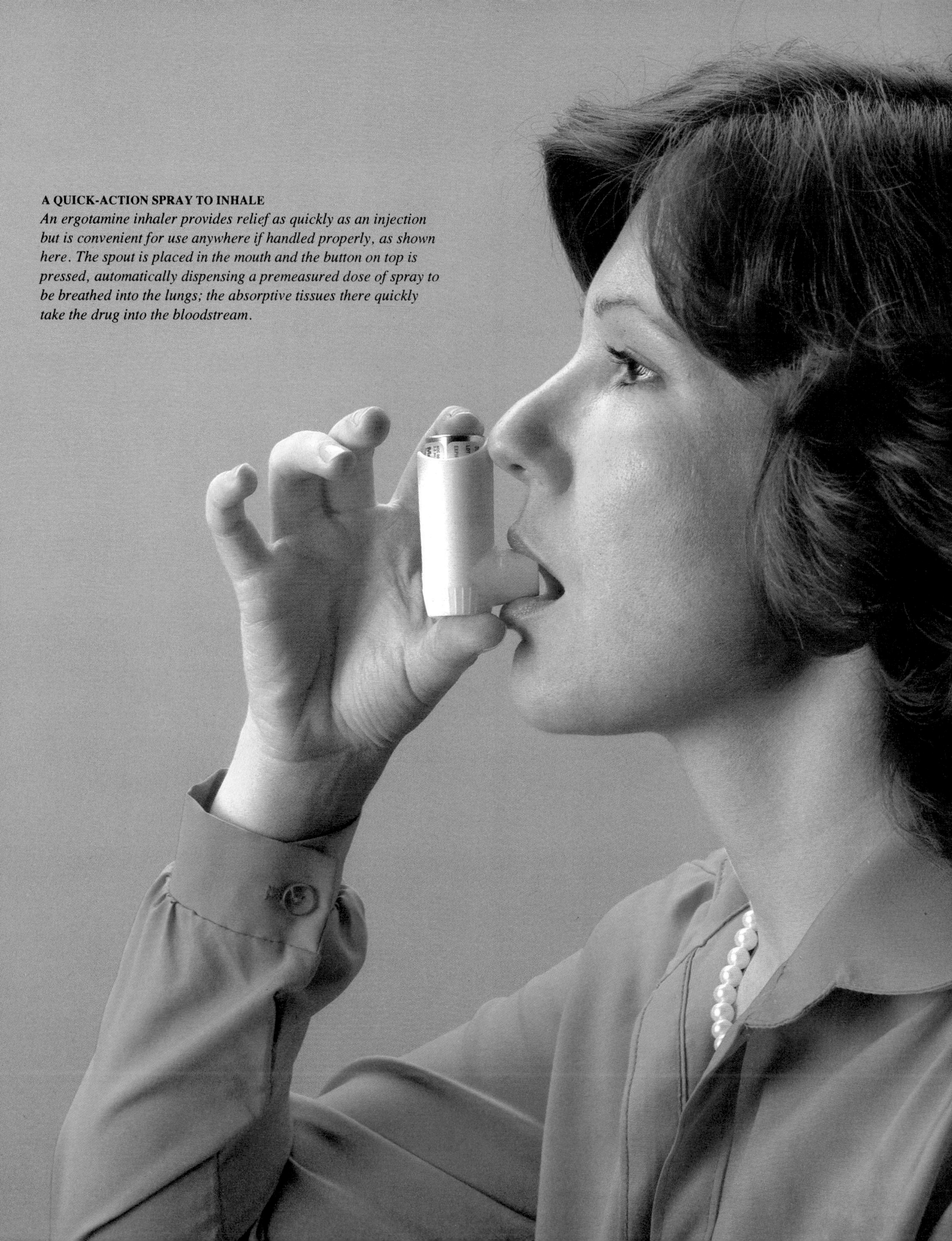

A QUICK-ACTION SPRAY TO INHALE
An ergotamine inhaler provides relief as quickly as an injection but is convenient for use anywhere if handled properly, as shown here. The spout is placed in the mouth and the button on top is pressed, automatically dispensing a premeasured dose of spray to be breathed into the lungs; the absorptive tissues there quickly take the drug into the bloodstream.

CHAPTER 5

How medicines stop the pain

The singular history of the painkillers
Drugs to relax mind and body
How ergotamine interrupts migraine
Four ways to fool the nerves
Where the ache begins
The brain's own narcotics

Of the treatments for headaches, the most useful are, not surprisingly, drugs—a vast and varied armamentarium of substances ranging from common aspirin to complex hormonal compounds. Many are as old as opium, others new. Until the middle of the 20th Century no one knew how any of them worked; little more could be said of them than that they stopped the pain. Then a series of discoveries revealed how, in headaches and other disorders, the body's own actions and chemicals initiate a nerve signal of pain. The way such a signal progresses along one nerve and crosses connections to another to reach the brain's computer was seen to be a complex combination of electrical and chemical operations.

The result was a new, detailed picture of the mechanisms of pain. Continually being filled in, it has finally explained how headache remedies stop the ache. It may even reveal why acupuncture helps. And more important, it has pointed the way to new, perhaps better, treatments. Already it has led to at least one promising type of medicine, the so-called beta blockers, introduced in 1965 for heart ailments but quickly shown to affect migraine.

Medicinal avenues of attack on headaches are almost as diverse as headache types and causes. Some, like aspirin, prevent the initiation of pain. Others, like narcotic analgesics, interrupt pain transmission. And many of the newest headache medicines work to alter the physical or emotional conditions that lead to headaches.

The most important headache drug is, of course, aspirin, which belongs to a long-used family of remedies known chemically as salicylates. Precursors of aspirin, prepared from the leaves and bark of willow and many other plants, have been employed as painkillers since prehistoric times. Hippocrates probably was drawing on long-established practice when he recommended some 2,400 years ago the chewing of willow leaves to counter pain.

Aspirin seems to work better against muscle-tension headaches than against the vascular headaches associated with food or atmospheric pollutants. It acts mainly on inflamed tissues, which are more prominent as a cause of pain in the tension type. It is often combined in patent remedies with other ingredients such as caffeine and phenacetin, but the additional value they confer is debatable. Some extra ingredients, such as caffeine, may be counterproductive; caffeine helps vascular headaches but may worsen tension headaches.

Because aspirin is so effective and so safe, it is the world's most widely used medicine—100,000 tons are consumed in a typical year. But because so much of it has been taken by so many different people over so many years, a great deal has been learned about its side effects. In this way, one of the least harmful medicines known has paradoxically acquired a rather long list of cautions. They generally do not apply to people who use aspirin occasionally for headaches, but they are worthwhile warnings against overuse.

Dr. Fred Sheftell, a Connecticut headache specialist, reported that some patients coming into his program said they were taking 100 aspirin tablets a week. Even in less extraordinary quantities, aspirin can cause ringing in the ears and

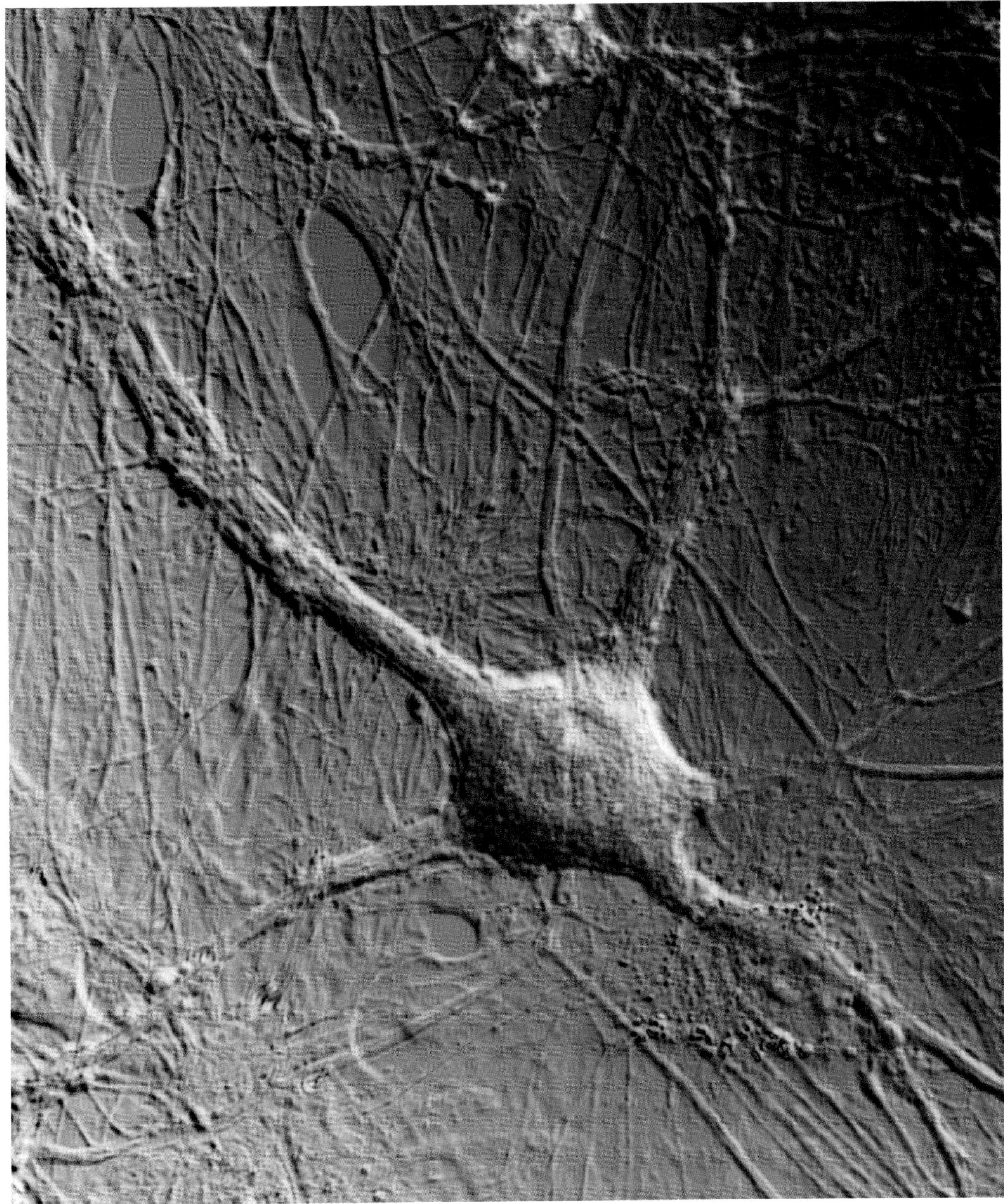

Typical of spinal-cord nerves that carry head pain to the brain in all mammals, this sample cell from a mouse is enlarged 600 times to reveal its spidery structure. The round lump is the cell body. Three of its four arms are message-receiving dendrites, and the other is the axon, which sends the impulse on to the next cell—but the two types are indistinguishable in photographs.

allergic reactions. It also prolongs bleeding and is sometimes prescribed to prevent blood clots; thus it should not be taken before surgery or extensive dental work. But its most common unwanted action is on the stomach. Aspirin is an acid. In many people it upsets digestion. In some it irritates the stomach lining or may even trigger an attack of ulcers.

The acid effects of aspirin can be lessened by use of the so-called buffered type, which contains balancing chemicals (taking plain aspirin with a glass of milk may serve the same purpose). But anyone with a sensitive stomach is probably better off using a different drug, acetaminophen, which achieves similar pain relief without digestive effects. It did not become a popular remedy for headaches until the 1950s, although it was used briefly before aspirin, in 1893.

The singular history of the painkillers

Aspirin and acetaminophen are not only the world's two leading headache remedies. They also have a strangely similar, convoluted history. Both were, in effect, invented by the same man, and in neither case did he have the slightest inkling of what he had wrought. Aspirin was compounded in 1853 by Charles-Frédéric Gerhardt, an obscure Alsatian chemist for whom it was just a curious chemical of no known value called acetylsalicylic acid. The formula languished as nothing more than an entry in his notebook for the next 40 years, until a Bayer company chemist resurrected the substance and found that it was miraculously effective against pain, fever and inflammation, and was much easier to tolerate than painkillers used up to that time.

Acetaminophen, too, lay ignored and unused for long periods. It is related to a drug called acetanilid, which was developed by the same Gerhardt in 1852, a year before he made aspirin. Like his aspirin, his acetanilid was nothing but a formula for many years, and might still be so except for a lucky accident. In 1886, an inexperienced pharmacist dispensed acetanilid by mistake to researchers testing another drug against intestinal parasites. They were surprised to find that the substance, though useless against parasites, reduced fever in test subjects. When the drug subsequently went on sale as a fever medicine, it was discovered to relieve pain, but it also proved to have serious side effects such as anemia and kidney damage.

Although acetanilid was used as an aspirin substitute well into the 20th Century, its side effects eventually caused this application to be discontinued. The drug was dropped from the semi-official American drug list—the *U.S. Pharmacopeia*—in 1955, and the Food and Drug Administration declared it unsafe as a headache medicine in 1977.

Its chemical relative, acetaminophen, is free of acetanilid's dangers. Pure acetaminophen was synthesized and recognized as an effective painkiller as long ago as 1893, but research on it was inexplicably dropped. Laboratory records of its invention, otherwise complete, are virtually silent on the advantages or disadvantages of acetaminophen. Not until the 1940s, when researchers demonstrated that Gerhardt's original acetanilid changed into acetaminophen in the body, was medical attention redirected to acetaminophen as a sovereign remedy for headache.

Although acetaminophen does not have aspirin's stomach-upsetting action, and although it is not as unsafe as acetanilid, it has disadvantages of its own. In prolonged heavy use, it can cause anemia and can harm kidneys and liver.

Narcotics, of course, are generally more powerful painkillers than aspirin or acetaminophen, but because their long-term use can lead to addiction, they are seldom used for treatment of persistent headaches. Among the few exceptions is the relatively mild opium derivative called codeine, which is sometimes used to help a patient get through a severe episode of pain while other forms of therapy *(Chapter 6)* are getting started. Codeine is considered to carry little risk of addiction when used on a temporary basis—but its superiority to aspirin as a painkiller has been questioned.

One controversial substance, dimethyl sulfoxide, known as DMSO, has been reported to provide striking relief for muscle-tension headache when brushed onto the back of the neck. DMSO, an extract of wood pulp, has been touted as a virtual panacea since its painkilling powers were first discovered in 1963. However, authorities, unconvinced of the drug's efficacy and safety—it is a very powerful chemical with still-unexplored effects—have moved slowly in permitting its use; in 1978 it was approved for use only to treat a rare bladder condition. But by the early 1980s many Americans were using a bootleg form of the drug—usually an undiluted, possibly impure, industrial version—for arthritis, bursitis, sprains and muscle strains. Ironically, DMSO's purported ability to block the pain of muscle-contraction headaches is accompanied by a tendency to promote blood-vessel dilation, and vascular headaches have been noted as a side effect.

None of these remedies, whether safe and effective or still unproved, may actually be needed to make a headache go away. Often the simple act of taking something—whatever it is—is enough to end the pain. This conclusion comes from a test conducted by doctors at the Mayo Clinic, who tried an assortment of painkillers, some of them real and some of them fakes, or placebos. All were disguised in tablet form to look and taste virtually identical. The study was carried out under double-blind conditions, meaning that neither patients nor doctors knew which substances were being given to whom until the test was over. The researchers found that 22 per cent of the participants experienced substantial pain relief after taking the placebo. Even such medium-strength narcotic analgesics as codeine and propoxyphene (Darvon) did not prove to be as necessary for relief as is often thought. In this study, the researchers found that neither was better than aspirin for the relief of pain.

Drugs to relax mind and body

Not all headaches can be alleviated so simply. Particularly in chronic headaches, emotions such as anxiety and depression often work in a vicious cycle with pain—pain feeding mood, mood exacerbating pain. In such cases a physician may prescribe one of the mood-altering drugs: a tranquilizer to reduce anxiety or an antidepressant to lift low spirits. To help combat anxiety, meprobamate (Miltown), diazepam (Valium) or chlordiazepoxide (Librium)—all so-called minor tranquilizers, as distinct from much more potent drugs used in severe emotional disorders—contribute to muscle relaxation and temporary alleviation of stress. However, when used for prolonged periods they may become habit-forming, with the body demanding higher and higher doses.

Drugs designed to fight depression have a useful role in preventing certain forms of recurring headache. Sometimes, as in chronic muscle-tension headaches, the depressive state of mind may well be the precipitating factor in touching off a series of headaches; in others, particularly migraine, the depression may come on as a secondary symptom of living with pain, interrupted sleep patterns and related miseries.

Antidepressant drugs are of two basic types—monoamine oxidase (MAO) inhibitors and tricyclic antidepressants. The MAO inhibitors banish depression, researchers believe, by keeping the enzyme called monoamine oxidase from breaking down two essential body chemicals: nerve-signal substances named norepinephrine and serotonin, which among other things help regulate blood pressure and emotional states. The resulting higher concentrations of norepinephrine and serotonin in the brain restore normal mood.

But excess monoamines can be harmful, causing sudden increases in blood pressure that may even bring on strokes. Some monoamines, such as tyramine, occur naturally in some foods, including aged cheeses, nuts, ripe bananas, red wines, beer and chocolate. Thus to prevent an excess of monoamines, anyone taking MAO inhibitors must avoid a whole list of tyramine-rich foods. Also banned are decongestant nasal sprays, nose drops and cold remedies, many of which contain norepinephrine or chemicals that release it.

The other category of antidepressants, compounds such as imipramine and amitriptyline, are called tricyclics because of their three-ringed molecular structure. They, too, appear to raise the levels of norepinephrine and serotonin, though at a slightly different stage than the MAO inhibitors. Their mood-altering effects may take as long as six weeks to reach the maximum level. Side effects are usually mild.

How ergotamine interrupts migraine

Neither ordinary painkillers nor mood-altering drugs can fight the suffering caused by severe cluster and migraine headaches. For them there is the unusual drug named ergotamine tartrate, made from ergot, a fungus that grows on rye and other grains *(pages 94-103)*. This drug acts as a powerful blood-vessel constrictor by causing prolonged contraction of

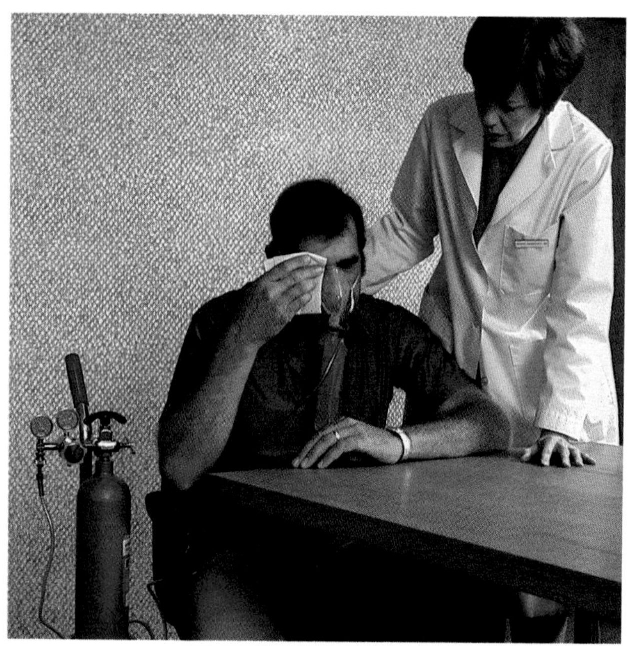

Handkerchief to his watering eye, a man suffering a cluster headache—so called because its symptoms recur repeatedly over a period of days, then vanish for months at a time—breathes oxygen from a tank at a Michigan clinic. Pure oxygen relieves the attack, probably by slowing production of chemicals that dilate blood vessels and are thought to cause cluster headaches.

smooth-muscle fibers, particularly the ones that control the size of the arteries involved in these serious headaches.

In a migraine attack, the arteries dilate because the nerves that serve their smooth-muscle fibers become less active than normal. In this state, the nerves give off less norepinephrine, and this allows the smooth muscles of the arteries to relax. This explains why migraine frequently occurs when a victim is resting—norepinephrine production decreases at rest. Ergotamine tartrate has the ability to mimic norepinephrine; it, too, stimulates the contraction of the blood vessel muscles.

The medical derivative of ergot, ergotamine tartrate, is generally taken at the first sign of head pain to reduce the intensity or duration of an acute attack. The dangers of constantly constricting the blood vessels, not to mention the risk of ergot poisoning, mean that the drug can be taken safely only once or twice a week and is thus not suitable for anyone with frequent attacks. For the same reason, ergotamine tartrate is not recommended as a preventive. However, a newer ergot compound, methysergide maleate, can be used as a preventive, fending off both migraine and cluster headaches.

Methysergide's actions, like the mechanisms of migraine itself, are strangely paradoxical. It works by first hindering, then helping, the action of serotonin. During the pre-pain phase of migraine, blood vessels that serve the brain become narrowed because blood platelets release excess amounts of serotonin, a constrictor of certain blood vessels. At this stage, methysergide plays an antagonist role, blocking the constricting effect of the serotonin.

During the headache phase of migraine, serotonin levels in the blood drop, causing vessels outside the brain to expand, distending the sensitive nerve endings within them and bringing about severe pain. In this situation methysergide reverses itself and substitutes for the missing serotonin, helping the blood vessels shrink back to normal size. In cluster headaches, methysergide also acts in this way, constricting severely dilated arteries.

Another effective medicine used in migraine and cluster headaches is a hormone called prednisone. Prescribed to relieve arthritis pain, allergic reactions, asthma and other ailments, prednisone works on these problems by reducing inflammation; in headache, it is believed to affect production of serotonin. The possible side effects of hormones—abnormal hair growth, ulcers, thrombophlebitis, obesity and mental effects, among others—rule out long-term use of prednisone for relatively minor headaches, but it can have striking results in preventing the onset of an episode of cluster headaches and in relieving migraine pain.

Also being tested for its effects on these severe headaches is cimetidine, better known by its trade name of Tagamet, the drug widely used for ulcers and other digestive ills. Cimetidine helps ulcers by blocking histamine, the body chemical that causes the release of stomach acid and also causes noses to be stuffed up and blood vessels to expand. Researchers testing the drug found that it also blocked the swelling of blood vessels in the head; presumably it could prevent the arterial dilation that causes migraine and cluster headaches.

In addition to these drugs, two special remedies are also used for cluster headaches. Victims suffering almost continuous pain may be given compounds of lithium—a common mineral that in 1949 was discovered to be a specific for certain types of depression. The other remedy is not even a drug: pure oxygen. The cluster victim dons a face mask at the first notice of an oncoming attack and breathes oxygen from a tank for 15 minutes. The pain usually diminishes to a dull ache or dissipates altogether—the oxygen inhibits production of a special dilation-causing type of prostaglandin in the walls of blood vessels. As the vessels return to normal, the stretched and twisted nerve endings embedded in them do the same, and stop sending pain signals.

Four ways to fool the nerves

These numerous headache drugs, from aspirin to lithium, share one basic trait: They relieve pain by interfering somehow with nerve signals. Aspirin and acetaminophen work at the pain site to prevent a pain signal from getting started. Opiates, the most powerful painkillers, stop pain signals from crossing connections between nerves. Tranquilizers and antidepressants operate at this point also, but block the signals that cause such painful reactions as muscle contraction. Some headache treatments that do not employ drugs—massage and the needle treatment, acupuncture—may stop pain signals at main nerve junctions in the spinal cord. Thus progress against headaches depends on progress in understanding how the nervous system brings on pain, generates pain signals and carries them to the brain to be perceived.

The nature of pain, the mechanisms that bring it on and the means of controlling it are still subjects of continuing controversy. To some extent, they will always be so, for no matter how much researchers learn about the physiology and chemistry of such sensations, they can never reduce these actions to simple cause and effect. Pain is, after all, subjective. What hurts one person may not be felt by another. Even the same person feels aches differently at different times.

Pain is so variable because it depends on a complex set of influences, of which the objective quantity and quality of pain-inducing stimuli are but a part. What did the person learn in childhood, for example, that might diminish or heighten present sensitivity to pain? Was the expression of pain rewarded with more sympathy? Does the individual have deep-seated memories of some long-ago hurt that has made him especially apprehensive of all subsequent painful experiences? What is his general state of mind—is he feeling vulnerable and depressed, or strong and positive? What is there in genetic make-up that might contribute to a unique response to pain? What time of day is it, what is the barometric pressure, what is the immediate environment? All are thought to play some role in determining a particular response to a particular pain stimulus.

Despite these many variables, all pains, whether in the head or elsewhere in the body, are in some respects much alike. The mechanisms by which they are initiated, communicated and felt are much the same regardless of their cause, location or type. No one is likely to confuse the pain of a broken leg with that of a headache, but the explanation of why each one hurts might differ only in small details.

Where the ache begins

Pain in its most essential form is a coded bit of information transmitted as an electric signal from the site of stimulus along nerve pathways to terminals in the brain. Each impulse

ARGENTINA

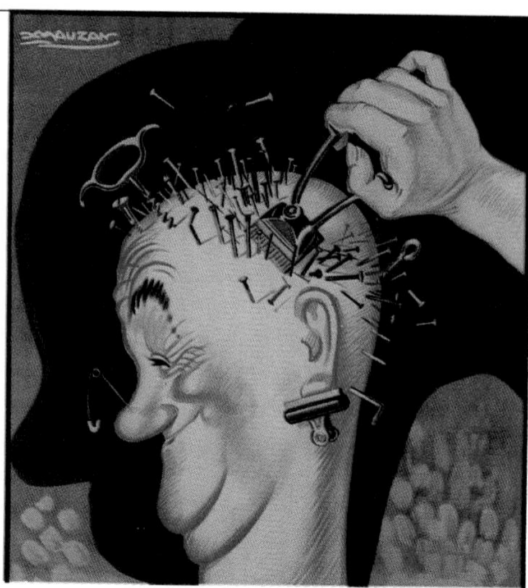

Images of head pain

Words and pictures describing various kinds of headache pain have become stereotyped over the years. Yet some artists commissioned to communicate these sensations in advertisements continue to surprise the eye, as is demonstrated by these four examples—each promoting a different remedy in a different country.

To suggest the grabbing, knifing pain of neuralgia, a Swiss advertisement depicts claws raking the facial nerves of an anguished victim *(below)*. Lightning bolts *(right, center)* represent sharp, quick head pain, while the viselike quality of many types of headaches is illustrated by giant fingers squeezing a poor sufferer's head *(far right)*. The illustration at near right, created in the 1930s by the noted French artist Lucien Mauzan, suggests relief rather than pain: The headache victim wears a grin as the hardware representing his suffering is clipped away.

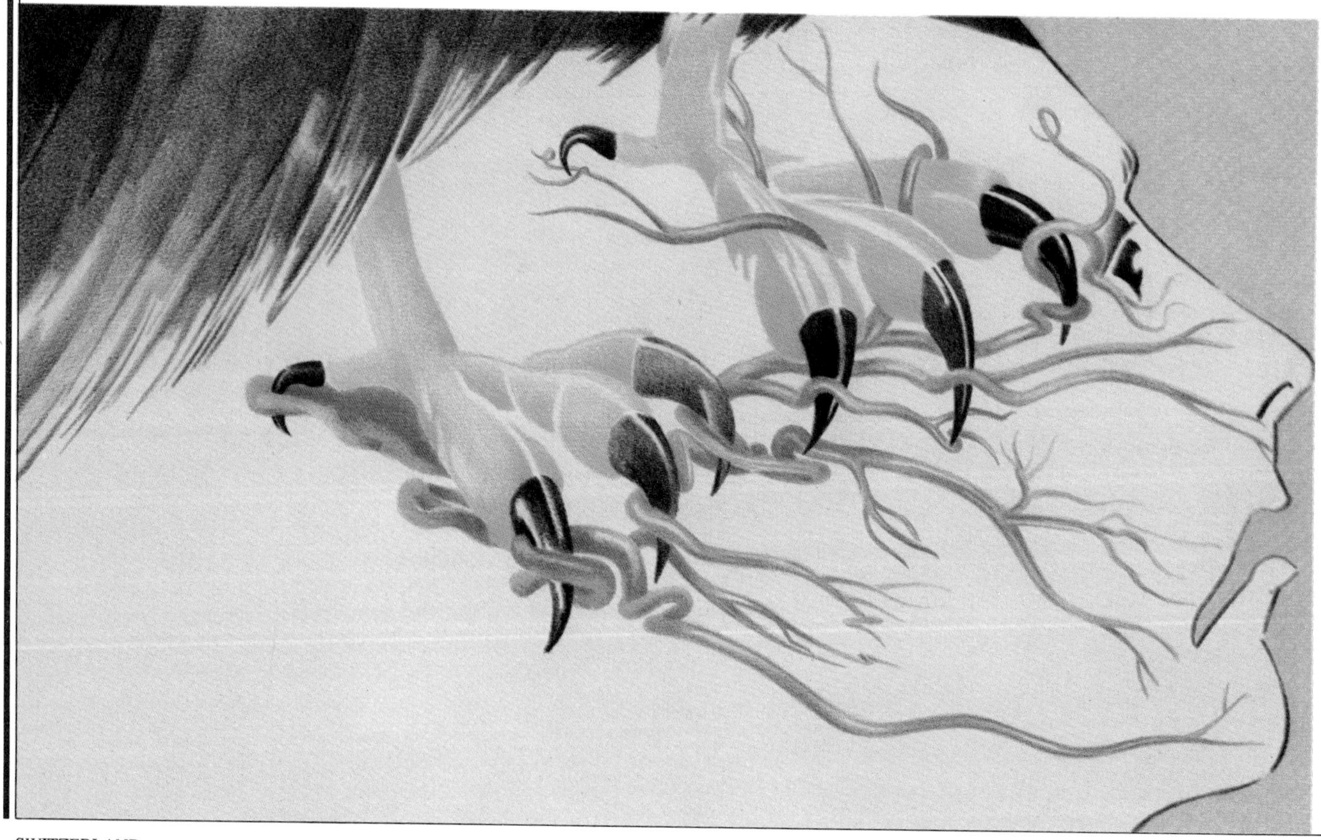

SWITZERLAND

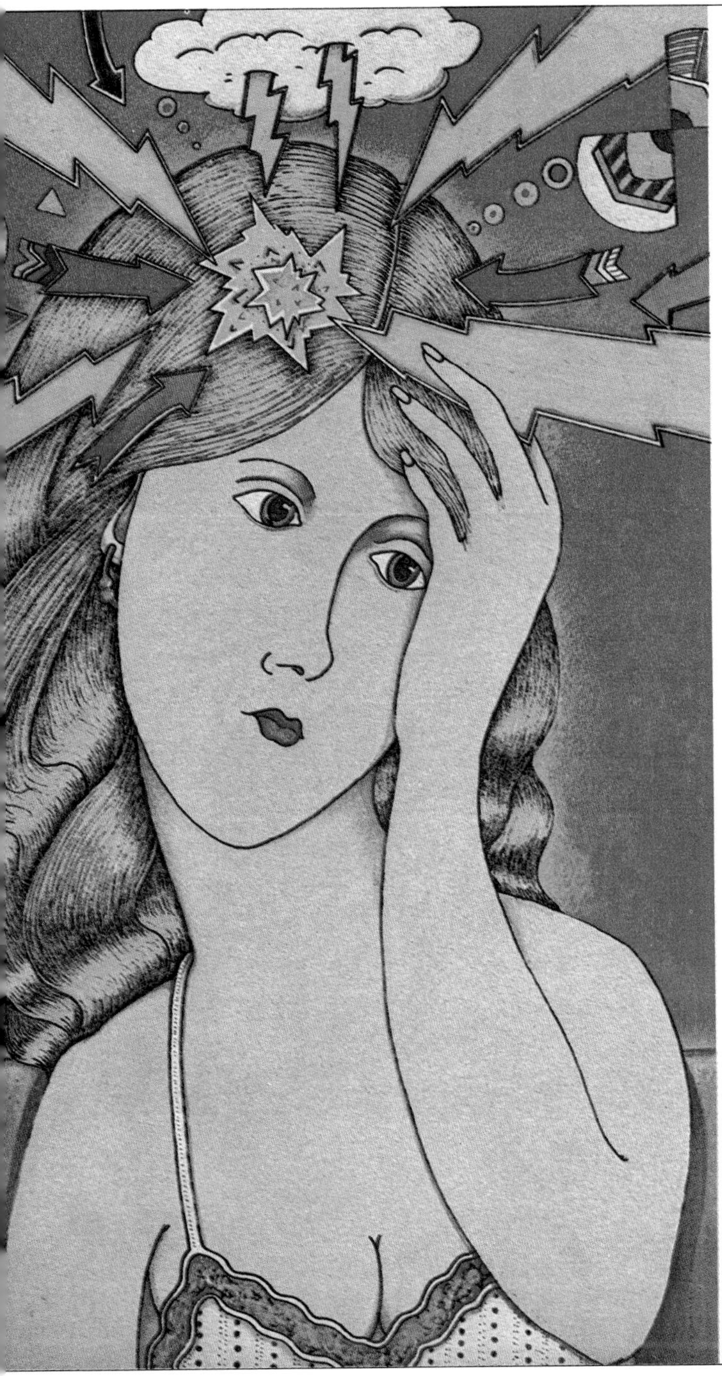

UNITED STATES

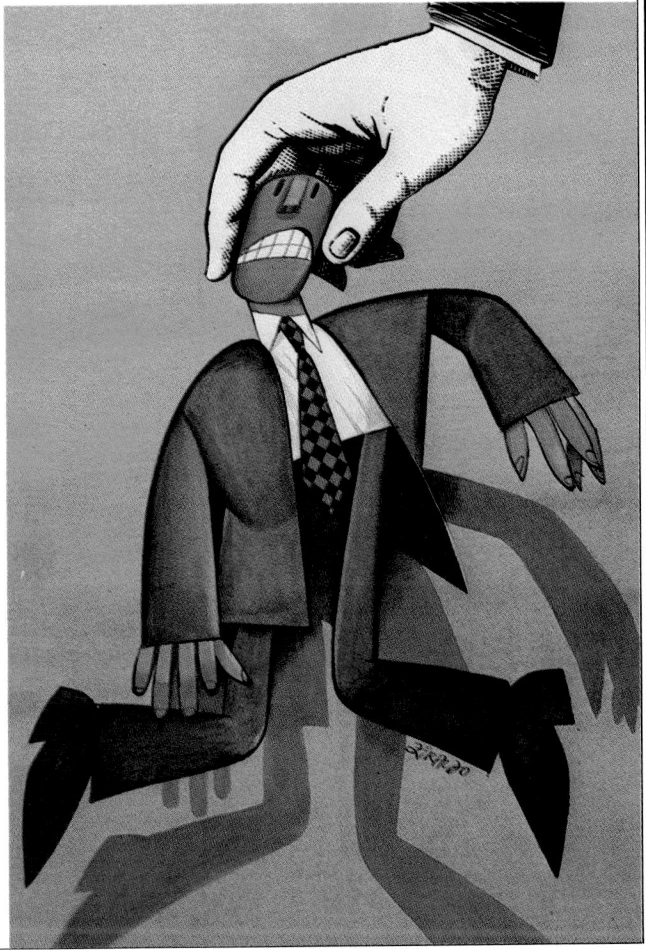

BRAZIL

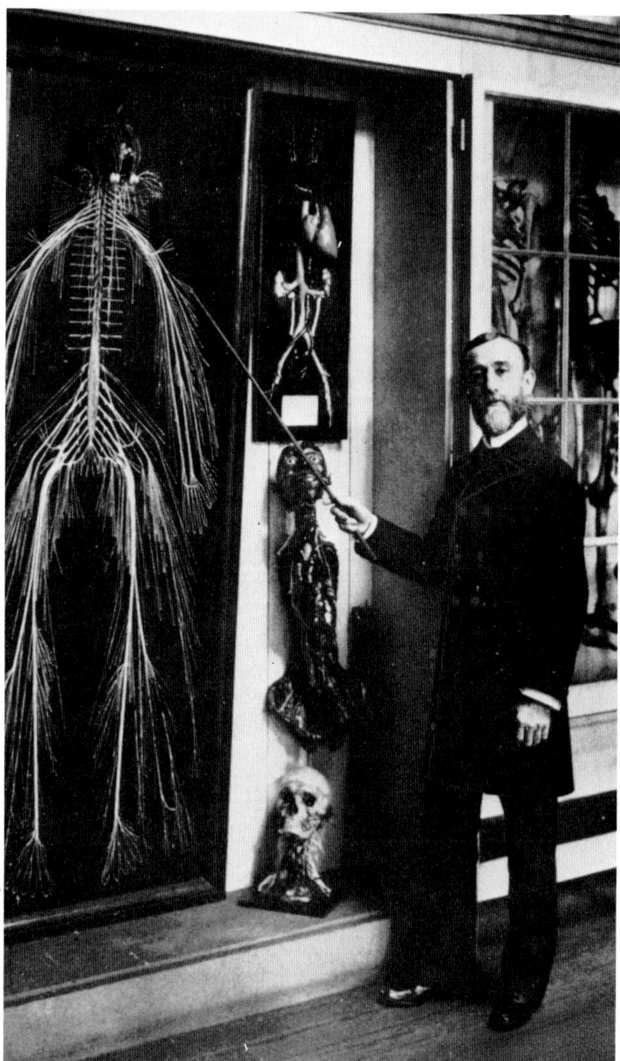

Dr. Rufus B. Weaver of Hahnemann Medical College of Philadelphia proudly points to the five-month labor of love with which he made medical history in 1888: the dissection and mounting of the nerves of Harriet Cole, a servant in Weaver's household who had asked that her body be used for science after her death, at 35, from tuberculosis. Clearly visible in the photograph above are the sheath that surrounded the spinal cord, the symmetrical sets of fibers that transmitted signals to and from the head, trunk and limbs, and the eyes, which have been preserved and left attached to the optic nerves.

originates in a single receptor at the end of a single nerve cell, or neuron, but it may pass through a few or many nerve cells to reach its destination. Only when it reaches the appropriate part of the brain is it perceived as pain.

The basic piece of equipment in this system is the nerve cell. It may be as short as a fraction of an inch in some parts of the brain or as long as four feet in an adult's leg. Looking somewhat like a tree—roots, trunk, branches—each nerve cell has at one end a root-like system of endings called dendrites, which receive stimuli from surrounding tissue or incoming impulses from other nerves. The bulbous base, called a cell body, contains the nucleus of the cell. From the cell body stretches the axon, a trunklike section that eventually branches out to pass impulses along to the next nerve in the chain of transmission.

The human body contains, according to one estimate, 15 billion of these nerve cells. Some are in the central nervous system, which includes the brain and its connections in the spinal cord, and the rest are in the peripheral nervous system—the network of nerve fibers that connects all the rest of the body to the spinal cord and thence to the brain. Both sections of the system carry messages to and from the brain, the outgoing signals ordering muscles and other organs to do their jobs, the incoming signals reporting back to the brain on conditions in and near the body. Thus the central nervous system transmits and interprets the messages that say something hurts, but only the peripheral nervous system picks up pain—the spinal-cord nerves and the brain are insensitive to it.

Pain begins at peripheral nerve endings that are designed to sense conditions around them and report to the brain. Some respond to temperature, others to pressure, chemicals, light or sound. For centuries, debate has raged over the possibility that similarly specialized nerve endings respond only to pain. If so, pain would have its own special network of nerves. If not, pain would be communicated by any sensory nerves that are overstimulated. Present-day belief is that both ideas are correct: The ends of some nerve cells apparently serve almost exclusively for the detection of pain, but other nerve endings that are sensitive to pressure, temperature and certain chemicals can also signal pain when stimulated strongly enough.

Headache pain, for example, might be touched off by chemicals or by pressure, depending on the type of headache. In a muscle-tension headache, researchers believe, tightening muscles of the scalp and neck restrict the flow of blood, and therefore oxygen, to these tissues, resulting in the oxygen starvation known as ischemia. As the muscle cells try to keep working while increasingly starved for oxygen, they become damaged.

One result of the damage is the release of a compound called arachidonic acid which, when activated by an enzyme normally present, combines with oxygen from the blood to produce the chemicals called prostaglandins. The prostaglandins affect the nerve endings so that they are more sensitive—lower the "firing threshold," in technical jargon. Then pain-inducers that normally activate nerves for various internal purposes—serotonin, bradykinin and many others—can more easily start a pain signal.

When the pain-inducers come into contact with the nerve endings, they set off disturbances in the normal electrical charge of the molecules in the nerve endings, generating electrical pain impulses. In 1971, some seven decades after aspirin came into general use, scientists finally discovered that the way this drug relieves muscle-tension headaches is by blocking the conversion of arachidonic acid into pain-sensitizing prostaglandins.

A somewhat different mechanism produces pain in the other common kinds of headaches, generally classed as vascular—they all involve some form of swelling of blood vessels in the head. Migraine and cluster headaches are the worst in this category, but it also includes various minor headaches caused by any number of triggers, ranging from the nitrites in hot dogs to high altitudes. In such headaches, swollen blood vessels distend nerve endings that are sensitive to deformation. Some headache specialists also speculate that a chemical called neurokinin—similar to the venom of a wasp—is released during blood vessel dilation and fires off impulses in chemical-sensitive nerves.

Chemical action on the nerve endings changes their elec-

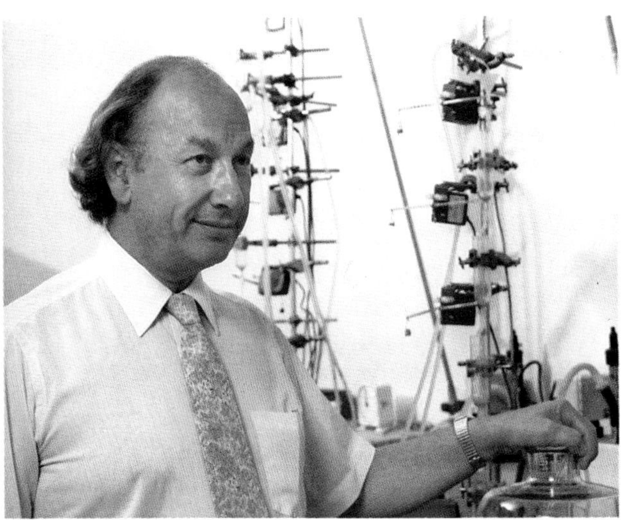

Dr. John Vane, the British pharmacologist who described in detail how aspirin may work chemically to relieve pain, stands beside an apparatus in his laboratory in London. Vane proposed that aspirin, by interfering with the chemical reaction illustrated below, blocks body cells from producing prostaglandins, compounds that help nerve endings to feel pain.

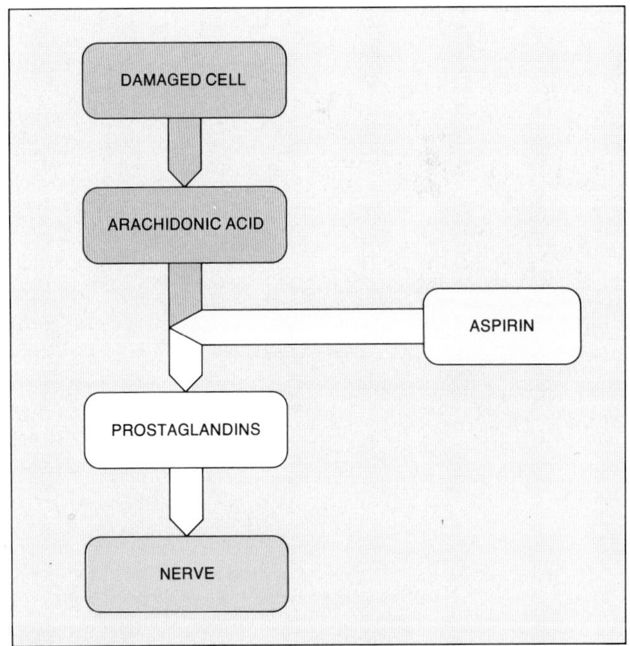

Aspirin interrupts a chain of reactions that produce chemicals called prostaglandins, which sensitize nerves to pain. In the absence of aspirin, an enzyme releases arachidonic acid from a damaged cell, and the acid joins with blood oxygen to create prostaglandins. When aspirin is taken, the enzyme combines the oxygen with aspirin, preventing formation of prostaglandins.

trical charges in much the way the chemicals in a battery alter the charges on its terminals. Pressure-caused deformation of nerve endings also produces electrical effects, but in a different way. The deformation changes the spacing of nerve endings; they always have some charges, and this movement of their charges changes the voltage between them. Thus, no matter how the nerve endings are stimulated, they generate an electrical voltage that travels from one end to the other. The nerve cell "fires."

When a nerve fires, it does so in only one way: all-or-nothing. There are no half signals, no weak ones or strong ones. No matter how great or small the stimulus that sets off the electrical impulse in a nerve cell, the cell always responds with an impulse of one particular voltage and duration. The intensity of the pain experience depends on how many individual nerve cells fire—and on how fast the impulses reach the brain.

The speed of a pain signal is determined by the type of nerve that picks it up and transmits it. There are two kinds, only one of which carries headache pains.

The complex nerves called A-delta—the name is arbitrary, assigned to differentiate this type from others—handle fast-pain signals. They warn the brain of immediate danger, not of the more subtle hazard of headaches. They carry only the sharp, pricking, highly localized sensation that is elicited at the instant of an injury. An A-delta fiber is identifiable by the curious-looking, thin sheath that surrounds it like insulation around a wire. The sheath, made of a fatty substance called myelin, is not a continuous insulating coat. It is interrupted at regular intervals by gaps, called nodes of Ranvier, after their discoverer, Louis-Antoine Ranvier, a 19th Century French scientist. Nerve impulses, instead of coursing along the fiber at a steady pace, skip rapidly along from one of these gaps to the next.

The second and simpler type of nerve cell, designated C-fibers, delivers slow pain—the dull, aching, burning, more diffuse and deeply felt sensation that lingers and is characteristic of headaches. C-fibers are unmyelinated—that is, they have no insulating coating; they are consequently perhaps a third smaller in diameter. They deliver pain messages at a considerably slower rate. Differences in the quality and time of arrival of the two kinds of pain are often subtle, but if you are looking for them you will in all likelihood recognize them. Try the simple experiment of pricking your finger with a sharp needle, for example; you should first feel the sharp, fast pain, followed at a distinctly later moment by the dull ache of the lingering, slow pain.

Not even the fast-pain messages, although carried by electrical impulses, travel at rates ordinarily associated with electricity. An electromagnetic wave in space goes 186,000 miles per second, but the fast-pain signals of the A-delta fibers lumber along at between 27 and 67 miles per hour—which is fast enough to tell your brain you stubbed your toe in about $^1/_{10}$ second. The signal of a headache, though it travels a shorter distance to your brain, takes longer because it goes by way of the C-fibers, which transmit signals only a tenth as fast, barely walking speed.

The existence of fast-pain and slow-pain fibers led two young scientists to put forth in 1965 a "gate-control theory" of pain, an idea that some specialists believe will have direct bearing on the future control and treatment of headaches. Neurologist Patrick D. Wall of the Massachusetts Institute of Technology and psychologist Ronald Melzack of McGill University, Montreal, proposed that the large (fast) and the small (slow) fiber networks operate together in a system of checks and balances to determine the transmission of pain messages to the brain.

As they described it, pain signals are added together at a way station along the spinal cord known as the substantia gelatinosa, where the networks of fast and slow nerve fibers meet and interact. Impulses arriving along the fast fibers have the effect of closing the gate to painful impulses traveling along the slow fibers. Slow fibers must work to open the gate. Impulses coming down from the brain also appear to figure in the summation, adding to or subtracting from the result.

Only if the total of these impulses exceeds the individual's pain threshold are they experienced as pain; the amount indicates a particular kind of pain. The researchers believe that their theory explains why people instinctively rub an injured area—in effect keeping up the flow of fast-pain impulses to block out the later-arriving deep-pain impulses. The concept may also throw light on the mechanisms of acupuncture and also of transcutaneous electrical nerve stimulation (TENS), a promising pain-relief technique that makes use of electrical impulses *(Chapter 6)*.

The relay stations

No nerve signal has an unbroken pathway to (or from) the brain. The electrical impulse generated at one end of a nerve travels only to the other end of that cell, where it stops. The signal then has to be regenerated in another nerve cell. Thus the signal must run in relay along a chain of cells, jumping from one cell to the next until it arrives at its destination. Transmission of a signal from one nerve to the next takes place across a specialized one-way junction known as a synapse, a minute gap between the axon of one cell and the dendrite of the other *(pages 120-123)*.

At the synapse the electrical energy of the impulse causes release of a chemical messenger called a neurotransmitter—norepinephrine, serotonin and certain other compounds affected by headache remedies are neurotransmitters. Stored in tiny sacs at the ends of the axon, the neurotransmitter diffuses into the synapse space each time an electrical impulse compels the sacs to release it.

The chemical crosses the space, and lodges in receptors on the surface of the next nerve cell's dendrites. When it enters the receptor, it changes the electrical charge there from negative to positive, creating a new electrical impulse that travels along the fiber to the other end and on toward the central nervous system and the brain. Work done, the neurotransmitter is then rapidly destroyed by enzymes, the charge at the nerve ending goes back to negative, and the synapse is cleared for the next message. Of the 30 or so different chemicals that play a neurotransmitter role in the nervous system, the two believed to have the strongest connection to headache pain are acetylcholine and norepinephrine, which normally control the size of blood vessels.

Neurotransmitters are of two opposite kinds: They either carry a nerve signal across a synapse, or they stop it from

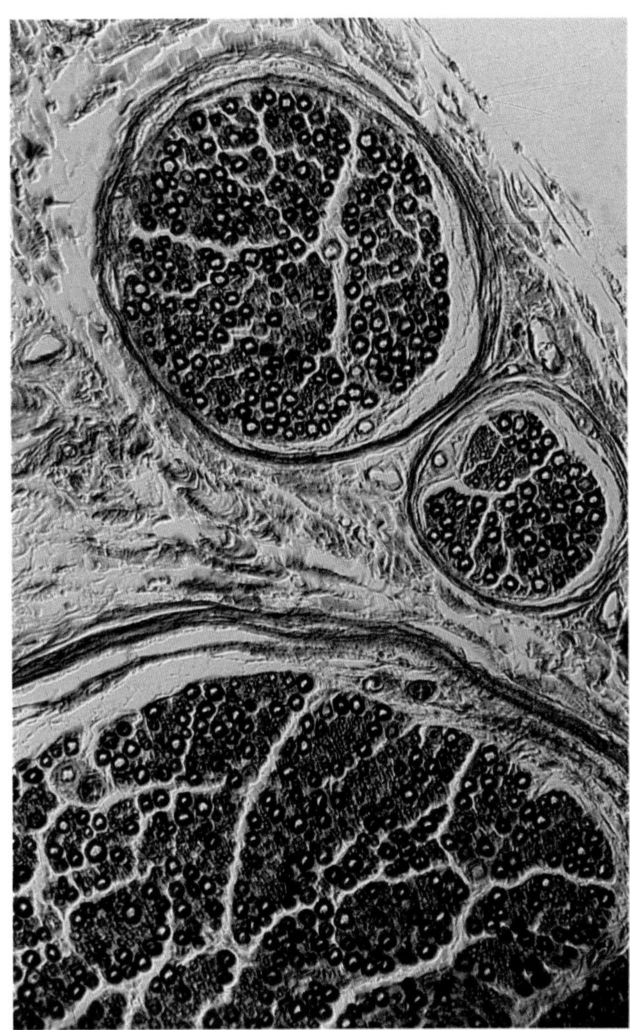

A magnified cross section of two nerve bundles and part of a third reveals the two main types of nerve fibers, resembling tiny wires inside a telephone cable, that transmit pain and other sensory information to the brain. In each bundle are black-rimmed fibers encased in sheaths of a fatty tissue called myelin; they transmit sharp, fast pains. Barely visible among these large fibers are smaller, grainier neighbors that lack myelin insulation and carry the dull, diffuse pain characteristic of many headaches.

crossing. Thus, manipulating neurotransmitters can interrupt pain. These chemicals can be made to carry signals to alleviate the cause of pain, such as the dilation or constriction of blood vessels; or they can be made to prevent the transmission of pain signals across a synapse. Such regulation of neurotransmitters is behind the action of those headache remedies, such as antidepressants, tranquilizers and ergotamine, that operate at synapses rather than, like aspirin, at the site of cell damage.

In 1973 Dr. Solomon H. Snyder and Candace B. Pert of Johns Hopkins University School of Medicine demonstrated that painkillers such as opiates work because they act like the inhibiting type of neurotransmitters. They found that the sending ends of nerve cells contained receptor areas so designed that they accepted the molecules of opiate painkillers. When opiate molecules fill these receptors, they prevent the pain neurotransmitters from being released; if enough opiate receptors are filled, too few pain neurotransmitters are released to fire a pain impulse and carry the signal onward.

The brain's own narcotics

The fact that some nerve cells had receptor sites specially designed to fit opiate drugs posed a puzzle: Why were the receptor sites there? Clearly their existence in the body predates the use of opiates, no matter how early in human history that practice began. There was only one possible answer. The body must contain natural opiates that use these receptors and that are capable of blocking pain. In 1975 Drs. John Hughes and Hans Kosterlitz of the University of Aberdeen became the first to locate a natural opiate chemical, and they found it in the brain of pigs.

Not one but several human opiates have since been identified; a type produced in the brain is called enkephalins; the pituitary gland and the hypothalamus, both near the bottom of the brain, produce another type called endorphins. (One of the endorphins has been found to be 48 times more powerful a painkiller than morphine in a comparative test.) They are believed to function as neurotransmitters, the kind that inhibit, rather than convey, pain signals. They are normally present at very low levels, but their production spontaneously increases under stress—one explanation for the battlefield phenomenon in which a severely wounded soldier is able to fight on, oblivious to his injuries. Some authorities speculate that human opiates are released by acupuncture.

The discovery of internal opiates raised hopes once again that a natural painkiller, powerful but nonaddictive, could be found. In the past, the story of this search has followed a familiar pattern: A new drug is developed and its makers proudly put it forward as a sovereign pain reliever that is not only nonaddictive but a cure for addiction to older narcotics. In as little time as it takes for its users to become hooked, the new miracle drug joins its predecessors as the latest addictive opiate.

In just such an instance, the Bayer company, seeking in 1898 a potent but safe painkiller for cases that were beyond the powers of its then-new wonder drug, aspirin, introduced a morphine derivative that seemingly presented no risk to the user: heroin. Its fall from grace was not long in coming, and this drug has been among the most abused narcotics. The first tests of molecular variations of human opiates were likewise disappointing. Heavy doses of enkephalins given to rats produced growing tolerance and, when the drugs were discontinued, withdrawal symptoms.

Later experiments with human subjects, however, demonstrated that natural opiates, addictive or not, may prove valuable in alleviating severe pain. Dr. Yoshiro Hosobuchi of the University of San Francisco School of Medicine injected endorphins directly into patients' brains and found that a fraction of a millionth of an ounce could stop pain for four or five hours. However, this procedure turned out to be as expensive as it was effective—a single dose of endorphins then cost about $3,000. So Dr. Hosobuchi turned to methods that would make the brain produce extra amounts of its own endorphins. He implanted platinum wires in the brains of victims of intractable pain, so that the patients, using radio controls, could electrically stimulate their own brains to release the painkilling endorphins.

The promise of new ways to control pain is only one practical result of the explosion of knowledge about neurotransmitters. The understanding of their operation has explained how several drugs work and has opened avenues to better drugs.

It is now believed, for example, that some of the tranquilizers used for headaches, such as diazepam and chlordiazepoxide, operate by assisting a natural neurotransmitter named gamma-aminobutyric acid, but usually known as GABA. GABA is a transmitter that stops nerves from firing—reducing the heavy load of nerve signals that accompanies the anxiety implicated in headaches. Its molecules stop signals by fitting into receptors on a nerve ending in such a way that the nerve ending becomes more accessible to atoms carrying a negative charge. Because a net positive charge is required to initiate a nerve signal, the addition of a negative charge prevents firing. The tranquilizer molecules help GABA by fitting into other receptors on the nerve ending, where they induce more GABA molecules to attach to the nerve ending, thus adding to the intake of negative charge and increasing the likelihood that firing will be stopped.

Now that researchers can tell which neurotransmitters cause which effect, they can look for chemicals that resemble them or act on them. From such efforts came propranolol, found through a deliberate search for a drug that would control norepinephrine, one of the neurotransmitters controlling the action of the heart muscle. Propranolol is a beta blocker; it fits into a so-called beta receptor (the migraine drug ergotamine works on an alpha receptor). When propranolol blocks norepinephrine from reaching the beta receptors of the heart, that muscle contracts more slowly, thus the drug's value as a relaxant for a damaged, vulnerable heart.

Quite by accident, another possible application of propranolol came to light: the use of the drug to prevent migraine. While being tested for its ability to ease severe heart pain—the symptom known as angina pectoris—propranolol given to one patient not only worked against his chest pain but also relieved his long-standing migraine headaches. When this patient was switched over to a dummy drug, his headaches returned.

Scientists seeking an explanation for this unexpected bonus effect found that when propranolol blocks norepinephrine from the beta receptors of arterial muscles, the outcome is just the opposite of its effect on the heart—propranolol makes these muscle fibers contract faster and thus constrict the arteries. Because of this paradoxical action, propranolol has great promise as a migraine preventive.

The switch from electrical impulse to chemical neurotransmitter and back takes place many times as a pain signal travels across synapses from nerve fiber to nerve fiber to reach the brain. The route may be roundabout. The ache of a headache is always in the head, perhaps half an inch from the brain, but in many cases it must go outside the head before it registers in the brain. Some head pains travel down along the slow C-fibers to the spinal cord in the neck. There they switch over to somewhat smaller nerve fibers called second-order neurons and travel up the cord, to be distributed to the various perceptual sections of the brain.

Only in the brain is a nerve impulse anything but a weak succession of electrical and chemical actions flashing along a chain of nerve cells. Once within the brain, it goes through a complex process of analysis by various components, each helping to fill in a picture of the pain's nature and to direct mental and physical reactions to it.

The first part of the brain to encounter the signal—the reticular formation of the brain stem—judges, from the speed of reception, whether it must command the body to get away from the cause of pain immediately. It makes this decision automatically. In the case of headaches, escape is impossible, and the reticular formation can only alert the rest of the brain that something hurts someplace. Other parts of the brain then locate the pain, assess its quality, check it against memories of past pains and trigger emotional reactions—all without conscious thought. Finally the thinking brain, the frontal cortex, reviews the data and interpretations and consciously decides what, if anything, to do.

What to do, generally, is take a painkiller. But now the better understanding of pain has shown new ways to relieve headaches and has revived interest in old ones. In modern headache clinics the most persistent headaches are being attacked with treatments that range from psychological counseling and biofeedback to yoga and acupuncture, in the hope that eventually the patient's own mind, rather than any external agent, will cure this insidious disorder. ❋

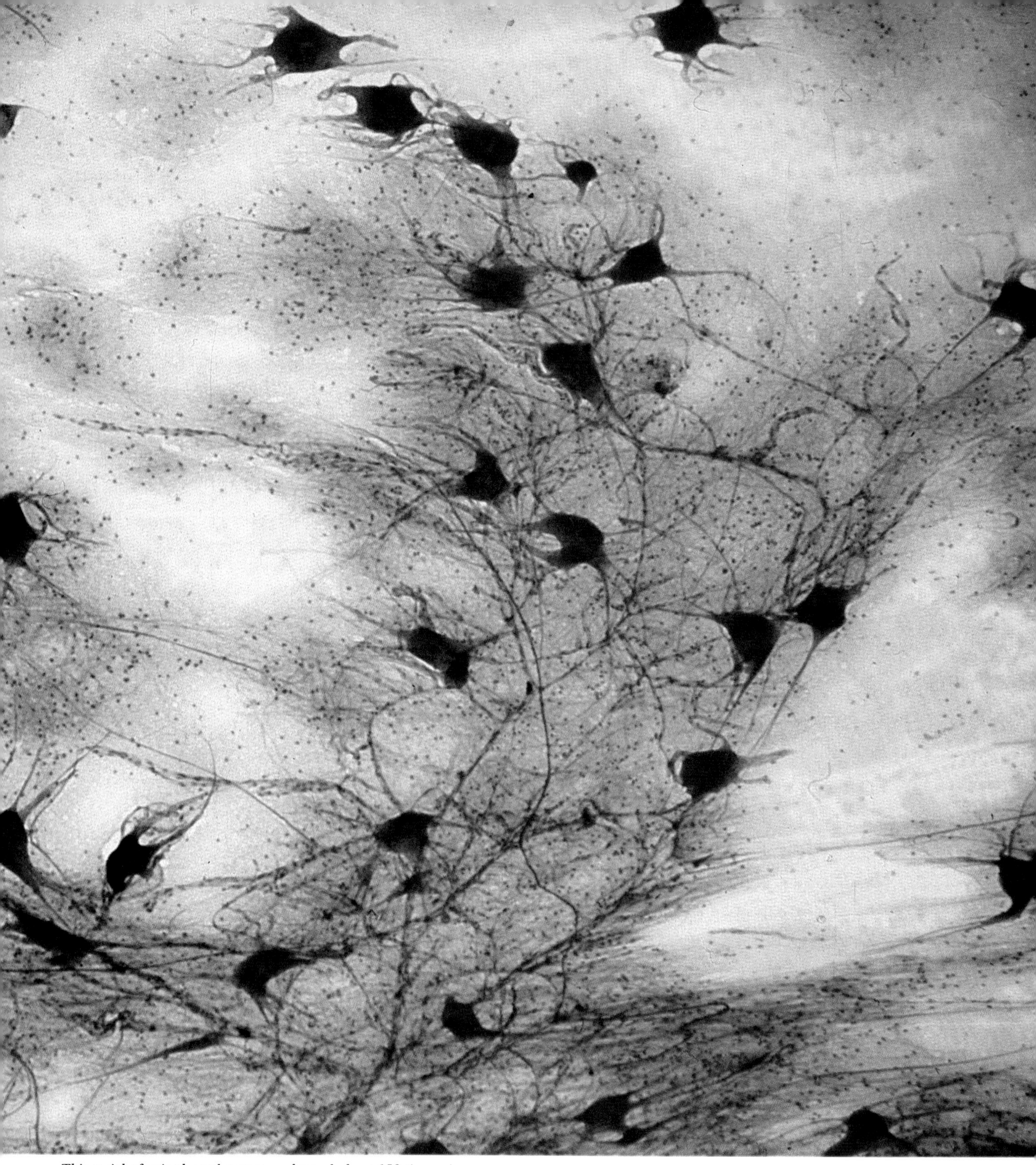

This swirl of spinal-cord nerves, enlarged about 150 times, is part of the complex circuitry for communicating sensations such as headache pain inward to the brain; it also carries commands outward to the muscles. The dark masses are cell bodies, the site of each nerve cell's nucleus. Many headache signals detour through the spinal cord on their way to the brain.

Tracking the ache in a headache

What makes your head ache is ultimately your brain. It responds to signals from some ailing section of your body with a feeling perceived as pain. How these signals are generated at the site of the ache, sent along the nerve circuits and finally read by the brain computer is far more complex than anyone imagined, but the intricacies are finally being unraveled.

With this new knowledge of the mechanism of pain come surprises. Different types of nerves transmit different types of pain at different speeds (headaches travel the slow route). A headache need not be in the head; it may come from the neck. Many aches originating in the head must send their signals by a roundabout route, outside the head and into the main nerve trunk in the spinal cord, before they can reach the brain to be perceived. But the most important surprise is the revelation of the workings of medicines that stop pain; in the great variety of their actions lies the promise of more effective remedies.

Whether a pain in the head stems from tensed muscles—the contraction headache, the type that is traced in micrographs and drawings on these and the following pages—or from swollen blood vessels, as in migraine and hangover headaches, the first step in the pain process is the stimulation of an electrical impulse in sensitive nerve endings.

The stimulation is partly chemical, partly electrical. It alters the electrical charge of molecules at the sensitive end of a nerve fiber. This change creates an electrical impulse that travels along the nerve fiber, somewhat like a telegraph signal traveling along a wire. At the other end of the nerve fiber, the impulse causes the release of more chemicals, stimulating the regeneration of the pain signal in the end of a neighboring fiber.

This relaying of chemical and electrical actions continues from nerve to nerve into the brain and through its centers of interpretation and perception. But at any of the relay points it can be blocked or canceled by a painkilling compound—whether a man-made drug or a natural opiate produced within the body.

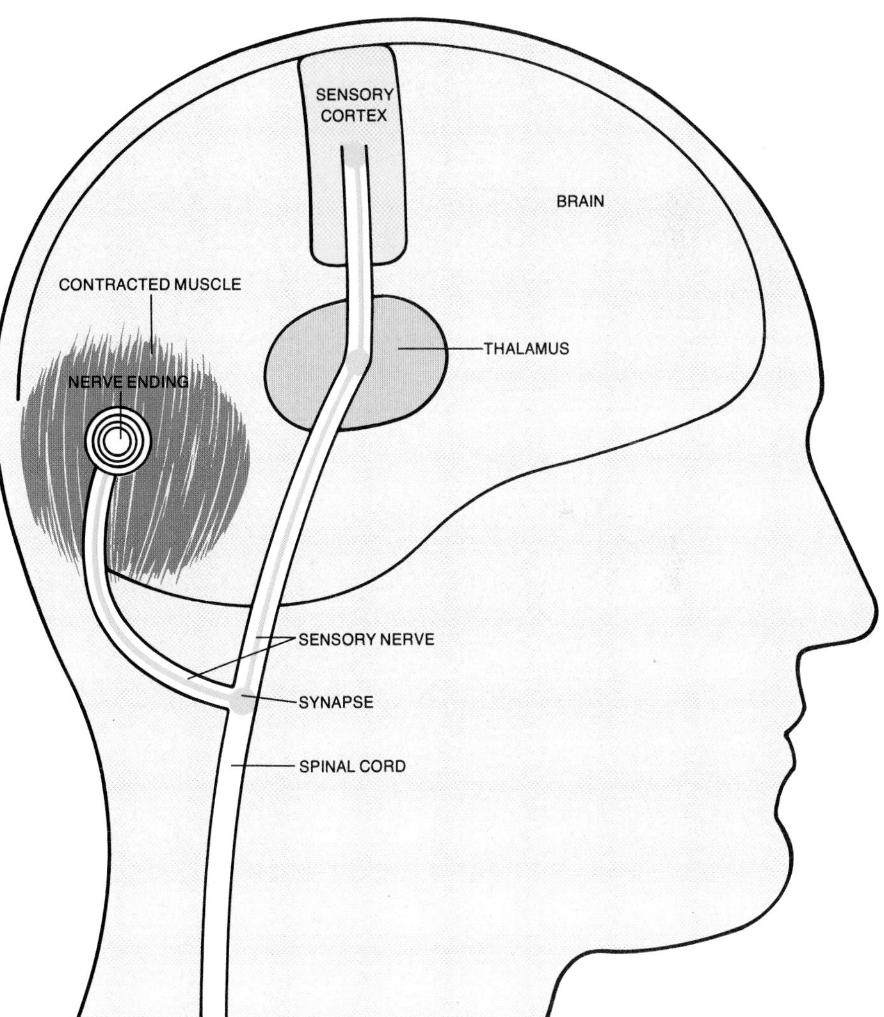

The pain of a typical tension headache originates at a nerve ending in a tensed muscle—in this case at the back of the head—then follows a sensory nerve to its junction, or synapse, with the spinal cord and up into the brain. There it is recognized in the thalamus as pain and sent to the cortex and other brain areas for analysis. Other headache pains follow a similar route.

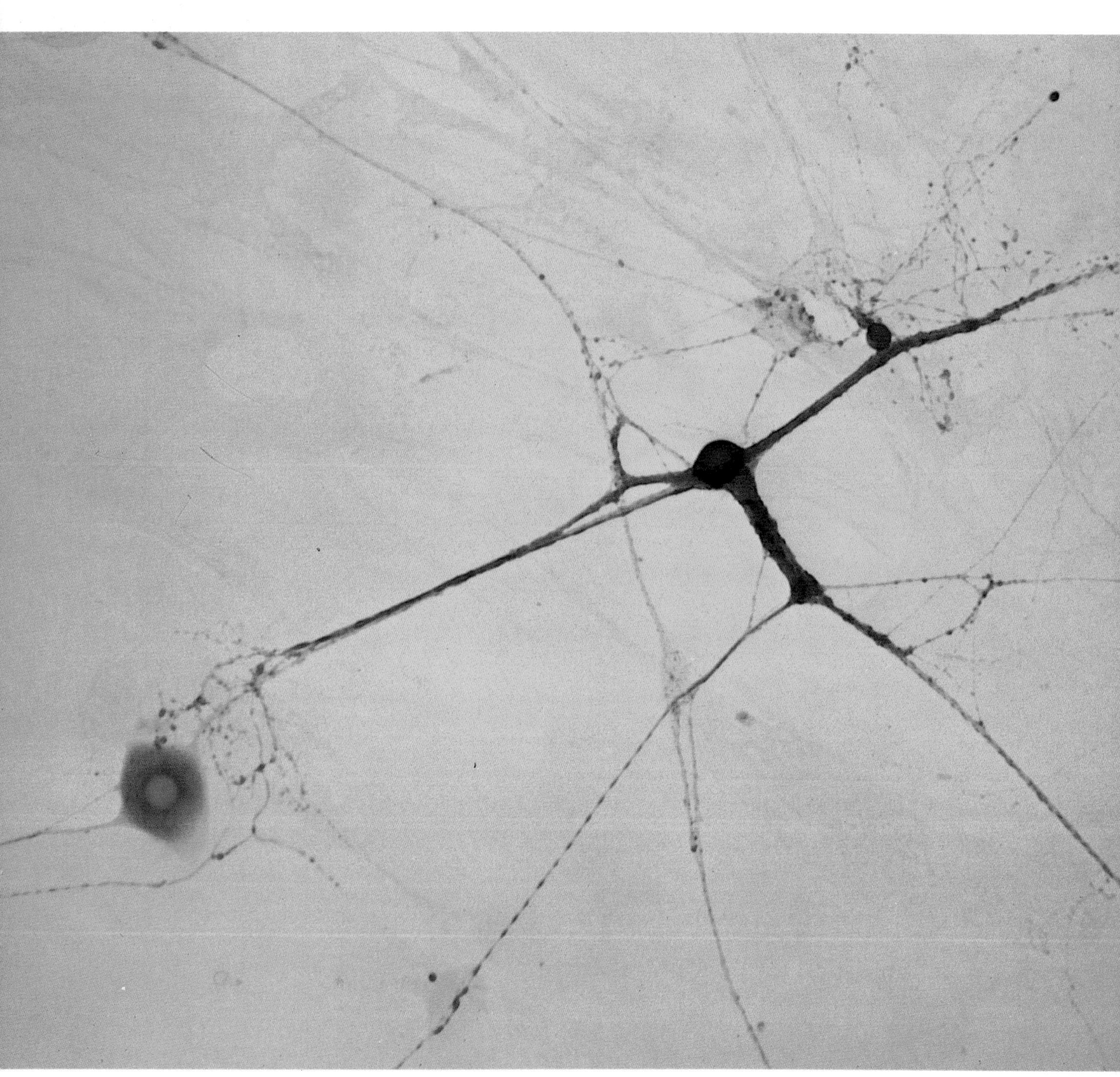

The connection of a sensory nerve (lower left), which picks up headache pains, to a spinal-cord nerve (center right), which sends it to the brain, is recorded in this photograph of mouse cells similar to human ones. The synapse gap that the signal must cross between the two nerve fibers is in the tangle of filaments near the round mass of the sensory nerve's cell body.

Sending off a pain message

Most scientists believe a tension headache begins with the release of chemicals *(drawing, left)* that start a pain signal along a sensory nerve *(bottom right)*. The signal must then cross a junction, or synapse, to a spinal-cord nerve and go up to the brain *(right)*. The signal can be blocked at the synapse by internal opiates from an interneuron.

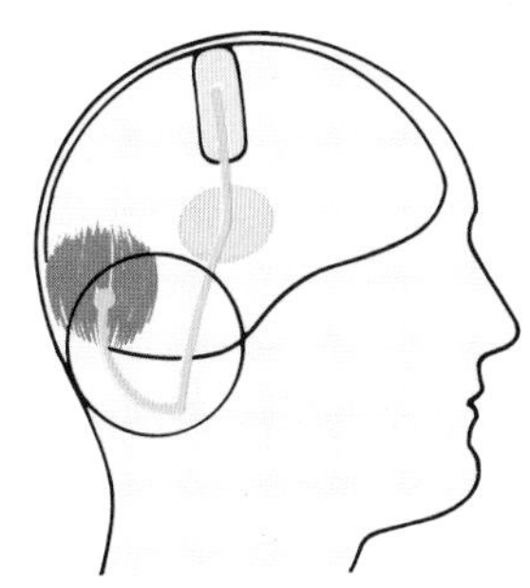

NERVE ENDING

HEALTHY CELL

DAMAGED CELL

PAIN-INDUCERS

PROSTAGLANDIN SENSITIZERS

PAIN-CAUSING CHEMICALS FROM DAMAGED CELLS

Contracted muscles squeeze shut the tiny vessels that supply them and surrounding tissue with oxygen-rich blood. As the cells continue working over prolonged periods without oxygen, they suffer temporary damage and begin giving off two different types of chemicals: pain-inducers such as bradykinin, serotonin, histamine and potassium (blue dots), and sensitizers such as prostaglandins (red dots), which make nerve endings embedded among the muscle cells respond to the inducers.

ASPIRIN TO STOP AN ACHE AT ITS SOURCE

When aspirin (yellow, left) is brought to the site, it blocks the damaged cells from giving off prostaglandins. Without the sensitizing effect of prostaglandins, the nerve endings do not react to the pain-inducing chemicals.

SIGNALS FROM ELECTRIFYING REACTIONS

Where no aspirin is present, the pain-inducing chemicals permeate the membrane coverings of the nerve endings sensitized by prostaglandins. There, they trigger chemical reactions that change the electrical charge on molecules in the area, generating a pain impulse.

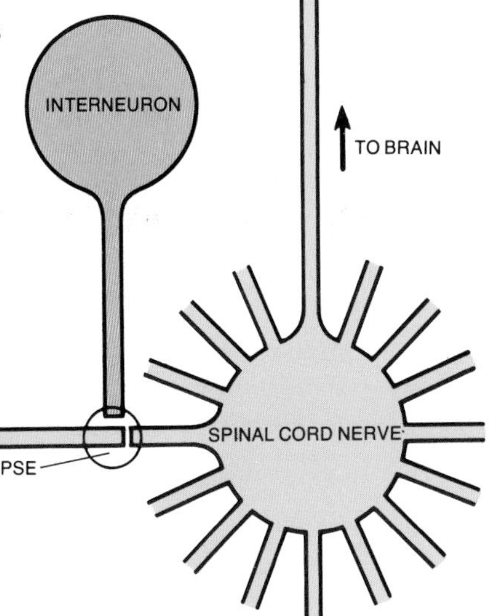

TO SPINAL CORD

SENSORY NERVE

ROADWAYS AND ROADBLOCKS ON THE WAY TO THE BRAIN

Once generated, a pain signal travels along a single sensory nerve until it meets another nerve in the spinal cord (above) or inside the brain. Also meeting at this synapse is a special type of nerve, an interneuron, which sometimes delivers substances to stop the signal there, as diagramed overleaf.

Crossing a synapse relay station

Like a telegraph message, a pain signal rarely travels over a direct connection. Along the way from origin to destination are relay stations where the message is taken from one wire and put onto another. The nervous system's relays even bear a striking resemblance to the old-time telegraph repeater, which employed a chemical battery and an automatic key to regenerate the message. At the nerve's relay—the synapse separating the end of one fiber from the beginning of the next—the nerve ending itself is both battery and key, using chemical reactions to send pain information to the brain.

The relay action occurs when an electrical pain signal, after traveling the length of a nerve fiber, arrives at a synapse. There the signal stimulates the nerve to release chemicals called neurotransmitters. A number of these compounds have been identified (many more presumably await discovery); among those believed to be principally responsible for pain transmission are glutamate and a compound called peptide substance P. These neurotransmitter molecules travel from the sender nerve ending across the gap of the synapse to the surface of the neighboring nerve ending, where they enter surface irregularities matching their shape. Once accepted into these receptors, they change the electrical charge in the receiving nerve.

If a large quantity of the neurotransmitter crosses the synapse, the electric charge generated will be sufficient to start that nerve carrying a pain signal of its own. If less crosses the synapse, the pain signal on that nerve fades away completely rather than weakening—nerve transmission is an all-or-nothing process. Opiates—whether compounds produced by the body or drugs taken as analgesics—lessen pain by controlling the flow of neurotransmitters across a synapse; the opiates can so reduce this flow that the signal is not regenerated and never gets to the brain.

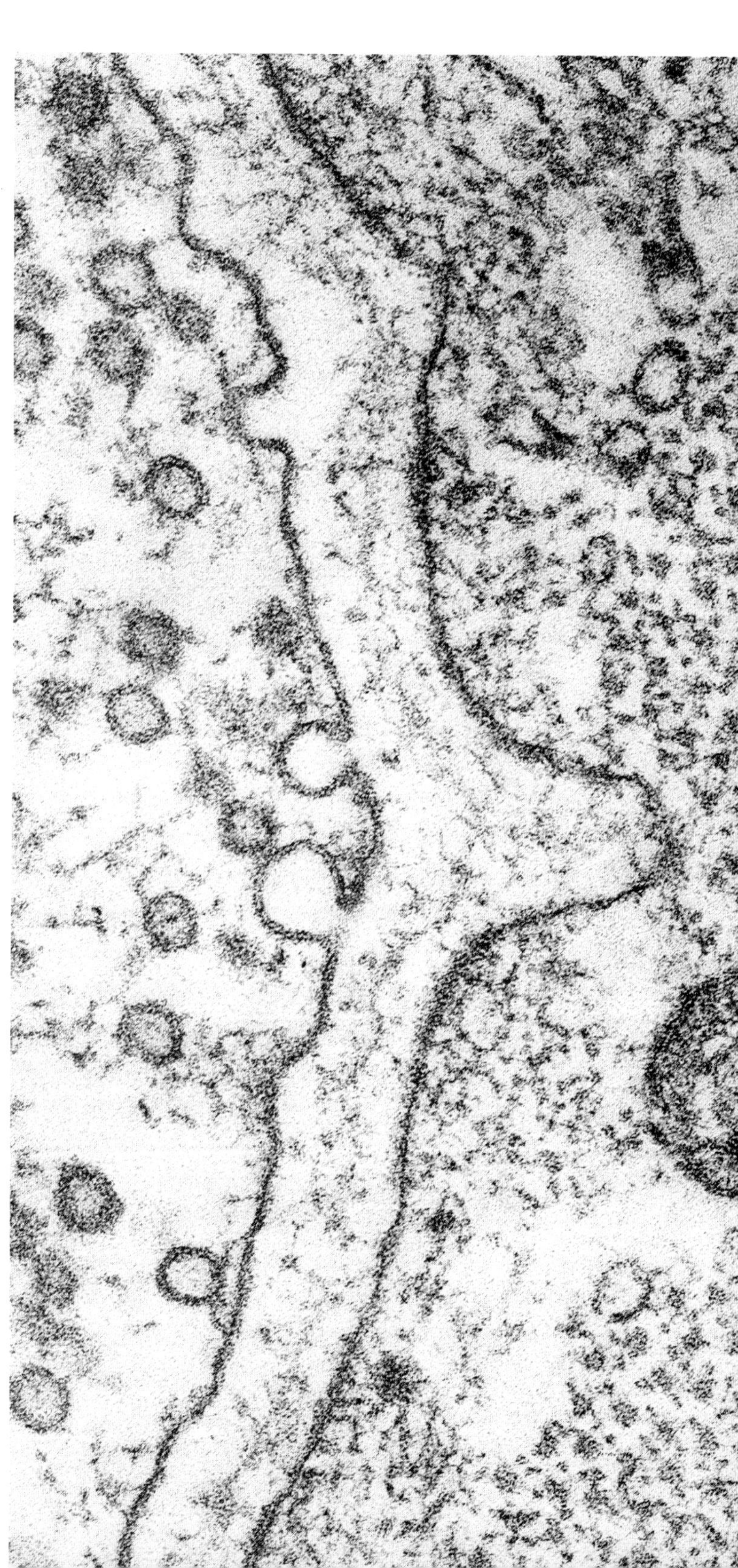

A synapse, here magnified 160,000 times, consists of, from left to right, the end of a sending nerve cell, a liquid-filled gap and a receiving surface. When an electrical nerve impulse reaches the end of the nerve, it induces the circular vesicles to move to the gap and spill their contents, chemicals called neurotransmitters. These cross the gap to the receiving surface, where they re-create the nerve impulse.

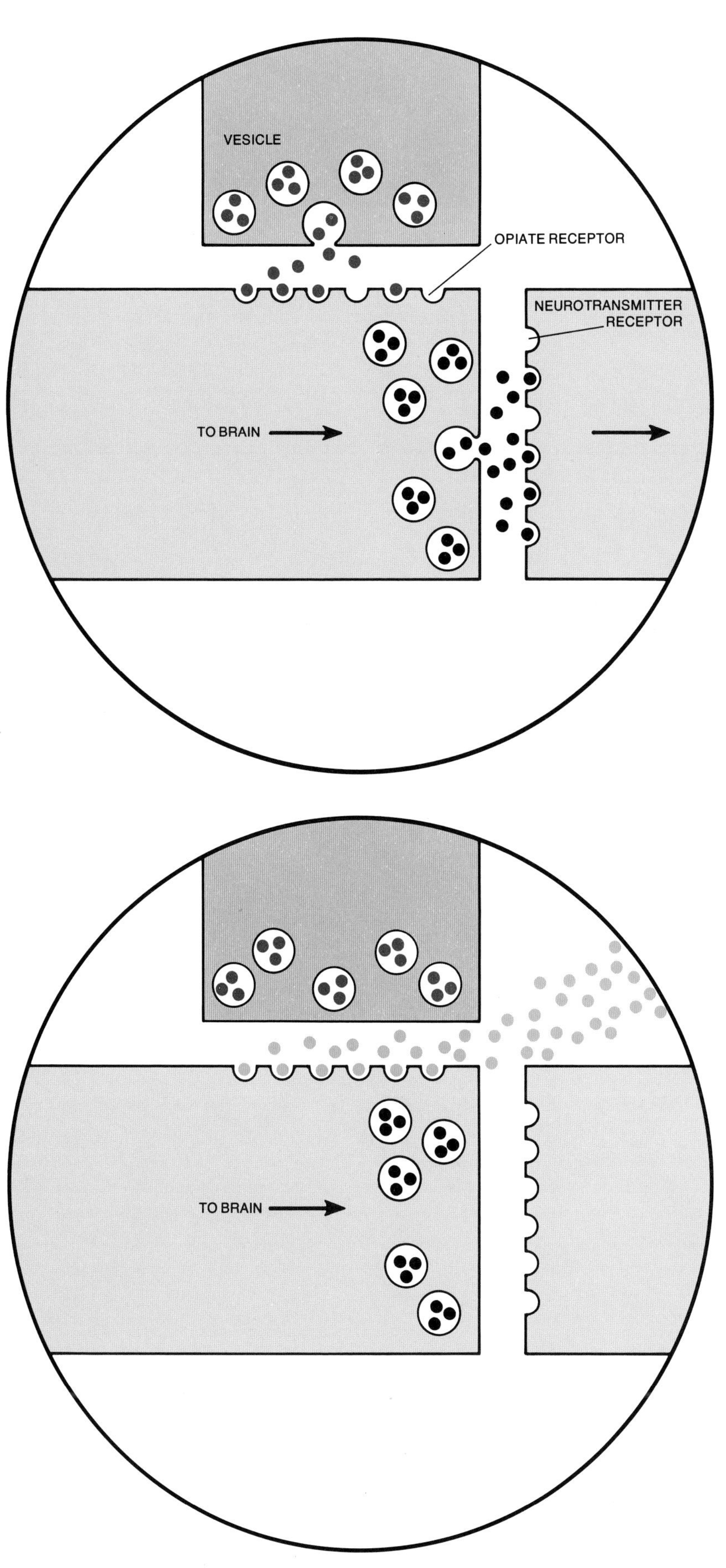

THE BODY'S OWN PAIN RELIEVERS
Two types of internal opiates (red dots)—enkephalins, produced in the brain, and endorphins, from the pituitary gland—are believed to act against headaches when released from vesicles (circles) in special nerves called interneurons (pink, left). The internal opiates cross to receptors on sensory nerves (green). They prevent the release of some neurotransmitters (black dots) that carry the pain message to receptors on the other side of the synapse; in this case, enough neurotransmitters get through to carry on the pain signal.

THE POWER OF OPIATE DRUGS
Opiate drugs (blue dots), such as the codeine often prescribed for severe headaches, are believed by many scientists to fit the same receptors on pain nerves as enkephalins and endorphins and to cause the same action. But unlike internal opiates, drugs can be brought to the synapse in such abundance that all the sending nerve's vesicles are prevented from releasing pain neurotransmitters. Since none of these chemicals cross the synapse, the pain signal is extinguished.

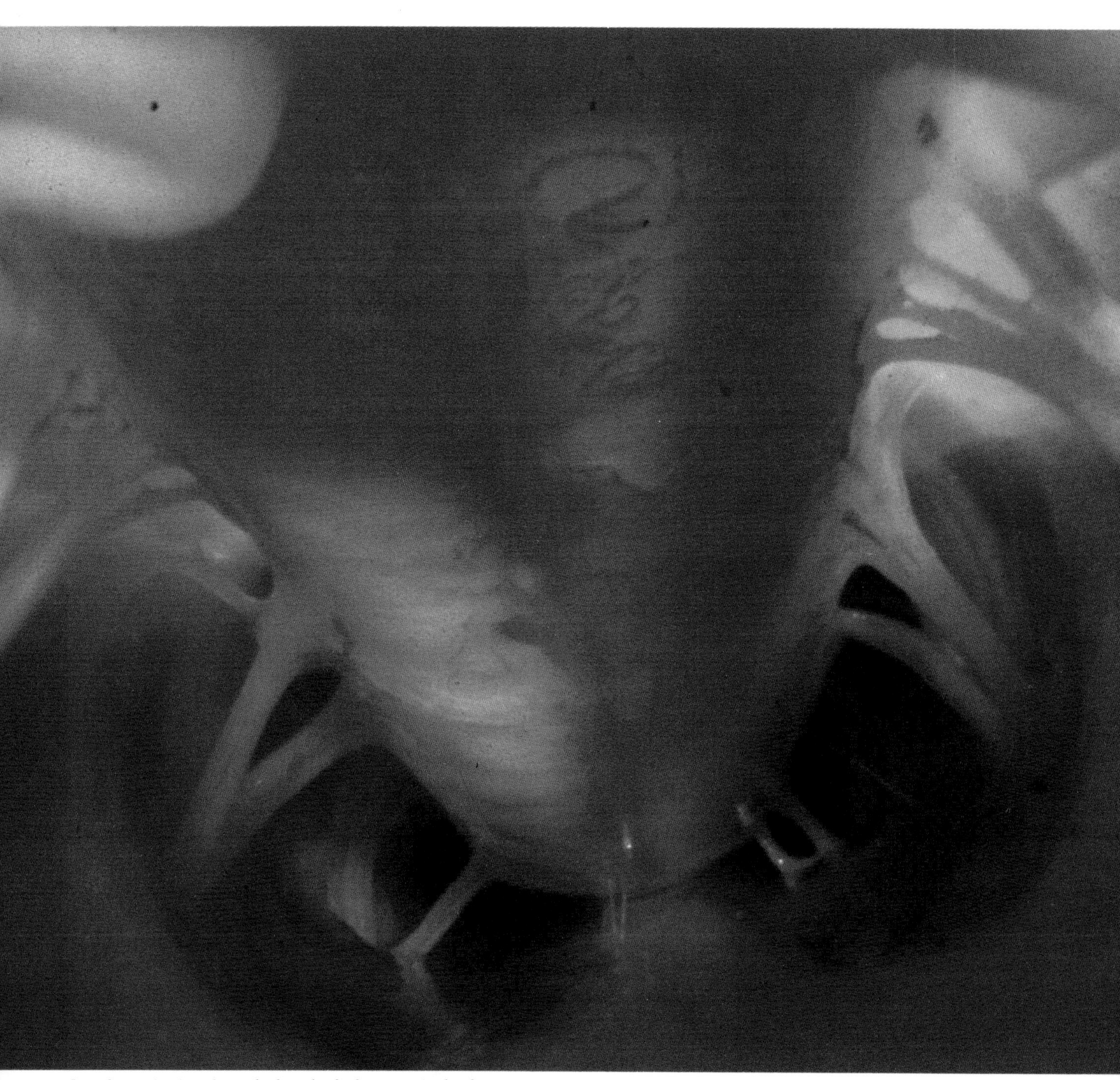

In a dramatic view down the length of a human spinal column, regularly spaced bundles of nerves enter the column and join the smoothly cylindrical spinal cord. The walls of the tunnel-like interior are formed by the vertebrae. Nerves carrying headache pain enter the spinal cord just below the base of the brain.

Reading signals in the brain

The brain cannot feel pain—it has no sensory nerve endings. Yet it is the sole organ in the body capable of making pain a reality. When the weak electrical impulses of sensory nerve signals enter the brain, they are run through a complex and interconnected series of readings in different parts of the brain, each adding to the interpretation of the signal and the coordination of responses by body and mind *(below)*.

The signals that denote headache are dull rather than sharp and pricking, and they come to the brain relatively slowly. These characteristics give the brain an important clue to the signals' nature: They are not an immediate threat to survival and, unlike the pain of a blow to the head, do not require instantaneous physical reaction to avert further harm. Rather, they call for a conscious response—the brain may instruct the body to rest or take a pill.

INSTANT RESPONSE TO STOP THE DAMAGE
Before consciousness of pain begins, the reticular formation of the brain reacts to crisis pains—not to headaches—by ordering muscles to remove the affected part of the body from harm.

IDENTIFYING PAIN AS PAIN
The main reception center for sensory signals, the thalamus, distinguishes an impulse as pain. Then it sends the signal on to other parts of the brain for further analysis.

FINDING PAIN A DISAGREEABLE EXPERIENCE
The limbic system, a group of bodies around the thalamus, creates an emotional response to pain and other sensory experiences. Rich in opiate receptors, this area of the brain may be where natural or drug-induced euphoria originates.

FIGURING OUT WHAT HURTS AND HOW
In the somatosensory cortex the brain recognizes where the pain is located and distinguishes the quality of the sensation—whether it is dull or sharp, steady or throbbing.

SCANNING MEMORY BANKS FOR COMPARISONS
The pain impulse triggers signals in the parietal cortex to register similarities to and differences from earlier pain experiences.

COORDINATING THE REACTION
Through complex connections with all other parts of the brain, the thinking part of the brain, the frontal cortex, orchestrates the analytical, emotional and protective responses to pain.

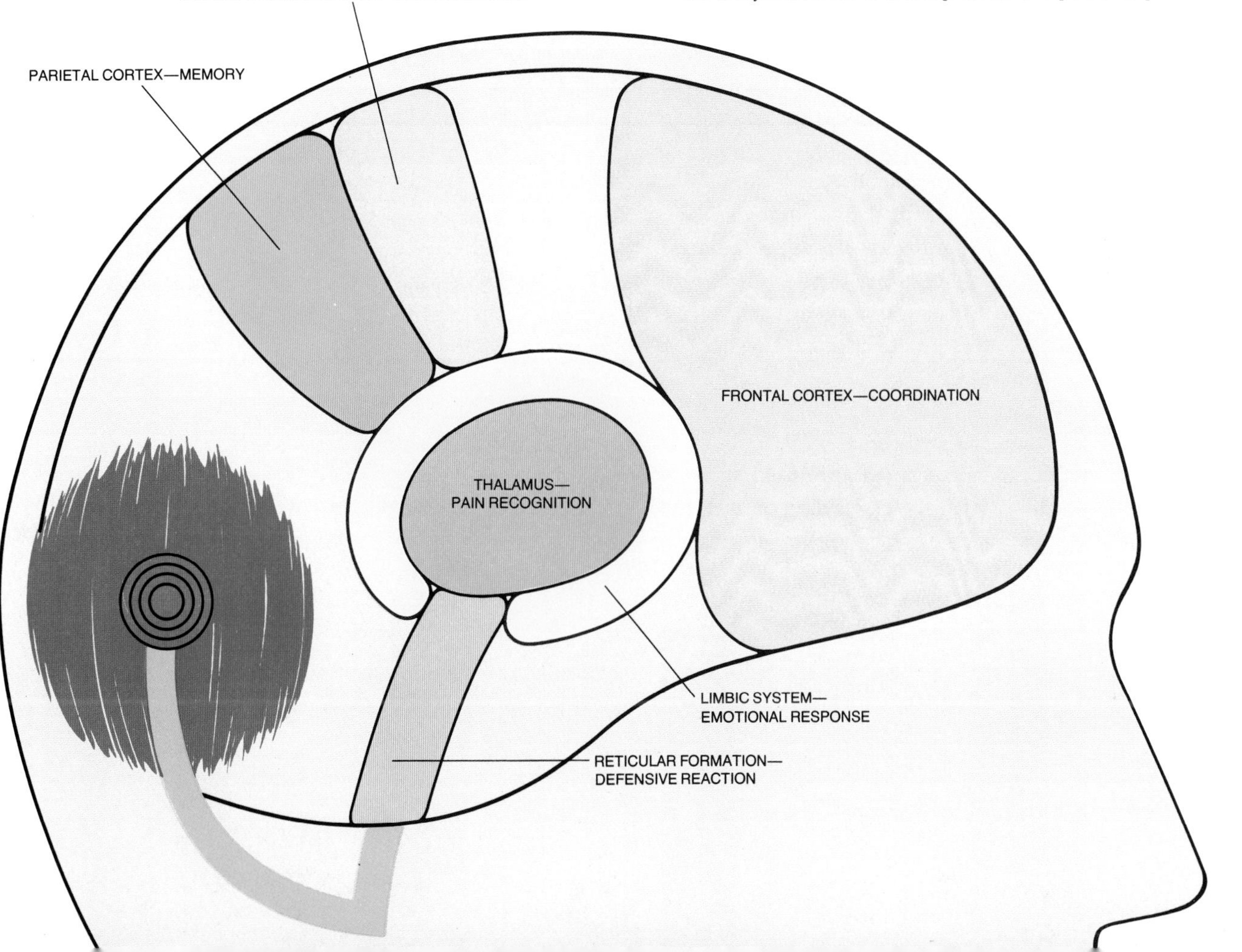

CHAPTER 6

Beyond drugs–the frontiers of treatment

Learning how not to have a headache
Teaching body and mind to relax
Controlling aches with biofeedback
The hot-hands treatment
Drowning pain in electricity
How acupuncture works

For those whose headaches refuse to give way to the standard cures of drugs, relaxation and sensible living habits, help may come from an astonishing variety of treatments at the frontier of medical acceptance. Some are new, the outgrowth of 20th Century research, with names that are modern buzz words: biofeedback, behavior modification, operant conditioning. Others are old: the ancient Chinese needle therapy of acupuncture and the bone and muscle manipulations of 19th Century chiropractic, as well as techniques for relaxation and mind-body control that are based on the practices of Indian yoga. Although their value continues to be debated, all seem to work—for some people, some of the time.

Many of these remedies are offered by practitioners who perform only one special kind of treatment and do nothing else; the patient must shop around, trying one after another until relief is found. The most advanced care—and generally the broadest, including many types of treatment—is provided by a small but growing group of medical specialists, physicians who concentrate on the causes and cures of headaches and not on any particular method of cure.

Many of these headache specialists practice in headache clinics, where talents drawn from diverse fields of the health sciences—neurology, psychiatry, psychology, ophthalmology and dentistry—can mount a combined attack on the complex origins of persistent headaches. Here can be applied the newest treatments, some of which, such as behavior modification, biofeedback and relaxation training, require sustained effort by doctor and patient. In these clinics delicate tests of the brain uncover hidden physical abnormalities that bring head pain—or rule out such organic causes, focusing attention on other factors.

The headache specialty is still relatively new in medical practice. Although headaches as a human affliction were specifically diagnosed millennia before Hippocrates hung out his shingle, the first medical facility devoted solely to this complaint did not appear until 1945. In that year, doctors at the Montefiore Hospital and Medical Center in New York City, confronted with a growing number of cases of post-traumatic headache syndrome *(Chapter 1)* among wounded veterans of World War II, created a special department to study and treat all aspects of headaches.

A generation and more later, clinics focusing on headaches or pain were still a rarity in the United States; perhaps a dozen or so centers qualified as full-time headache clinics, to which might be added perhaps another dozen or two major pain clinics that treat headache along with other types of intractable pain, such as backache.

In the United Kingdom, headache clinics have been operated by a charitable organization, The Migraine Trust. Unlike their American counterparts, the clinics of The Migraine Trust do little work with behavior modification and relaxation techniques—fringe medicine, in the eyes of many British practitioners. Instead, they emphasize drug therapy and research into the biochemistry of migraine. At one Migraine Trust facility, the Princess Margaret Migraine Clinic in London, migraine patients are studied while their attacks are

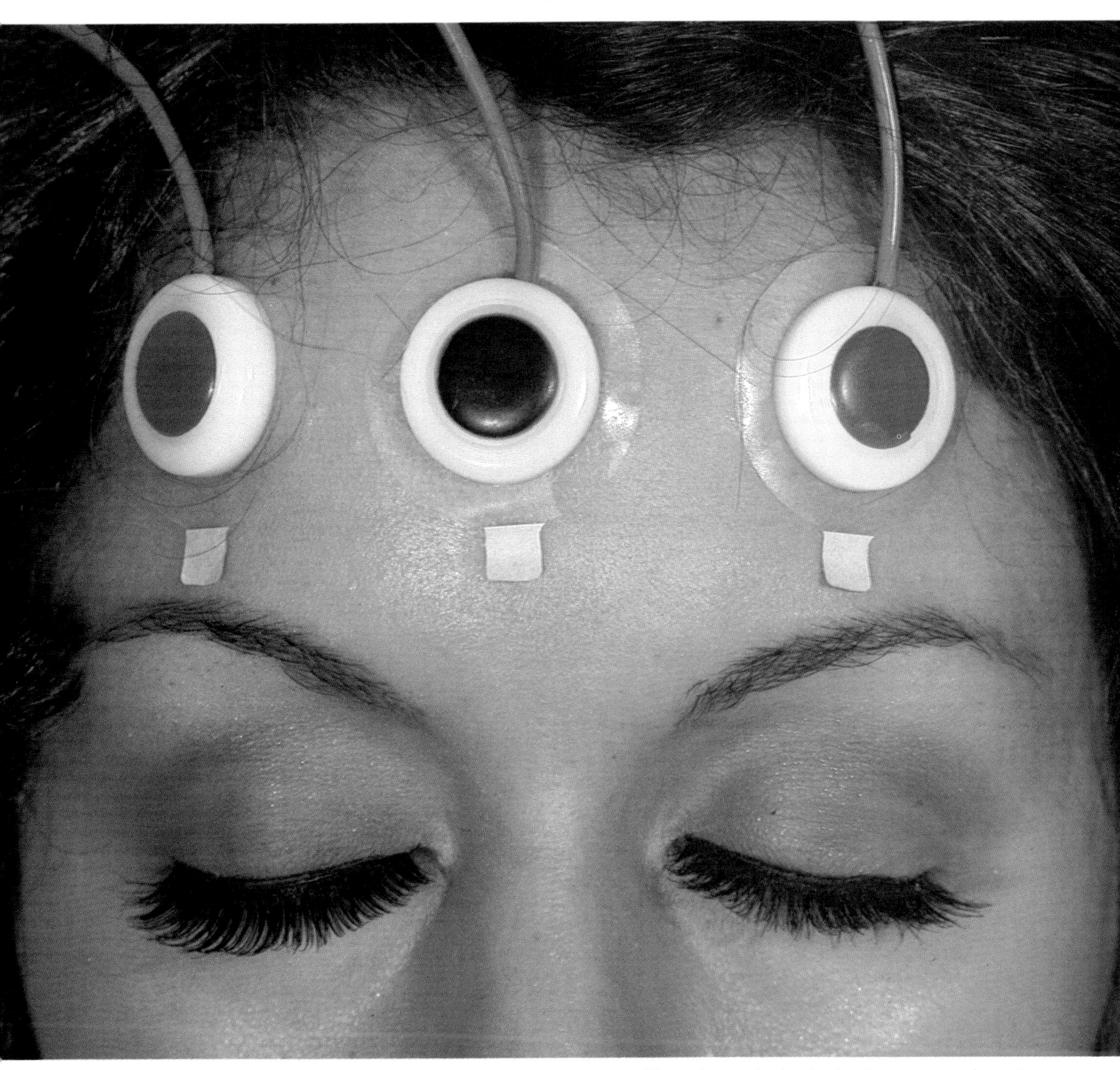

Electrodes taped to her forehead to gauge muscle tension, a patient relaxes away a tension headache by means of biofeedback. The electrode measurements control a tone emitted by a nearby machine—the louder the tone, the more tension. Using sound as a monitor, the subject learns mental techniques—such as imagining a tranquil scene—that lessen tension and relieve headaches.

going on—some rush to the clinic by taxi or ambulance whenever they perceive the warning signals preceding head pain. The trust also supports investigation of blood platelets—their behavior and their role in migraine—along with experimentation on new migraine drugs and research into diet as a cause of headache.

Physical exams with psychological twists

In the United States, headache specialists probe deep for causes, seeking clues in body and mind. A new patient gets the physical checks, blood tests, X-rays and medical history-taking common to the management of any serious disorder. But then he goes on to tests less common, some to determine the physical health of the brain and nervous system, others to investigate family relationships, attitudes toward work, and feelings of anxiety, anger or frustration.

Many specialists administer paper-and-pencil tests to evaluate the patient's psychological profile. Perhaps the most commonly used is the Minnesota Multiphasic Personality Inventory (MMPI), a list of about 550 statements the patient marks true or false as he thinks they apply to him—"I daydream very little"; "My mother and/or father made me obey even when I thought it was unreasonable." This self-evaluation is compared with the results obtained from other people in order to detect behavior that might be implicated in the patient's chronic headaches.

Another commonly used psychological test searches for personal crises that may be related to headaches. A grading of stress prepared by Dr. Thomas H. Holmes of the University of Washington, it lists 42 "life-change" crises—positive as well as negative—ranging in seriousness from a ticket for jaywalking, through getting married or taking on a large mortgage, to death of a spouse or parent. Each crisis the patient has experienced is given a numerical value, depending partly on how recently it occurred, and the cumulative score indicates the likelihood that stress plays some role in the individual's head pain.

Serious organic causes of head pain—brain injury, a blood clot, infection—generally reveal themselves by specific symptoms in addition to headache, but in some cases of inexplicably persistent pain, extensive testing may be needed to rule them out entirely. Detecting the presence or absence of such organic problems requires some of the most complex procedures and machines of modern medicine. The skull and brain may be examined with a CAT scanner or with radioactive tracers; brain waves may be studied with an electroencephalograph, or EEG for short.

The CAT—for computerized axial tomography—scanner, a device that almost fills a good-sized room, takes detailed X-ray pictures of the body interior. Its size and method of use—the patient is left alone in the room with his head inside a giant circle of machinery *(page 147)*—make it frightening, but it is basically an X-ray machine and the patient feels nothing during or after the scan. In a scan that takes five minutes and circles the entire head, some 28,800 X-ray measurements are taken, each of a microscopically thin slice of the brain. A computer processes the measurements, calculating tissue density from the strength of the X-ray beam detected during the scan and comparing it with normal density for each measurement; by this means abnormal conditions are picked up and diagnosed with remarkable accuracy. A CAT scan can, for example, distinguish a brain hemorrhage from a tumor by the differences in the density recorded.

If cancer is deemed a possibility, a test using mildly radioactive technetium may seek it out in a so-called brain scan. The technetium, its radiation too weak to harm the normal body but detectable by electronic sensors, is injected in tiny amounts into the bloodstream, which carries it to the brain. It is known to accumulate wherever there are many small blood vessels, and such dense growth of vessels is a characteristic of cancerous tissue; consequently, a scan that picks up high concentrations of the material suggests the presence of a brain tumor.

Clues in brain waves

When headaches do not fit any particular pattern, or when suspected brain injury cannot be located, physicians may turn to a study of the natural electrical activity of the nerves making up the brain. This is done with the electroencephalograph, or EEG, a sensitive measuring instrument originally devised in Germany in 1924 by Dr. Hans Berger, a University of Jena psychiatrist. Dr. Berger devoted his life to an attempt to connect physical actions within the body to the thinking processes of the brain. He made finicky measurements of every quantity he could think of—temperature, blood circulation, electrical activity. That there was electricity in the brain had long been known—Dr. Luigi Galvani discovered the electrical action in nerves in 1791—but Dr. Berger found that the electrical voltages generated by the nerves of the brain changed in distinctive ways. They came in waves, and the kinds of waves depended on mental state.

Subsequent research has identified four patterns of brain waves, each roughly indicating a different level of mental activity. The pattern Dr. Berger found first, designated alpha waves, is made up of crests of voltage peaking at an average rate of about 10 per second; it usually occurs in an awake but relaxed person whose eyes are closed so that few visual signals are sent to the brain. A person involved in some mental activity or operating under pressure is likely to give off beta waves, in which the peaks have lower voltage and come with greater frequency—at a rate of 13 to 28 per second. Drowsiness or dreaming might produce theta waves, which are rather slow, alternating at a rate of three to six per second—but paradoxically, theta waves also appear when an individual is alert, particularly at moments of creative thinking or sudden insight. The lowest-frequency waves, called delta, at three per second or less, come with deep sleep. (The absence of any voltage peaks—a "flat" brain wave—is one legal definition of death.)

Variations from the normal EEG patterns offer clues to injury inside the brain or to malfunctions in its operation. Instead of an alpha pattern, for example, an awake but relaxed patient may produce the slower delta or theta waves. Or mixed into a normal pattern may be bursts of peaks of unusually high or low voltage. Almost complete disruption of a normal pattern may occur during an attack of epilepsy, the disorder that brings severe headaches as well as convulsions. Epilepsy is distinguished by a frenzy of electrical discharges within the brain—the nerve cells are firing at random rather than in their normal, orderly sequence—and this abnormal activity shows up as a characteristically chaotic pattern on an EEG recording.

The instrument that measures such waves causes no pain and sends no outside electricity into the body; it only measures the electricity that the body naturally makes on its own. But an EEG may seem formidable to a patient experiencing it for the first time because he gets all wired up. He is likely to be seated in a comfortable reclining chair while a technician roughens selected spots on his head, dabs them with conducting jelly, then secures eight to 16 electrodes around his head from front to back and over the top from side to side. A wire from each electrode sends the signals to the EEG unit itself, an extremely sensitive voltmeter approximately the size and shape of a home videotape recorder, and this instrument prints the signals out as zigzag lines on a continuous strip of paper *(page 147)*.

Each electrode picks up signals from the brain area nearest to it and produces a separate tracing on the printout. The separate signals indicate where an injury may be; unusual waves from one part of the head may point to the location there of a blood clot, tumor or sharply constricted arteries. Because the functions of different parts of the brain have now been mapped—the visual cortex, in the back of the head, for example, registers sight—the separate signals also provide clues to types of malfunctions.

To obtain readings of different kinds of brain activity, the EEG operator will ask the patient to participate in various exercises while hooked up to the machine. In addition to relaxing with closed eyes to produce alpha waves, for example, the patient may be asked to breathe deeply and rapidly. Such breathing will "blow off" extra carbon dioxide, a compound that helps control the size of arteries; its reduction causes arteries to contract, limiting blood flow and producing characteristic brain-wave patterns. Such waves are one feature of a migraine attack, which starts with constricted arteries in the head—the abnormal waves are picked up on the side of the head that hurts.

The patient may also be exposed to flashing lights, music, conversation or sudden noises as part of the EEG testing. As

TYPE OF TREATMENT	EFFECTIVENESS			
	Excellent	Fair	Poor	Adverse Effect
Chiropractic	15	36	44	5
Yoga	8	50	33	9
Acupuncture	26	23	48	3
Physiotherapy	10	38	46	6
Exercise	22	39	27	12
Psychotherapy	12	34	50	4
Hypnosis	19	31	50	0
Relaxation	17	46	36	1
Meditation	13	50	37	0
Biofeedback	22	29	47	2
Osteopathy	11	33	54	2

RATING TREATMENTS: EASY CURES BEST
Telling a headache victim to relax may be sound advice, as the Canadian Migraine Foundation discovered from 1,500 migraine sufferers who rated their success with nondrug treatments (listed by frequency of use in the table above). Although the Oriental needle techniques of acupuncture produced the greatest percentage of excellent results, some benefit—excellent or fair—was most often reported for the physical and mental workouts frequently recommended for relieving tensions: meditation, relaxation, exercise and yoga.

the brain responds to these stimuli, there are fluctuations in the frequency and voltage of the waves of electricity. Once again the EEG pattern changes in ways that are characteristic for people who have some kinds of headaches. When migraine sufferers watch a flickering light, for example, their brain waves react to a wide range of flicker frequencies; people who do not suffer from migraine also show brain-wave changes in response to flashing lights, but not over such a wide range of flickering. Epilepsy produces an effect similar to that of migraine, and the EEG traces produced by the two ailments are not easily distinguished.

The electroencephalograph offers up its data only grudgingly. The multiple rows of squiggly lines on an EEG printout are difficult to make sense of under the best of circumstances. But a new method of computerized imaging of the electrical signals picked up by an EEG may make the machine much more informative. Computerized imaging replaces the customary squiggles with a video-screen display of a brightly colored map of the brain as seen from directly overhead. The signals are assigned colors according to their strength and frequency, and the signals from each electrode are displayed in these colors inside the head outline on the screen, in the location corresponding to the electrode position. From the appearance and location of these colored shapes, the diagnostician can see immediately what is going on where inside the brain. For example, when this type of computer transformation was applied to the EEG of one 12-year-old boy with epilepsy, the center of nerve disturbance was revealed on the screen as a bright red spot on the right side of the brain.

Learning how not to have a headache

Assuming no serious underlying disorder is found, the headache itself becomes the focus of treatment. Drugs are prescribed, of course. As an adjunct, the therapy favored by American specialists, and the one showing the greatest promise, is behavior modification.

Behavior modification means exactly that—changing a pattern of conscious or unconscious actions. It can be achieved in many ways. Its value in controlling headaches is based on the view that many disorders, both mental and physical, strike because the victim either fails to develop healthful responses to the challenges in the environment or else learns faulty ones, that is, responses that somehow answer the immediate challenge but do so at a cost to health—excess muscle tension in the scalp is one such faulty response. Either way, the problem is seen as one of learning unhealthful behavior, the solution one of unlearning the unhealthful response and learning responses that are beneficial or at least less costly to health.

In the treatment of headaches, the retraining focuses on varieties of stress management—teaching an individual to rein in inappropriate physiological responses and to consciously downplay situations that have given rise to unnecessary anxiety in the past. One physician said that the patient learns to stop giving each 10-cent problem a dollar's worth of emotion. Because many chronic headaches are wholly or partly stress-induced, and because the remainder generally come to have a secondary component of stress by virtue of the anguish they cause, reducing stress through behavior modification often helps headaches.

The various techniques of behavior modification are at least distantly related to ancient Oriental systems of thought, such as yoga and Zen Buddhism. They hold that an individual can, by mental concentration, regulate many of his thoughts and actions—including bodily actions that ordinarily are beyond conscious control, such as heart rate and blood pressure.

The idea that the mind could be trained to control such automatic actions was long scoffed at by Western physicians, and its acceptance has been slow. Yet as long ago as 1901, self-regulation of seemingly inaccessible body functions was demonstrated in a crude way by psychologist Joseph H. Bair, who put on a curious, almost whimsical, experiment for one of his advanced classes. He attached electrodes to the ears of student volunteers and instructed them to press a button wired to deliver a mild electrical charge. Just as Bair expected, the low-level shock initiated muscle contraction and the volunteers' ears wiggled.

Professor Bair then told his subjects to repeat the shock several times; next he asked them to reproduce the wiggle on their own without the electric shocks to help. At first they experimented with all manner of grimacing, jaw clenching and brow furrowing in efforts to move their ears; gradually they were able to focus on the specific events involved in wiggling and to dispense with the rest. Having earlier been passive participants in ear wiggling, having experienced the subtle sensations and inventoried the musculature and nervous equipment needed, they were able to take control of a previously uncontrollable process; they had learned to wiggle their ears at will.

No serious application of Bair's observations occurred until many years later, although his use of electricity to train subjects to command their muscles in new ways foreshadowed some modern methods of behavior modification. Operant conditioning and its outgrowth, biofeedback, for example, employ somewhat similar techniques to extend and refine the learning of inner control. But simpler methods, much closer to yoga, are also widely used as an initial step in training people to alleviate their headaches.

Teaching body and mind to relax

One relatively simple form of inner control of headaches—relaxation training—was developed in Germany and the United States in the 1920s. The German form, called autogenic training, was devised in Berlin by psychiatrist Johannes Schultz and remains the most widely used relaxation technique in Europe. Dr. Schultz's method helps the patient achieve physical and mental relaxation through an almost hypnotic process of self-persuasion or, as psychologists call it, autosuggestion. The patient is instructed to relax and close his eyes. He then says to himself, "I am at peace," and then continues systematically through a list of short phrases, repeating each one and at the same time trying to visualize and concentrate on the condition he is describing: "My arms and legs are heavy. . . . My arms and legs are warm. . . . My heartbeat is calm and regular. . . . My breathing is relaxed and comfortable. . . . My abdomen is warm. . . . My forehead is cool."

Dr. Schultz and his followers found that with extensive

Beyond headaches: B.F.Skinner and the "baby in a box"

The career of Burrhus Frederic Skinner, the Harvard psychologist whose techniques of behavior modification underlie such headache therapies as biofeedback, took more twists in its 60-odd years than a winding backwoods road. In his childhood Skinner devised a flotation device to separate ripe elderberries from green ones, then made money selling it door-to-door. As a college student, he submitted poems and short stories to a literary giant—the poet Robert Frost—and won fond praise for them. As a scientist studying behavior, he taught pigeons how to walk in figure eights, how to play a kind of ping-pong with their beaks and, during World War II, how to guide a missile. His books stirred controversy: In the didactic novel *Walden Two* and in his philosophical tract *Beyond Freedom and Dignity,* he proposed reshaping human beings and their culture through operant conditioning—rewarding benevolent and socially constructive behavior. Yet it was as a parent, in 1945, that B. F. Skinner earned his first public recognition.

That year his baby daughter was America's most talked-about infant—the so-called baby in a box, featured in an article in *Ladies' Home Journal.* Indeed, Skinner was raising Deborah, then 11 months old, in a box—a glassed-in, insulated, air-controlled crib that he thought would revolutionize child rearing and produce happier, healthier children.

The box, about the size of a normal crib, bore striking similarities, at least in theory, to the little "Skinner boxes" that the behaviorist used in his laboratory to confine, study and teach pigeons. Air entered the box through filters, keeping the child free of germs and so clean that she needed only one bath a week. She was taken out of the box for meals, for diaper changes and for cuddling and play, but the "air crib" remained her primary environment for two and a half years. Horrified critics complained that the crib seemed a goldfish bowl. Yet some 25 years later, Deborah Skinner, then an art student in London, laid the criticism to rest: "I think I was a very happy baby." Although Deborah's air crib never gained broad acceptance, the operant conditioning techniques her father invented have found wide practical application in helping people free themselves of snake phobias, quit smoking and rehabilitate injured muscles as well as stop headaches.

practice—often a matter of many months—a patient could increase skin temperature in his hands and feet by one or two degrees and could lower his blood pressure and pulse rate by as much as 10 per cent. As an accompaniment to such changes, the patient's brain-wave activity and breathing also slowed, with beneficial results in a wide variety of stress-related afflictions, such as sleeplessness and ulcers. For headache sufferers, such physiological changes are a means to an end; the emphasis in autogenic training is on the relaxation of muscles and arteries.

The other formal relaxation-training method that is widely used, particularly in headache clinics in the United States, is known as progressive relaxation. It was devised by Dr. Edmund Jacobson of the University of Chicago, who began his work in mind-muscle communication at about the same time that Dr. Schultz began his experiments. Dr. Jacobson's technique is based on the simple act of contrasting tension with relaxation. It takes the patient through a series of exercises in which he first tenses certain muscle groups until he is fully aware of the tension; then he slowly relaxes the muscles while trying to discriminate between the different sensations produced by muscle tension and muscle relaxation. In later sessions, the degree of deliberate tension and relaxation is reduced. As the patient continues to practice, he gradually learns to recognize infinitesimal changes in tension and relaxation of single groups of muscles.

Dr. Jacobson was able to show that imagination alone was often enough to produce muscle tension or relaxation. In one experiment he had subjects pretend in their minds that they were operating an old-fashioned telegraph key with their middle fingers—they were instructed not to move any muscles in the experiment, only to imagine that they did. Tests showed that the muscles normally involved in manipulating the middle finger were being bombarded with the same nerve impulses that would be involved in actual movement. Dr. Jacobson went on to propose that anxiety is a construct of "muscle tension-image patterns," that muscles become tense when the person imagines a stressful situation. Headache therapists, using this principle, encourage patients to imagine the kinds of situations or memories that will induce warmth, heaviness and relaxation. Regular use of this simple procedure can prevent many head pains, but it must be practiced for some time to be effective.

Lessons from dogs and pigeons

Some years before Dr. Schultz and Dr. Jacobson developed their methods for training the mind to will body actions, Russian physiologist Ivan Pavlov began the Nobel prize-winning experiments on dogs that showed how outside influences could help in this training. Working off dogs' instinctive desire to eat when hungry and their reflexive salivating when presented with food, Dr. Pavlov first offered the dogs small amounts of meat (called, in the parlance of psychologists, an unconditioned stimulus) and measured the quantities of saliva (an automatic, normally uncontrollable reaction, or "unconditioned response") that the sight of food produced in their mouths.

Then, in a second series of feedings, he rang a bell before giving each dog its plate of food. Soon the dog was salivating when it heard the bell, even before the food appeared. Pavlov had thus demonstrated that a seemingly automatic reaction to the stimulus of food—salivating—could be triggered by a substitute, and previously neutral, stimulus such as a bell. The ringing bell he termed a conditioned stimulus because its ability to stimulate the response was conditional upon the dog's associating it with food. Similarly, the act of salivating to the sound of the bell was a conditioned response. Dr. Pavlov subsequently proved that if the conditioned salivation went unrewarded repeatedly—if no food followed—the association between the two events, the bell and the food, was soon forgotten and the conditioned response, salivation at the sound of the bell, was unlearned or "extinguished."

Dr. Pavlov's revolutionary theory applies to involuntary actions. Later it was refined and extended by several psychologists, notably B. F. Skinner of Harvard, to include voluntary actions. Skinner's theory of "operant conditioning" became the psychological basis for biofeedback training and many other therapies that are used to relieve headaches. The theory of operant conditioning presumes that a subject presented with an unconditioned stimulus may often have not just one but a number of responses to choose from.

In animal studies, for example, a pigeon might be given a ball. It can ignore the ball, peck at it or push it one way or another. Various environmental influences help determine, or condition, the choice of response. Choices that are "right"—not necessarily good or healthful—are the ones that are rewarded in some way, satisfying a physical or emotional need. A pigeon that pushed the ball into a hole might be given some food. Choices that are less right are the ones that go unrewarded.

In the same way, human beings can find rewards for certain choices. Because the individual naturally seeks rewards, he gradually learns what behavior is the right, or rewarded, response to a recurring stimulus. Ultimately his response ceases to be a matter of voluntary selection and settles in as ingrained, habitual, automatic behavior, something that will persist until some other process of operant conditioning causes him to replace it or erase it.

Skinner, working mainly with pigeons (and in one fascinating though inconclusive experiment in scientific parenthood, with his baby daughter), demonstrated how the giving or withholding of rewards could train a subject to develop an automatic habit. People can even train themselves, through operant conditioning, to learn to have pains, including head pains; many environmental forces work quite innocently to reinforce and sustain the pain.

Dr. Richard Sternbach, Director of the Pain Treatment Center at the Scripps Clinic and Research Foundation in La Jolla, California, counted off some of the classic kinds of reinforcing behavior that may begin as natural responses to physical pain and then go on to gain permanent status in the individual's total pain performance: "moaning behavior, rewarded by attention from the family; taking analgesics, rewarded by a decrease in pain; being bedridden, rewarded by respite from unpleasant work . . . or attention from an otherwise negligent spouse."

In these and countless other ways, Dr. Sternbach maintained, chronic-pain victims often come to have a heavy investment in their problems, so that simple relief from the original disorder becomes difficult to obtain. Such a person's chances of returning to good health will be extremely slim unless treatment makes him aware of how he has come to depend on costly negative rewards in his daily life, then helps him unlearn such responses, and finally leads him to learn new responses that positively reinforce recovery and the maintenance of good health.

Controlling aches with biofeedback

Skinner's experiments focused on external, visible responses to stimuli, such as choosing between two selections or making one kind of movement instead of another. But beginning in the 1960s a number of researchers, particularly in the United States, began using variations of his techniques to teach subjects to alter unconscious, internal bodily functions, such as those that are intimately tied to tension and relaxation. They called their method biofeedback.

The practice of biofeedback involves the use of mechanical and electrical devices to monitor, amplify, record and report back to the subject a more-or-less continuous, instantaneous description of changes in a particular biological function—heartbeat, muscle contraction, brain activity, temperature regulation—that is going on inside him. The instruments used are specialized versions of the equipment employed in hospitals, doctors' offices and laboratories to record certain bodily responses, the difference being that with the biofeedback equipment, the information gathered is shared immediately with the patient. He sees or hears the signals from the instrument, and he knows what they mean.

Usually the patient sees a light or hears a sound that varies in some simple manner to let him know how well he is succeeding in his attempt to change some physiological process. The signal of success is in effect a reward. The patient

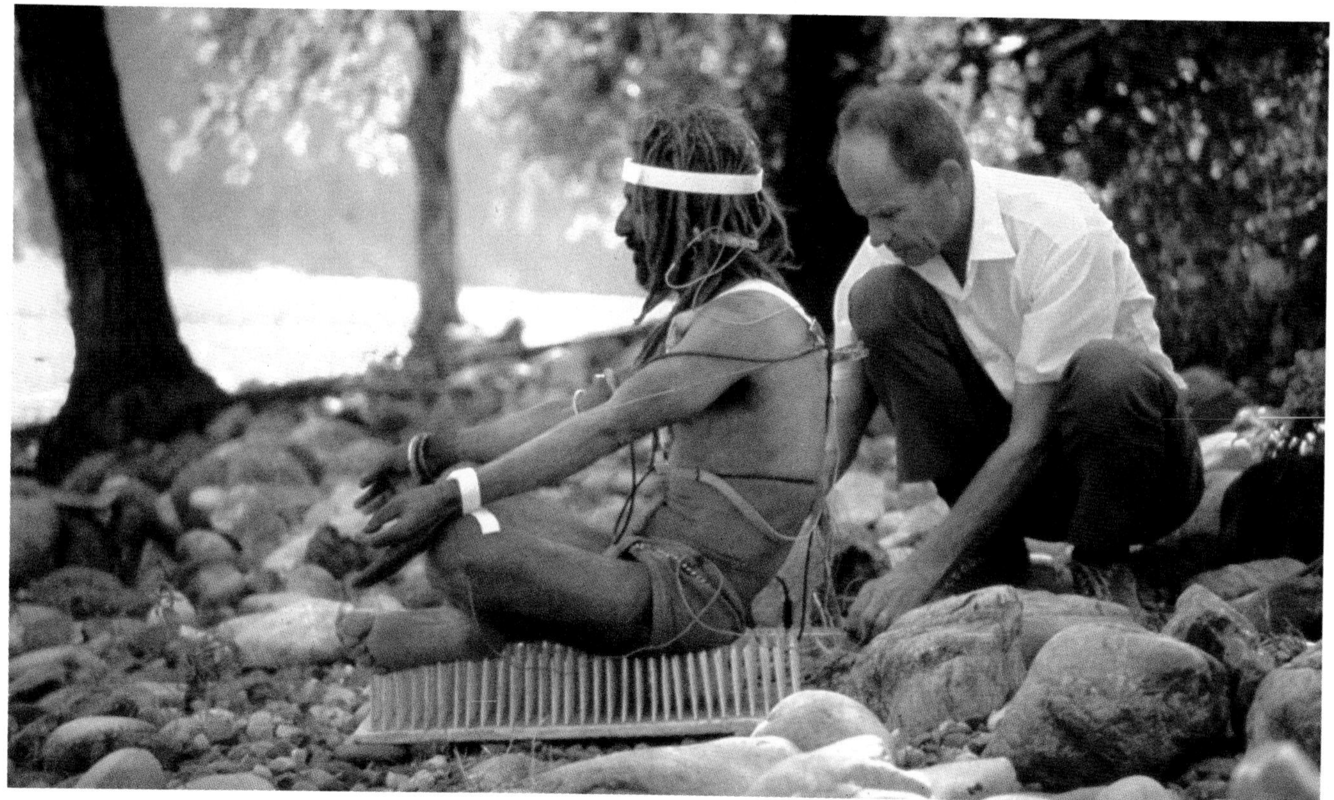

Feeling no pain on a bed of nails, a yogi in India is checked for brain activity, pulse, breathing rate and temperature by Dr. Elmer Green of the Menninger Foundation during research into mental control over headache. The readings were low, indicating that the yogi's concentration had blocked normal responses to pain—a technique applied by Dr. Green to headache treatments.

can, with practice, begin to make a mental association between the information feedback and the sensations attending the physiological change. From that awareness it is theoretically only a matter of repeated practice before the patient is able to exert conscious control over a particular internal process—for example, the bunched scalp muscles of a chronic tension headache—without the need for external signals, without instrumental monitors and outside the clinical setting. Like the simpler relaxation exercises, biofeedback training is not an end in itself but a means to self-awareness and self-regulation; once those are readily accessible, the technological supports can be abandoned.

Biofeedback training differs in equipment and techniques according to the body function being monitored. Muscle tension, the most frequent target, is tracked by an electromyograph, or EMG. The EMG, like the EEG, is a very sensitive gauge of electrical voltage, but it measures electrical activity in muscles rather than in the brain. It picks up the voltages generated within motor units—groups of muscle fibers that contract in unison under the command of a single nerve cell. A fully relaxed muscle gives off no electrical signals, but living muscle is never completely relaxed; it constantly alternates between contraction and relaxation to maintain normal muscle tone.

When an EMG is used for biofeedback training, two disc-shaped electrodes, set within cuplike plastic holders, are taped to the skin over an appropriate muscle; a third electrode is placed between the two to serve as a point of comparison. The signals picked up in this way are amplified and filtered, then sent to some form of feedback display—a speaker producing a variable click or hum, an oscillating needle on a dial, or a variable light. Simultaneously, the EMG records the activity on a graph so that patient and technician can note progress from one session to the next.

To monitor headache-related muscle tension, the EMG sensors are typically attached over the frontalis muscle, which is in the forehead. When the frontalis muscle relaxes, the muscles of the scalp, neck and upper body often relax, too, so monitoring here generally gives the patient a report on the status of all the muscles implicated in tension headache. If neck muscles are believed to be involved, the sensors will be placed there instead.

At first the technician sets the machine to feed signals back only when the subject is doing the task correctly; movement in the opposite direction—heightened muscle tension—is not reported back, on the grounds that it will discourage the novice. At the beginning, also, the machine is adjusted to reward even the slightest improvement with a positive signal. Later on, as the patient progresses, the technician readjusts the machine to require larger and larger decreases in muscle tension for the same rewarding signal and also to give negative signals to indicate when tension has gone up instead of down. The biofeedback sessions typically take place in a minimally furnished cubicle with a couch or comfortable chair on which the patient rests, eyes closed. To minimize distractions, the therapist may withdraw to an adjoining room and monitor the session from there.

Biofeedback is used not only to help a patient control muscle tension directly but also to regulate the blood-flow changes blamed for muscle-tension and migraine pains. Blood circulation is gauged by measuring skin temperature, which varies according to the amount of blood in the area. The potential value of skin-temperature biofeedback was first suggested in 1964 at the Menninger Clinic in Topeka, Kansas, by Dr. Elmer Green, who also studied the mind-control abilities of a number of yogis in India *(opposite)*. Dr. Green and his associates recognized effects on migraine while working with volunteers in a training program designed to teach control of brain waves, muscle tension, and blood flow in forearms. They noted that one of their subjects, a migraine sufferer, experienced spontaneous relief from her headache pain when the rising temperature of her hands indicated increased blood flow there.

The hot-hands treatment

After further testing, Dr. Green and his team proposed what they called the hot-hands theory for treating headaches. They proposed that if constriction of blood vessels in the fingers can be stopped when a migraine attack appears imminent, the technique that the person is using will simultaneously stop the constriction of head arteries that leads to tension-headache pain and also initiates the first step in the sequence leading to the headache of common migraine. However, some migraine specialists hold to an opposite, "hydraulic," explanation for the effectiveness of skin-temperature biofeedback in migraine headaches. They believe that warming the hands leads to partial draining of the arteries of the head, thereby preventing arterial dilation, the second, pain-inducing part of the migraine sequence.

With the aid of signals from a temperature-measuring biofeedback device hooked up to his finger, a headache sufferer can eventually teach himself to change from a person who habitually has cold hands to one whose hands are usually warm. And he learns to will his hands warmer by as much as 15 degrees, deliberately inhibiting blood-vessel constriction, when he feels he is under stress. Patients are usually given

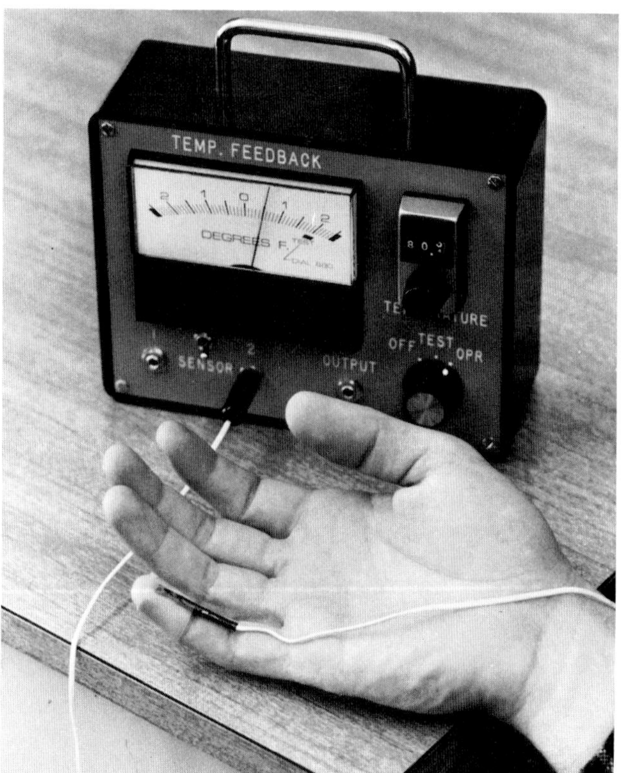

An electric thermometer taped to his finger helps a migraine victim learn to will blood into his hands and warm them, preventing headache—according to one theory—by draining cranial blood vessels. The digital readout (right) shows temperature, the meter temperature change. Watching the gauges, a patient can learn to control bloodflow and stop attacks.

homework in the form of practice sessions with a small portable temperature trainer, a device that changes color with variations in finger temperature.

You can experiment with finger-temperature control yourself by using a standard wall thermometer. Place it face down along the length of your middle finger, setting the bulb against the inside fat pad nearest the palm. Tape it in place, firmly in contact with your finger but not so tightly that the tape will constrict blood flow or prevent you from lifting the upper part of the thermometer to take readings. Next settle down in a comfortable chair and wait five minutes, to let the thermometer adjust to your finger temperature. Make a note of this baseline measurement.

Then, while still seated and with your eyes closed to promote concentration, repeat some of the phrases used in Dr. Schultz's autogenic training—"I feel relaxed. . . . My hands feel warm. . . . My hands feel heavy. . . ."—trying as you do so to visualize each sensation. Or simply picture in your mind warm, relaxing imagery—taking a warm bath, lying on a beach in the sun, savoring a bowl of hot soup, whatever notions have particular appeal. After 15 minutes of this, check the temperature reading a second time. Unless you are one of the small minority resistant to such techniques, you will, after some practice, be able to warm your finger three or four degrees.

One other type of biofeedback instrument is sometimes used by specialists, not so much to train patients in managing headaches as to demonstrate the interaction between mind and body. Many patients, explained Dr. Steven Baskin of The New England Center for Headache, find it very hard to embrace the idea of mind-body control. To convince them such control is practical, he uses an instrument similar to a lie detector, which gauges emotion, excitement or anxiety—all conditions that prevent relaxation. A pair of electrodes transmitting a weak current of electricity is affixed to the palm of the hand, which sweats when the mind is aroused. Excess sweat on the palms permits the current to flow across the skin from one electrode to the other more freely than when the person is relatively calm.

"Once in a great while," explained Dr. Baskin, "we will

see patients who claim not to feel strongly about things, to be rather matter-of-fact, about issues we suspect they actually are very responsive to internally. If you can hook them up briefly, talk to them a little bit about the subject and let them see for themselves, you can get them to be more open to the whole idea of mind and body being one. Once the fundamental skepticism is gone, then, you can start discussing the bigger subject of self control.''

Drowning pain in electricity

Self-control is the goal of much of the treatment provided by headache specialists. But there are other advanced remedies that attack head pain more directly. One of these techniques is nerve stimulation by electricity—actually a modern version of a treatment that can be traced back at least to Scribonius Largus, a Roman physician. In 46 A.D., he described the use of a live torpedo fish—a type of ray that stuns or kills its prey with electrical discharges—to cure, among other things, headache *(right, top)*.

Wrote Scribonius in his influential textbook, *Compositiones Medicae,* ''Headache, even if it is chronic and unbearable, is taken away and remedied, forever, by a live black torpedo placed on the spot that is in pain.'' Electrostimulation cropped up again in the 19th Century in a variety of dubious forms that were supposed to aid headaches and almost every other ill known or imagined. Such quackery eventually drove the use of electricity into disrepute and obscurity until the 1960s, when Melzack and Wall's gate-control theory of pain *(Chapter 5)* suggested that pain might be drowned out by applications of electricity.

It was then that electrical stimulation began to be reassessed. Drs. C. Norman Shealy and Blaine S. Nashville of the Pain and Health Rehabilitation Center, in La Crosse, Wisconsin, reopened the subject by experimenting with stimulation of large nerve pathways in the spinal cords of people afflicted with chronic pain. They found that small, safe amounts of electrical current could so reduce the pain that drugs were not needed. They developed a small portable device that they called a dorsal-column stimulator, part of which was implanted in the body near the spinal column and

An ancient Greek vase is adorned with a torpedo fish—a ray that paralyzes prey with electricity and was used as a headache cure. The live fish, placed on the patient's head, produced a charge to block pain much as electrical nerve stimulators do today (bottom).

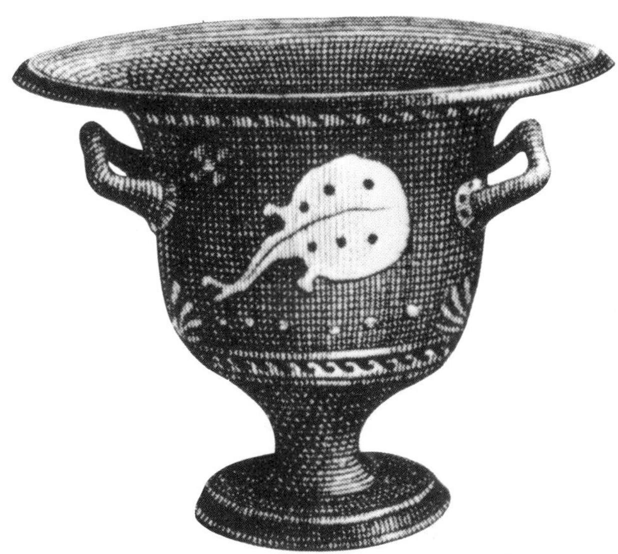

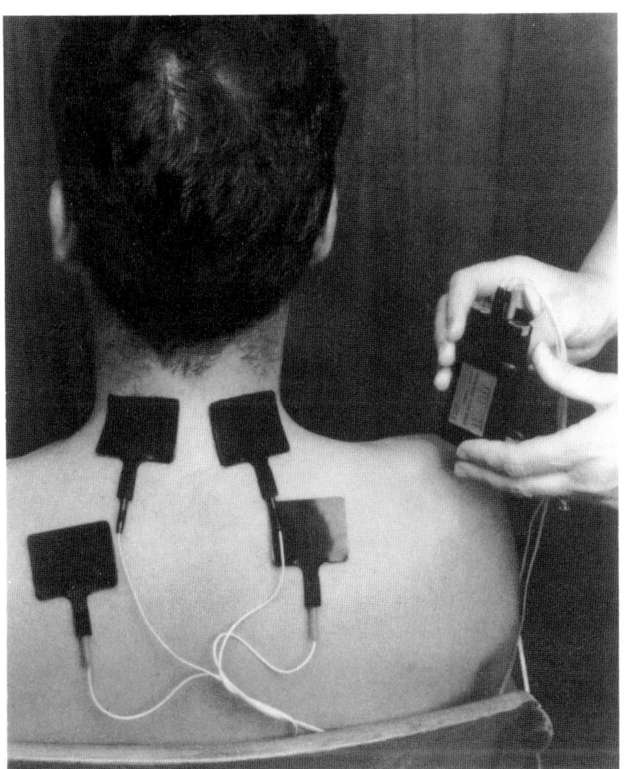

A cluster-headache patient is treated with a mild charge from a battery pack the doctor holds. The current goes through electrodes to stimulate nerves in the neck and shoulders. According to one theory, nerve impulses spurred by electricity—whether from the fish or from the battery—reach the brain faster than pain signals, blocking them by monopolizing the channels of access.

part of which was worn on the patient's belt. When pain erupted, the patient could send electrical signals from the belt unit to the implanted device and stimulate the spinal cord, blocking the pain messages.

Later an electrical device that did not have to be implanted surgically, a transcutaneous electrical nerve stimulator, or TENS, was devised. It has small electrodes that are taped to the skin over the area of discomfort. The electrodes are connected to a portable unit that generates a pulsating current to block pain. Some specialists anticipate that it may help that small percentage of headache patients not reached by the usual mix of drugs, biofeedback and behavior modification.

The value of electric stimulation is the subject of a continuing debate among headache specialists. Dr. Joel Saper of the Michigan Headache and Neurological Institute assessed it as "a fad." Yet this treatment is provided to patients at Dr. Saper's own institute because, he explained, it makes some of them better.

The same judgment can be applied to many of the special treatments sought out by victims of severe chronic headaches. They work sometimes; sometimes they do not. And no one is sure whether they really work—or whether the relief they provide is owed to the reassurance and psychological support of a skillful practitioner, or possibly to the placebo effect, the curative power of doing something for pain, no matter what.

How acupuncture works

Among the remedies that are considered miraculous by many patients but questioned by many physicians are acupuncture and chiropractic. Acupuncture, an ancient Chinese system used both to cure disease and to maintain health *(right),* is based on the theory that disease is some sort of imbalance in a life force; this imbalance can be set right, according to the theory, by needles placed at specified places in the body so as to intercept a wrongful flow of the force to or from various organs, thus redirecting it and restoring the balance. In modern practice, fine needles of stainless steel are pressed against or inserted into the skin at these special locations.

There are, depending on the particular school of acupunc-

The age-old needle cure

The art of acupuncture, which employs needles inserted into the flesh to kill pain and cure disease, appears to relieve headaches for many millions in the Orient and is finding increasing acceptance in the West. The treatment is based on the belief that a two-part life force, called *ch'i,* travels throughout the body along 12 major pathways, or meridians *(opposite);* if the two parts of *ch'i,* masculine and feminine, are out of balance, pain and illness result.

To restore the healthy balance, acupuncturists slip hair-thin needles about half an inch into the meridians influencing the affected organ. Two very long meridians are believed to control the head: One runs across the forehead and down to the small toe, the other extends from the ear down to another toe. The acupuncturist chooses his points by the location and character of the pain. Each point is supposed to affect the flow of *ch'i* and need not be near the site of the disorder. But acupuncturists differ on the number, location and purpose of points—a disagreement reflected in the various charts and models *(right)* used by acupuncture students.

Most Western doctors question the scientific validity of acupuncture, but they find it difficult to dismiss a technique that often seems to work. And recent research on pain mechanisms suggests physical explanations—unconnected to masculine or feminine life forces—for the effects of the needle treatment: The sharp pricks may prompt nerve signals that override pain sensations, or they may release the body's own painkilling chemicals.

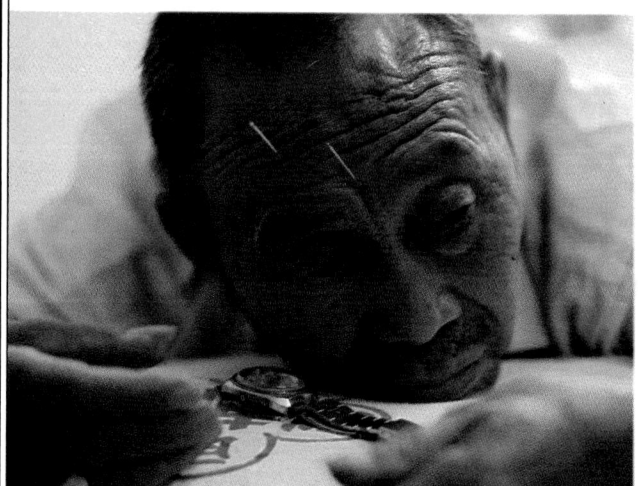

Two needles protrude from an elderly migraine patient's forehead as he uses his wristwatch to time a 15-minute acupuncture session at a Taiwan hospital. The needle above his eyebrow is intended to improve his vision—often impaired just before the onset of a migraine headache—while the needle above the bridge of his nose is positioned to relieve his pain.

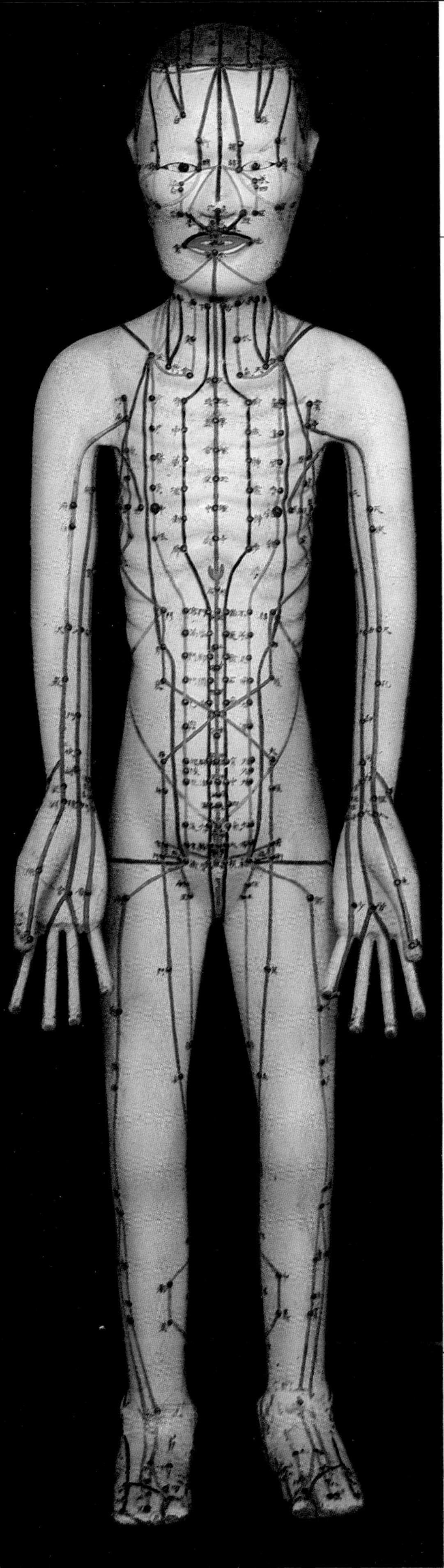

1880 PAPIER-MÂCHÉ MODEL DISPLAYING ACUPUNCTURE POINTS (JAPAN)

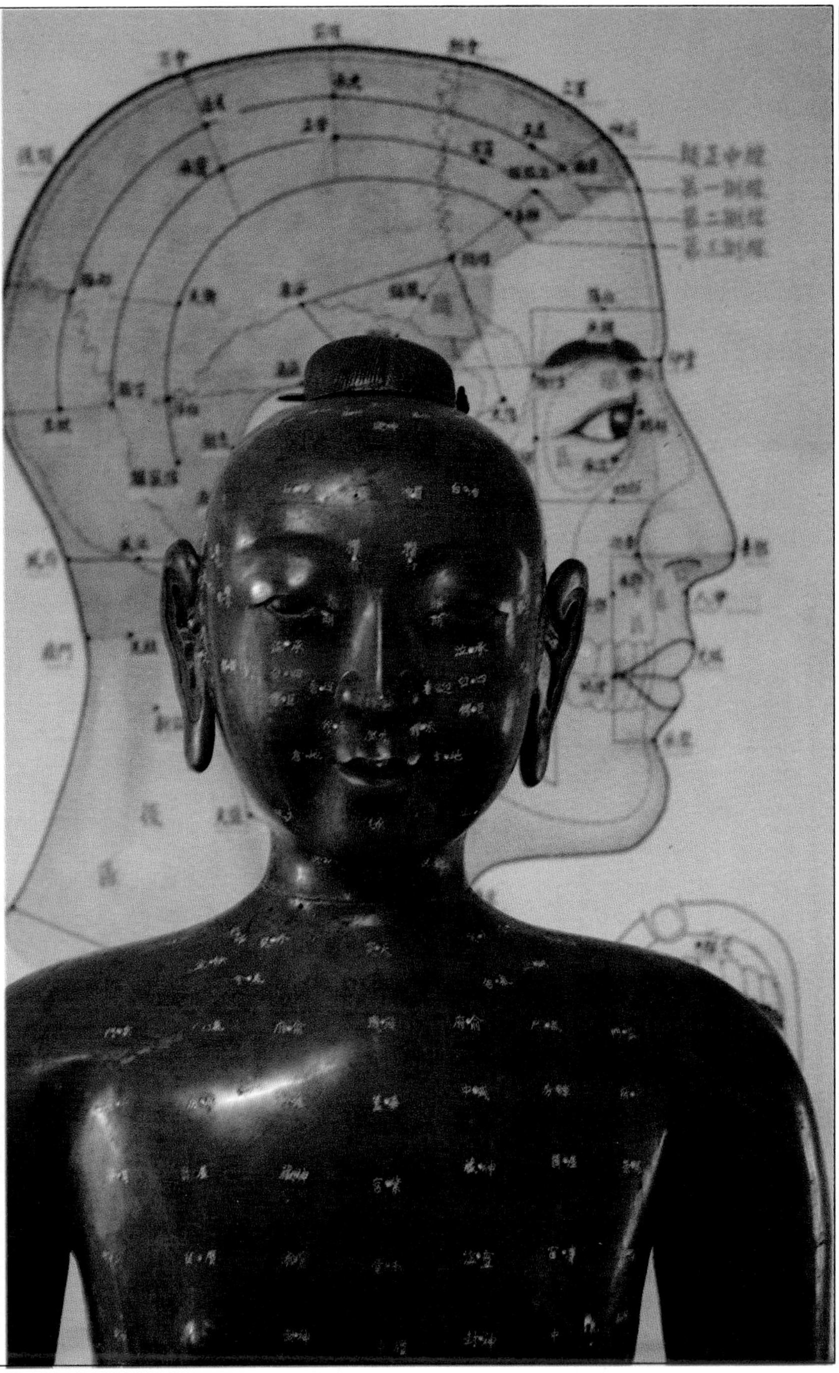

16TH CENTURY BRONZE ACUPUNCTURE GUIDE AND MODERN CHART (CHINA)

ture followed, between 500 and 800 acupuncture points, which the skilled acupuncturist commits to memory, or checks by referring to charts or models. To treat a particular complaint, he must know the prescribed combination of points (by no means are their locations necessarily suggested by the location of the disorder) and he must be adroit in manipulating his needles, applying the right pressure or inserting them to the precise depth.

The Chinese claim a high degree of success for acupuncture in the treatment of headache and many other disorders, and some tests in the West have confirmed their experience. Dr. Jaakko Laitinen of Finland reported that he had found significant reduction in head pain among volunteers who submitted to periodic acupuncture treatment. California pain specialist Dr. David E. Bresler also reported obtaining good results with acupuncture.

"On the basis of my experience with it," wrote Dr. Bresler, "I have found it particularly effective in treating a variety of chronic pain problems"; among them he included muscle-contraction headaches and migraines. "There is no conclusive data yet available as to its effectiveness in treating allergic headaches," he noted, but added, "Acupuncture may also be effective in treating psychological as well as physical pain. I have cared for many patients suffering from anxiety and severe depression, some of whom have been helped by acupuncture when accompanied by appropriate psychotherapeutic care." Dr. Bresler reported that, following success with acupuncture in one case, he had treated "approximately twenty-five severely depressed patients in a similar manner. Almost all of them have shown at least some degree of improvement."

As the great complexity of the nervous system's pain mechanisms has become more evident, some Western pain researchers are beginning to believe that a neurological explanation for acupuncture may yet be found. Dr. Donald J. Dalessio of the Scripps Clinic in La Jolla and Dr. Seymour Diamond, Executive Director of the National Migraine Foundation, related the success of acupuncture to the gate-control theory of pain, proposing that the insertion of needles may have a counterirritating effect on the skin, and this counterirritation could send pain signals to the gate and block the slower pain of headaches.

Three variations of acupuncture—*shiatzu (below), G-jo* and *jin shin do*—employ finger pressure rather than needle pricks to relieve headaches and are often called acupressure techniques. Long used in China and Japan, these methods have found new popularity in the United States, partly because treatment does not always require a professional practi-

Pressing the ache away

Of all the treatments said to cure headaches without drugs or long relaxation training, one of the easiest to try yourself is the Japanese massage known as *shiatzu*. The practice depends on pressure; for headaches, the fingers, thumbs and palms are pushed and moved mainly over the face, scalp and neck.

The movements at right are among the most common of those used for headaches. Separately or together, they relax muscles involved in tension headaches. Some migraine victims report the pressure helps them too.

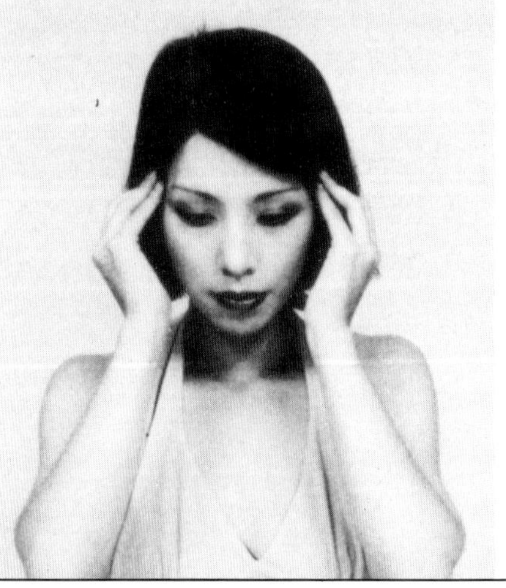

In this treatment pressure is applied to the temples with the fingers of each hand while the thumbs rest along the jawbone. A pressure of 15 pounds is recommended; the feel of the weight can be learned by practicing on a bathroom scale.

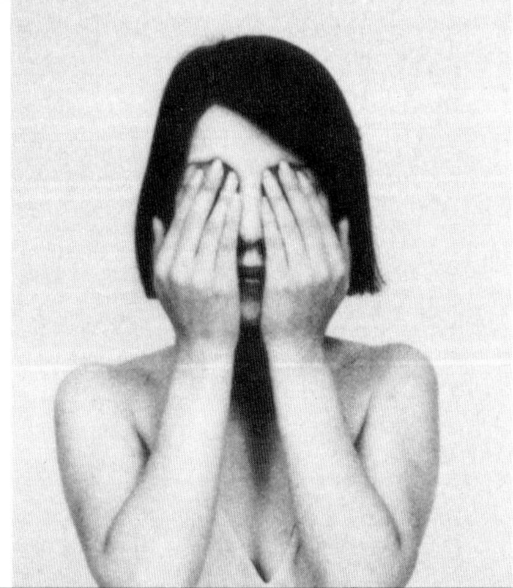

This exercise is recommended for relieving headache caused by eyestrain. It is accomplished not by pressing the eyes with the fingers but by bringing the face gently to the fingers. Hold the position for three to five seconds.

tioner. A number of illustrated books published in English provide detailed instructions so that a headache sufferer can learn where and how to apply the pain-relieving pressure to his own body.

Acupressure is also recommended by Dr. Bresler. "When a trial of acupuncture proves helpful, I will teach my patients how to massage their own acupuncture points so that they can assume greater responsibility for their own care," he wrote. "In my opinion, nearly every person in pain can significantly benefit by learning a few simple acupressure techniques. When you hurt at 2 a.m., pressing the appropriate acupuncture points can often provide immediate relief."

These Oriental techniques are, in effect, forms of massage, somewhat different from the peculiarly American type of massage that also is both praised and damned as a headache remedy: chiropractic. It was developed in 1898 by an Iowa healer named Daniel David Palmer, who asserted that disease is due to some dislocation of the vertebrae. This "spinal subluxation," chiropractors maintain, leads to pressure on spinal nerves that produces health disorders, headaches among them. Chiropractic treatment involves manual manipulation of the vertebrae to correct the misalignment and thereby cure the disease.

The American Medical Association takes a dim view of chiropractic, condemning it as "an unscientific cult whose practitioners lack the necessary training and background to diagnose and treat human disease," and stating flatly that the treatment has never been found to have any relevance to any of the diseases it purports to relieve. However, Dr. Bresler pointed out, "In-depth studies of chiropractic by unbiased investigators are rare." And chiropractic treatments, like many others, get enthusiastic support from numbers of satisfied patients.

Chiropractic can sometimes aggravate physical ailments that are the cause of pain. And any single type of treatment, whatever it is, may bring hazards if it is relied on exclusively. Patients whose headaches have a hidden physiological basis may fail to get the care they urgently need. Others with persistent but nonthreatening headaches may miss the opportunity for the full relief possible from the headache specialists' multiple attack.

Despite all the new knowledge of the mechanisms of headache pain, curing this pain remains as much art as science. Even the worst of headaches can be eased. But getting relief depends on skillful choice among the many kinds of treatments now available—and determined effort by the sufferer. Anyone who wants to get better, said one physician, can get better.

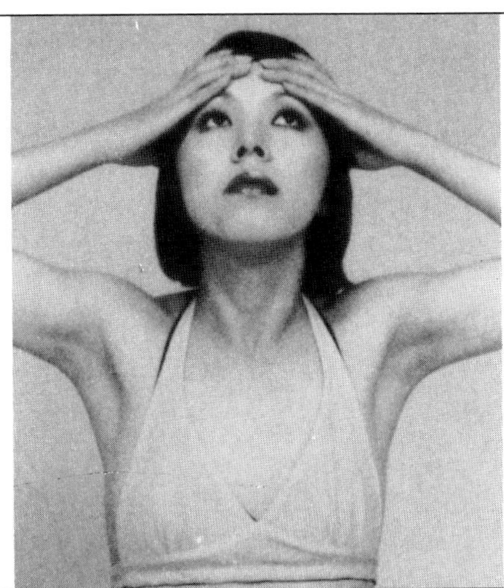

With fingertips pressing gently on the forehead, the hands are drawn toward the ears. In Chinese and Japanese medicine, such movements are believed to influence body processes along lines that are called meridians (page 138).

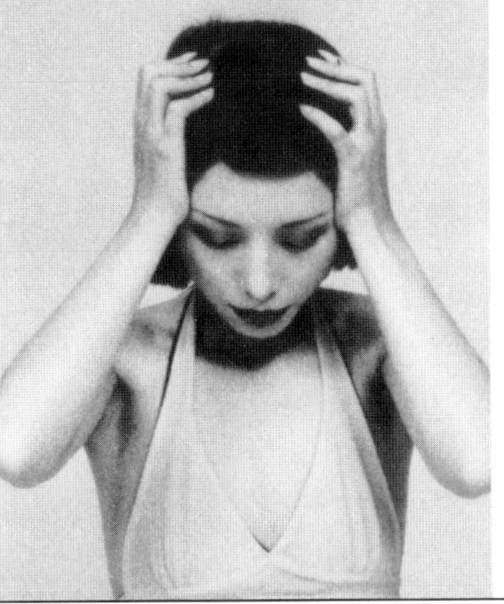

In a movement that is said to be particularly effective for headaches, the fingers and the palms begin the application of pressure at the forehead and temples and then proceed up and back along the head to the position shown above.

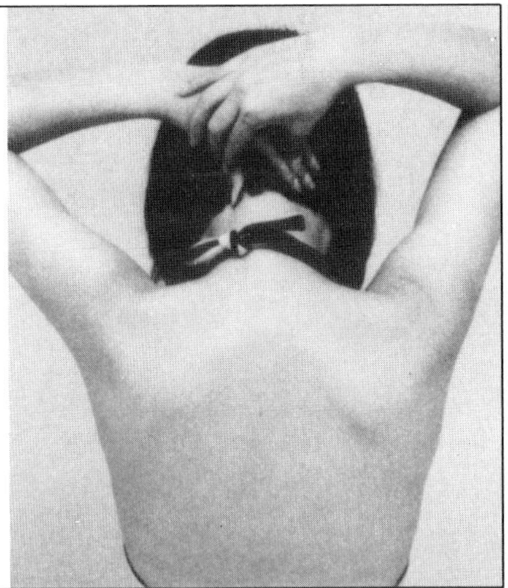

Before doing the massage above, which is designed to loosen tight neck muscles, place a hot towel on the back of the neck. Then press the neck muscles with the thumbs, each thumb's pressure reinforced by the fingers of the opposite hand.

The headache clinic: not by pills alone

The patient at right is in obvious headache pain, but with the aid of a headache clinic she has already taken the first step toward a new way of fighting it—attacking its causes rather than merely its symptoms. In contrast to conventional treatment, which covers up headaches with pain-dulling pills, the clinic's program aims for prevention and control. Head pain is viewed as a reaction to underlying imbalances—involving diet, emotional anxiety, organic illness, even bad posture—which must first be diagnosed before the aches can be countered.

At a typical clinic, such as the Michigan Headache and Neurological Institute in Ann Arbor, where the photographs on these pages were taken, a patient's case can command the attention of a small army of medical specialists. Many disciplines are called for: The complexity of isolating the basic causes requires a huge variety of physical and psychological tests. Once the evaluation is completed, treatment begins. It includes some drugs but places greater emphasis on other therapies. "You can't cure pain," said the Michigan clinic director, Dr. Joel R. Saper; rather, he and his associates try to teach patients ways of coping with headache triggers such as tension and stress, so that they can avoid an episode altogether or at least minimize its severity.

Some treatments involve direct physical therapy—a massage, say, for the tight neck muscles that can lead to a muscle-tension headache. Others rely on mental or physical exercises that enable patients to relax tense muscles by themselves *(pages 152-153)*. Still others emphasize the simple pleasures of individual and group activities *(pages 154-157)*—a straightforward way to ease the stress that underlies so many headaches.

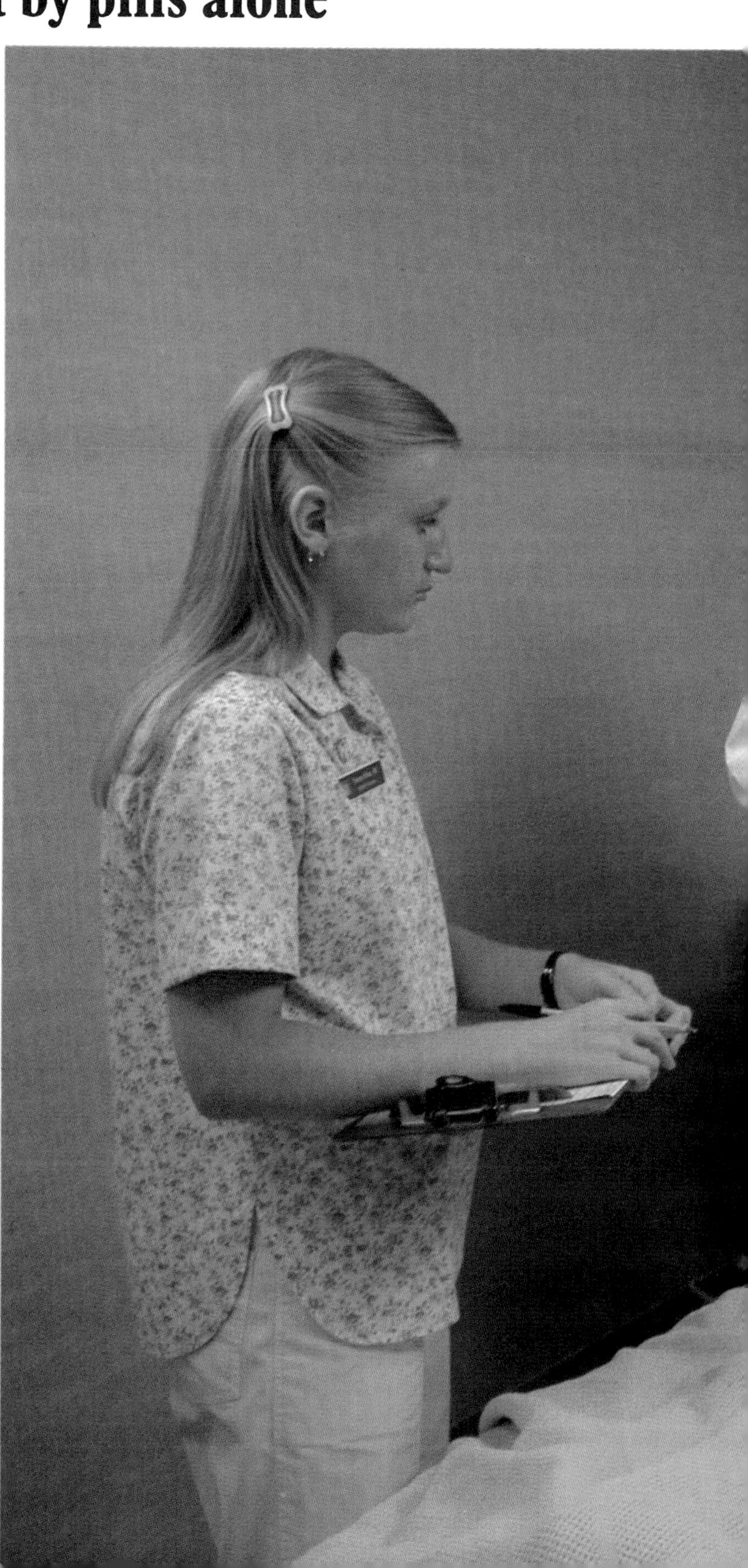

Pressing a moist-heat pad to her temples, a newly admitted patient describes her pain to Dr. Joel Saper (center), Director of the Michigan Headache and Neurological Institute, who is accompanied by three nurses and staff neurologist Dr. Neill Hirst.

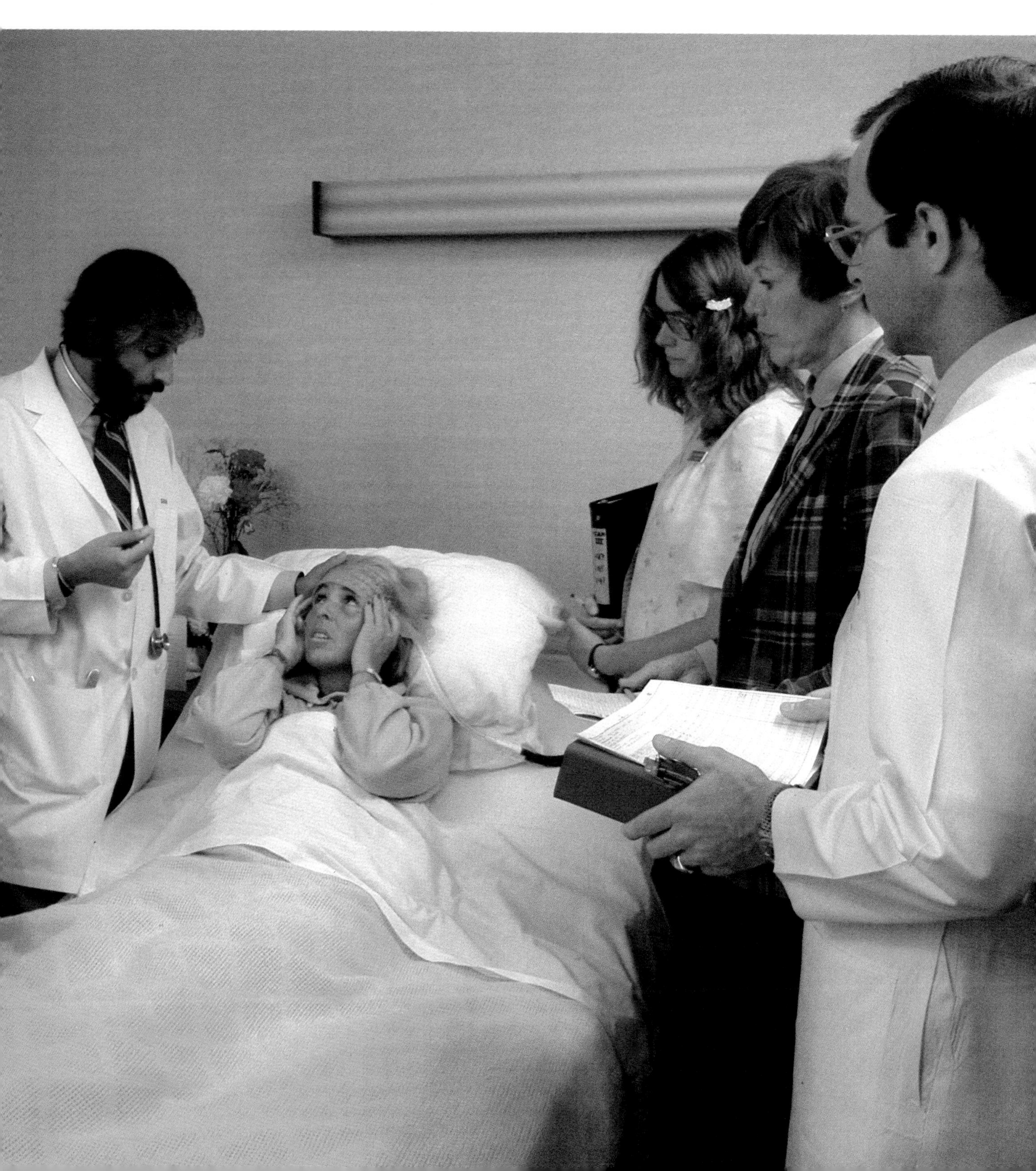

Getting to know the patient

Because most headaches are symptoms of deeper problems, new patients are examined for personal stresses that may be a factor. Family members are encouraged to participate in such reviews, for conflict and stress often begin at home. One woman, for example, discovered through counseling that she was using headache complaints to force her workaholic husband to return home early from his job. After the couple began to talk out the problem, her headaches virtually vanished. At the same time, new patients are weaned off painkilling drugs—most are overmedicated when they arrive.

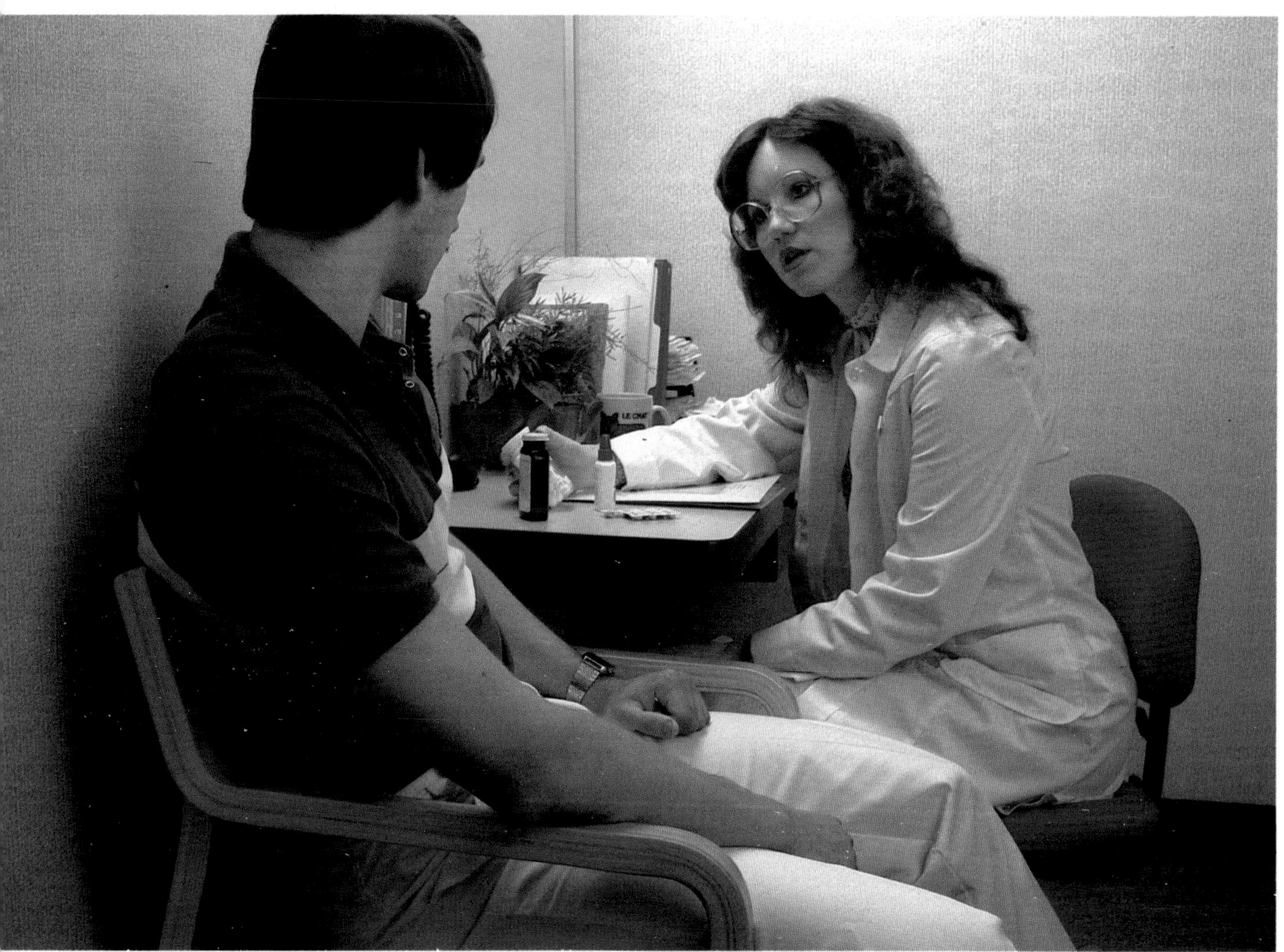

Interviewing an incoming patient, nurse Davida Lee notes the pill bottles he has brought in to show her the amounts and types of drugs he has used. One patient reported he had been taking 35 aspirin tablets a day. "That's like turning the lights off in a dirty room," commented Dr. Saper. "You're just covering up the problem, not really making it go away."

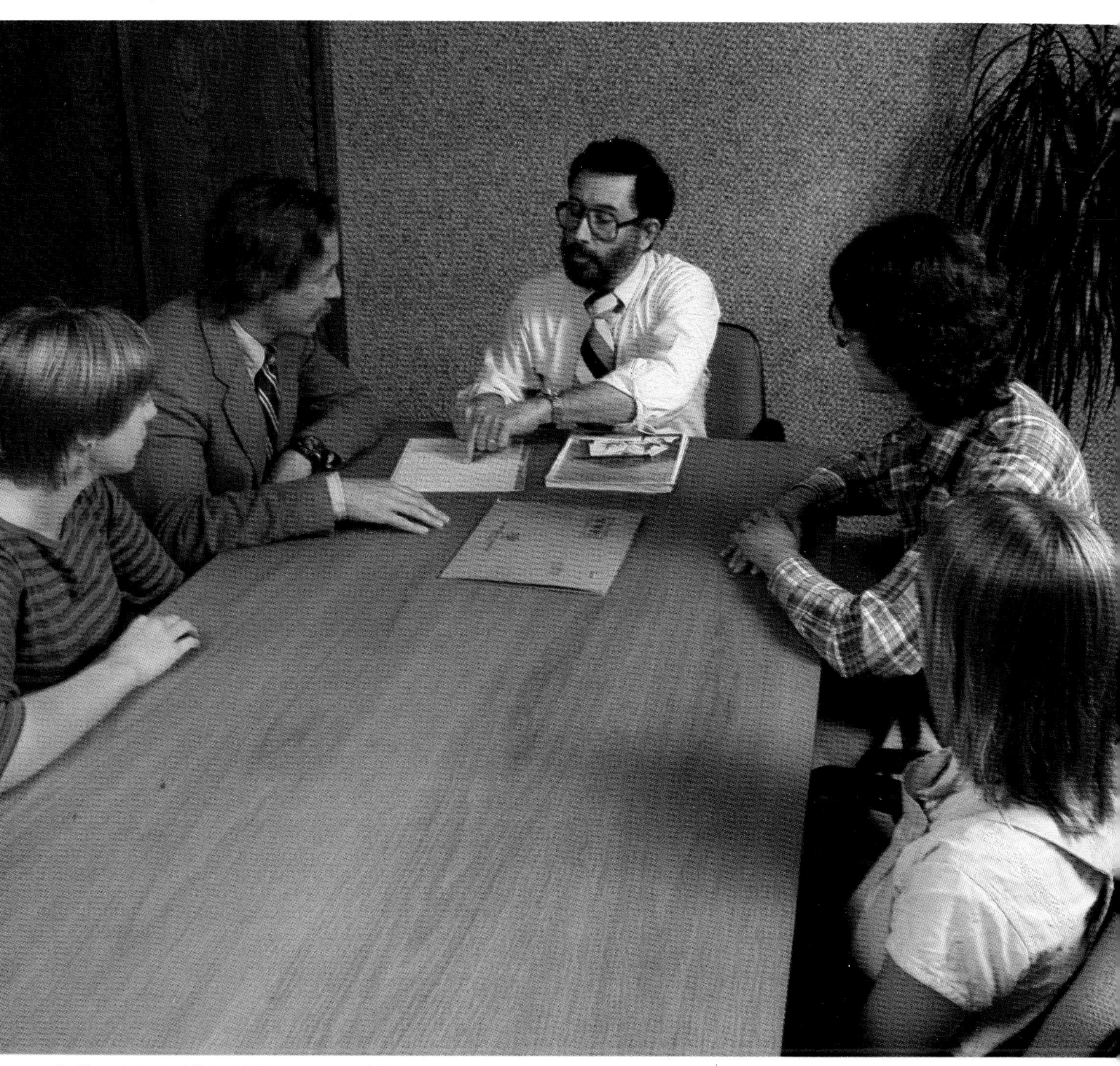

Staff psychologist Michael R. Barnat (center) discusses a psychological test with a patient and his wife and children. True-false responses to hundreds of statements like ''My sleep is fitful and disturbed'' help doctors pick up signs of anxiety, depression and other emotional problems that may find physical expression in the form of a headache.

Looking for flaws in the brain

In rare cases, headaches are caused by serious brain disorders—tumors, strokes or nerve-damaging diseases—and all patients undergo neurological tests to check for that possibility. Most are simple and routine *(near right and below)*. For the few patients whose symptoms or routine tests suggest serious ailments, more sophisticated procedures may be required *(opposite)*. In one of the most widely used, brain waves are recorded with an electroencephalograph, or EEG *(top)*. Variations from established norms can suggest brain injury or disease—or migraine.

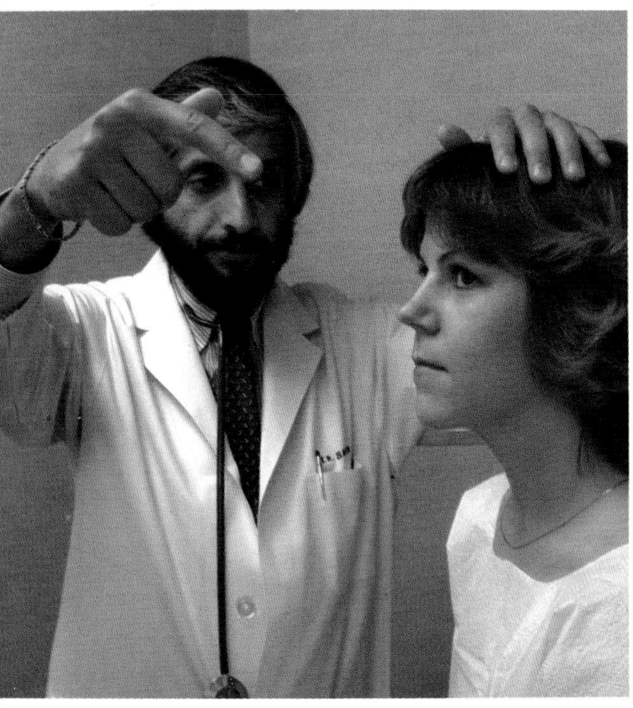

In a simple eye-coordination test, a subject's eyes follow the zigzag motions of Dr. Saper's finger. Eyes that wander from side to side, independently of each other, may indicate paralysis of certain eye muscles or nerves—a condition frequently related to tumors, strokes or the brain infection of meningitis.

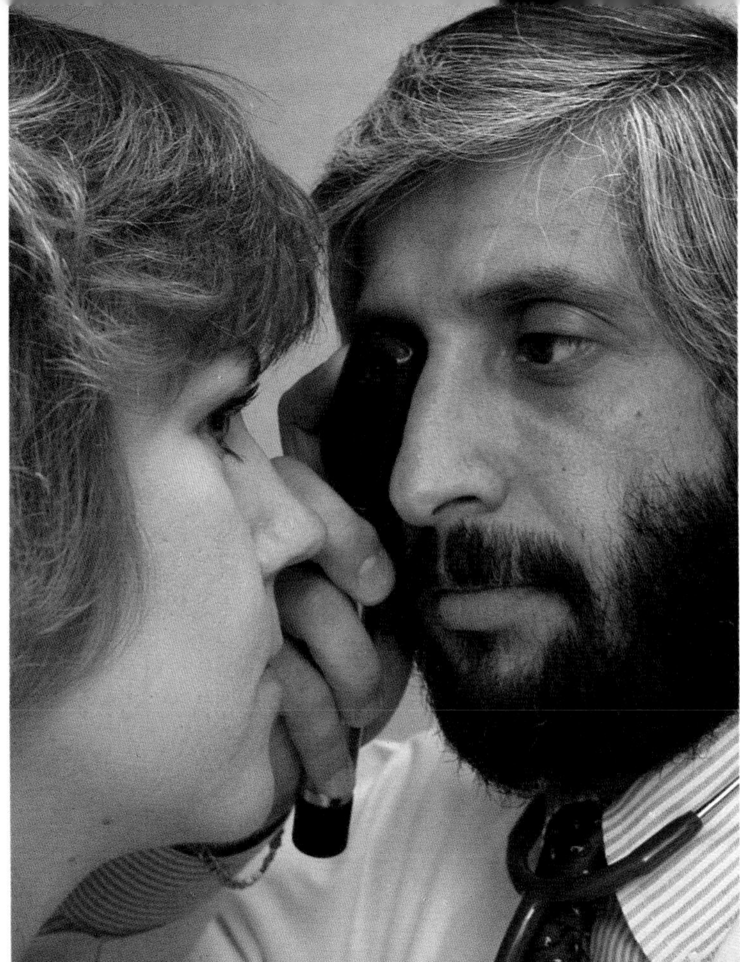

Dr. Saper peers through a familiar medical tool—an ophthalmoscope, whose bright light and magnifying lens enable him to examine blood vessels inside a patient's eye; their condition may indicate thickened or hardened blood vessels in the brain.

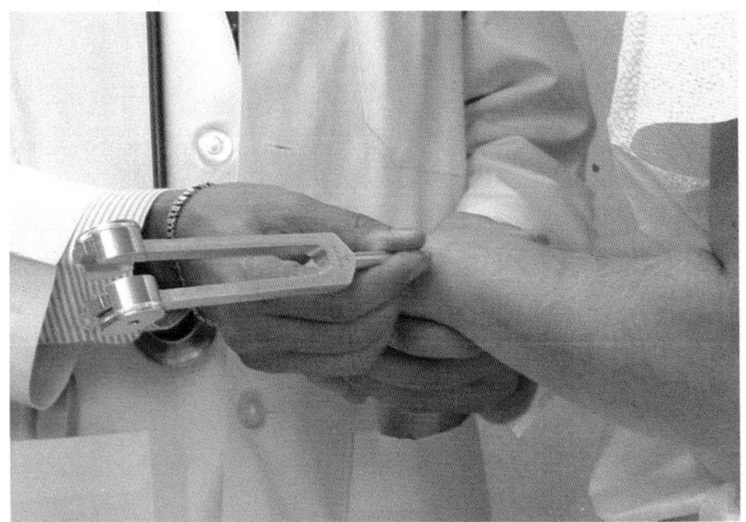

In a test designed to measure and compare nerve responses, the handle of a vibrating tuning fork is placed on a bone—in this case the wrist. In one test, a patient who feels the vibrations more strongly on one side than the other may have a nervous system that sends distorted or imagined pain impulses to the brain.

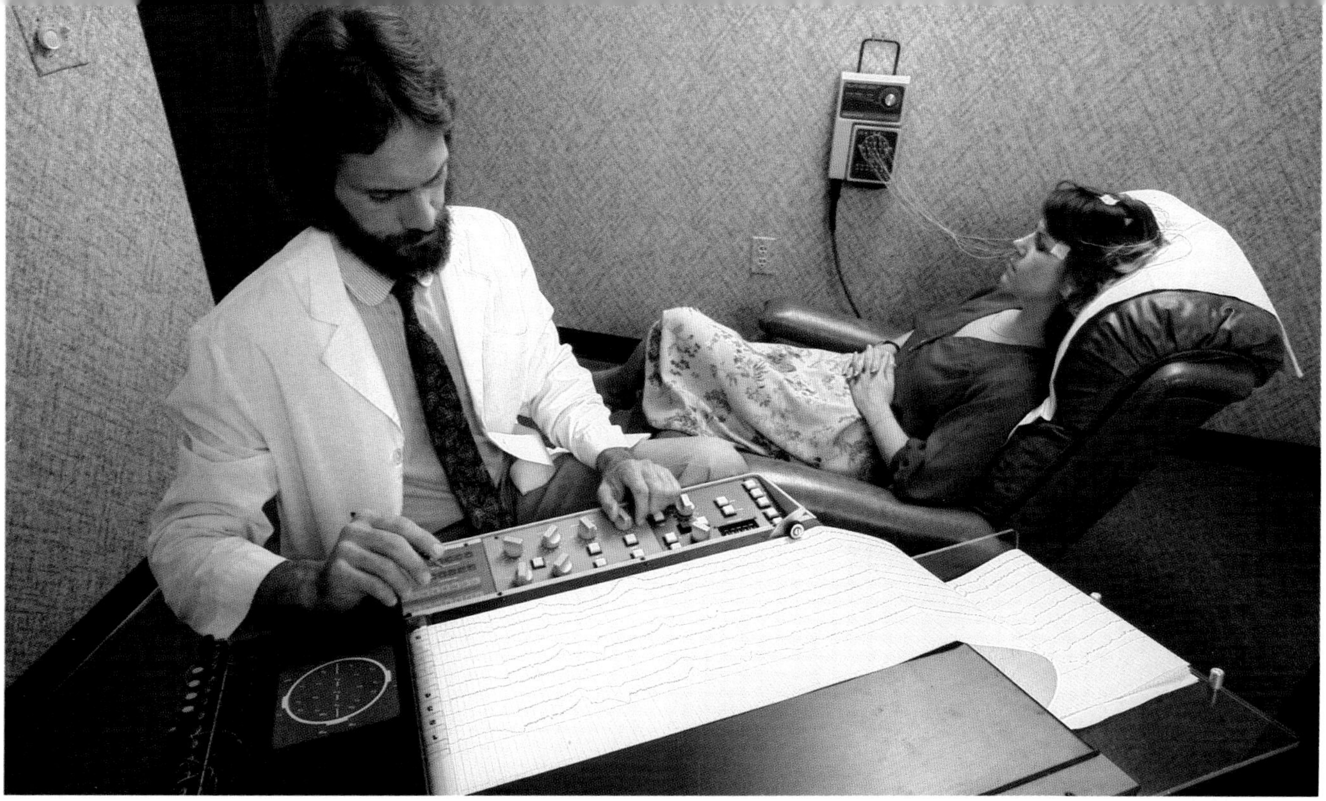

A technician uses an EEG to monitor a woman's brain waves, picked up by scalp electrodes and printed out as squiggly lines on the paper.

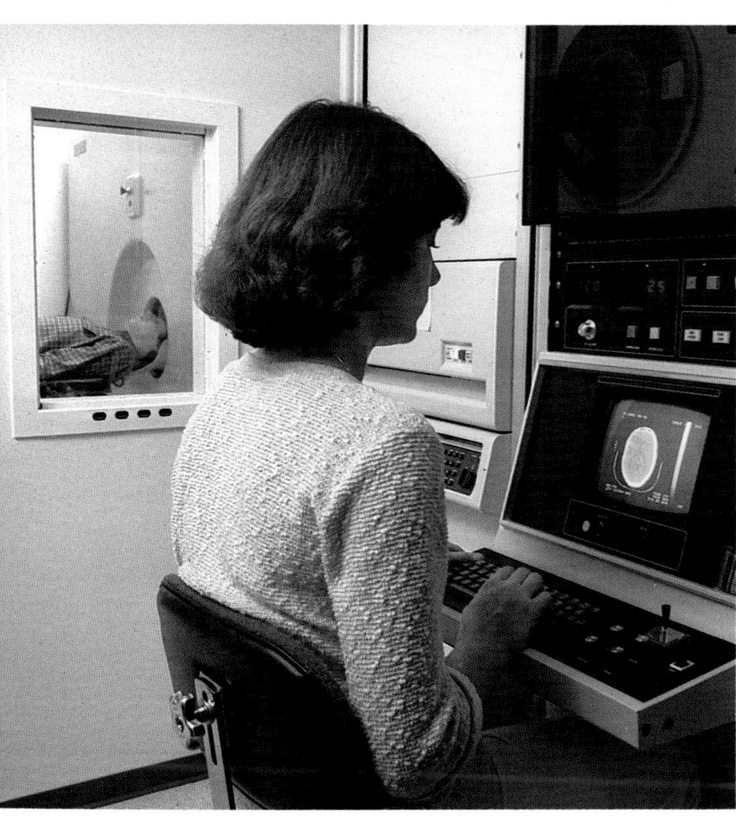

In a CAT scan, demonstrated above, a technician at a computer console controls a special X-ray machine (behind window) that takes multiple shots of a patient's head from different angles. The many views are combined by the computer to produce a series of pictures that can reveal the location and shape of tumors.

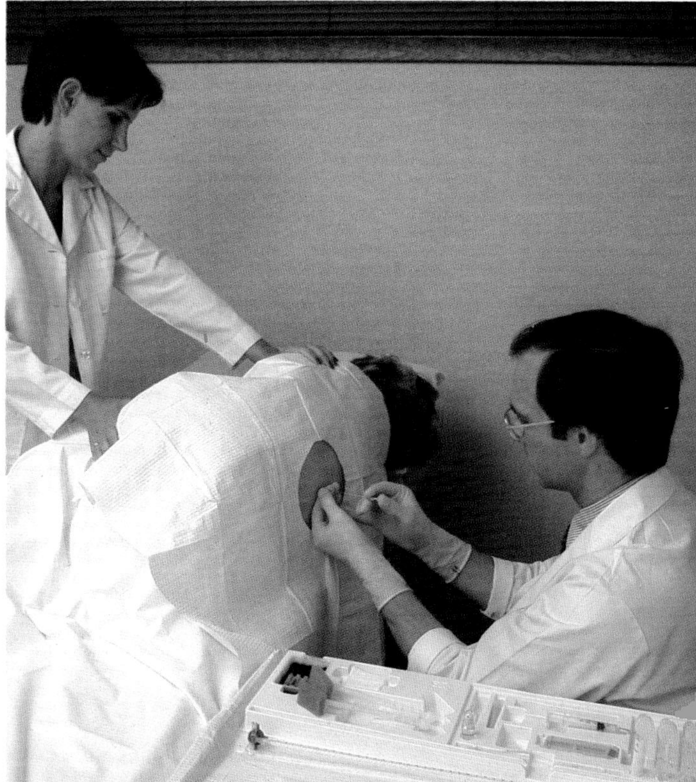

In this demonstration of a spinal tap, staff neurologist Neill Hirst prepares a needle to draw out a sample of the fluid that cushions the spinal cord. The fluid can then be examined under a microscope for signs of meningitis or other diseases that might be provoking the patient's headaches.

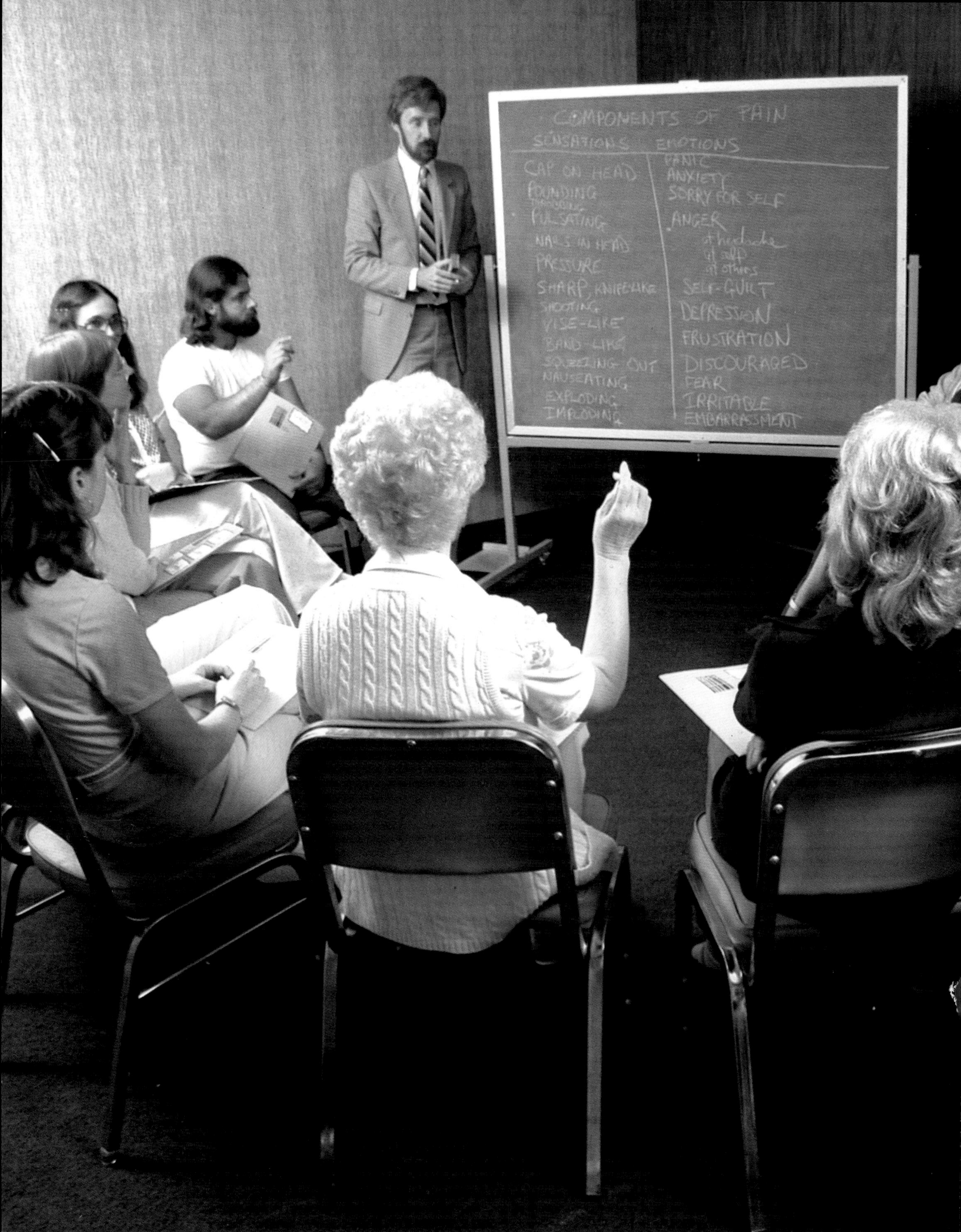

COMPONENTS OF PAIN
SENSATIONS
EMOTIONS
CAP ON HEAD
POUNDING
PULSATING
NAILS IN HEAD
PRESSURE
SHARP, KNIFELIKE
SHOOTING
VISE-LIKE
BAND-LIKE
SQUEEZING OUT
NAUSEATING
EXPLODING
IMPLODING
PANIC
ANXIETY
SORRY FOR SELF
ANGER
at headache
at self
at others
SELF-GUILT
DEPRESSION
FRUSTRATION
DISCOURAGED
FEAR
IRRITABLE
EMBARRASSMENT

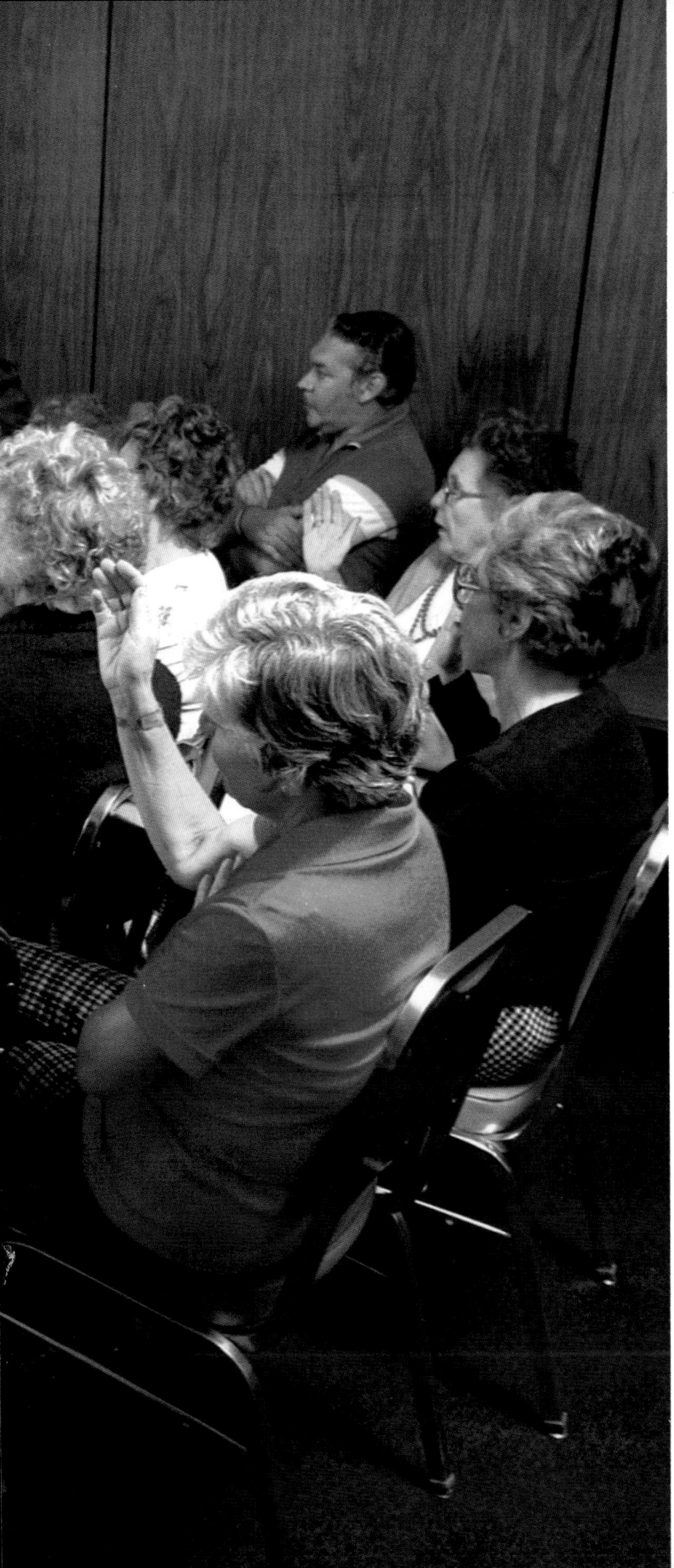

Misery finds company

About 10 per cent of headache-clinic patients spend a few days in a hospital, where doctors can monitor them around the clock and evaluate therapies as they are being tried. Most are admitted because they suffer from severe daily head pain, because illnesses or emotional problems such as chronic depression underlie their headaches, or because they have become dangerously dependent on drugs.

The confinement also demonstrates to headache victims, perhaps for the first time, that they do not suffer alone. "For many," said Dr. Saper, "the camaraderie with others in the same fix is therapeutic in itself."

Newly hospitalized headache patients gather with psychologist Alvin E. Lake (standing) for a seminar on pain. At this session, the doctor urges patients to describe the personal sensations, emotions and fears headaches provoke in them.

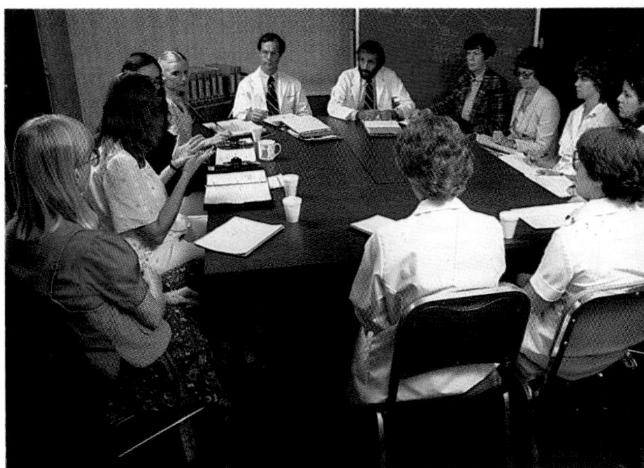

Proceeding case by case, Dr. Saper (center) pools observations of clinic and hospital staff members on the progress of the hospitalized patients. Such meetings take place twice weekly, and smaller conferences are held daily.

Physical therapist Laura Dale positions one of the clinic's patients behind a transparent posture chart. Viewing the woman's stance through the grid and determining just how her body differs from the norm—stooped shoulders, say, or an unnaturally curved spine—will enable the therapist to prescribe for her a program of corrective exercises.

Workouts for muscles and nerves

The pulling and probing of physical therapy may prevent some muscle-tension headaches from occurring and can lessen the severity of many that do. Even improvements in a patient's posture *(left)* can have similar effects, for faulty carriage can place stress on muscles, passing tension along to the head and aggravating headache.

In addition to such established therapies are experimental methods that rely on mild electrical stimulation of nerves *(far right)*. One explanation holds that the shocks, when applied to one part of the body, alter perception of pain in another.

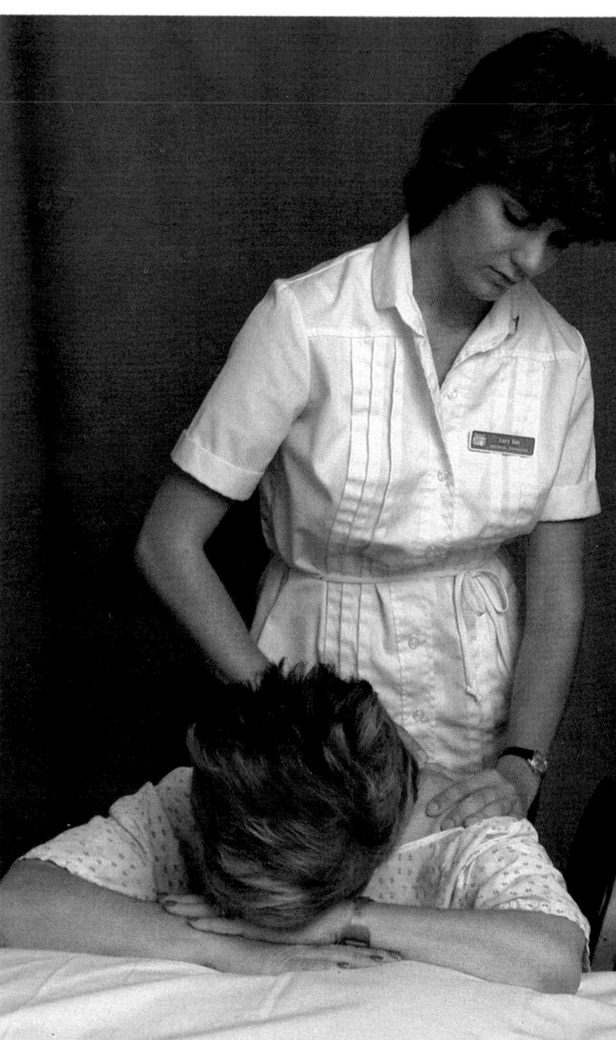

A patient rests her head on a table for a relaxing massage of her head, neck and upper-back muscles. As the kneading action loosens muscles, some may get immediate—if temporary—relief from the "tight-cap" feeling of muscle-tension headaches.

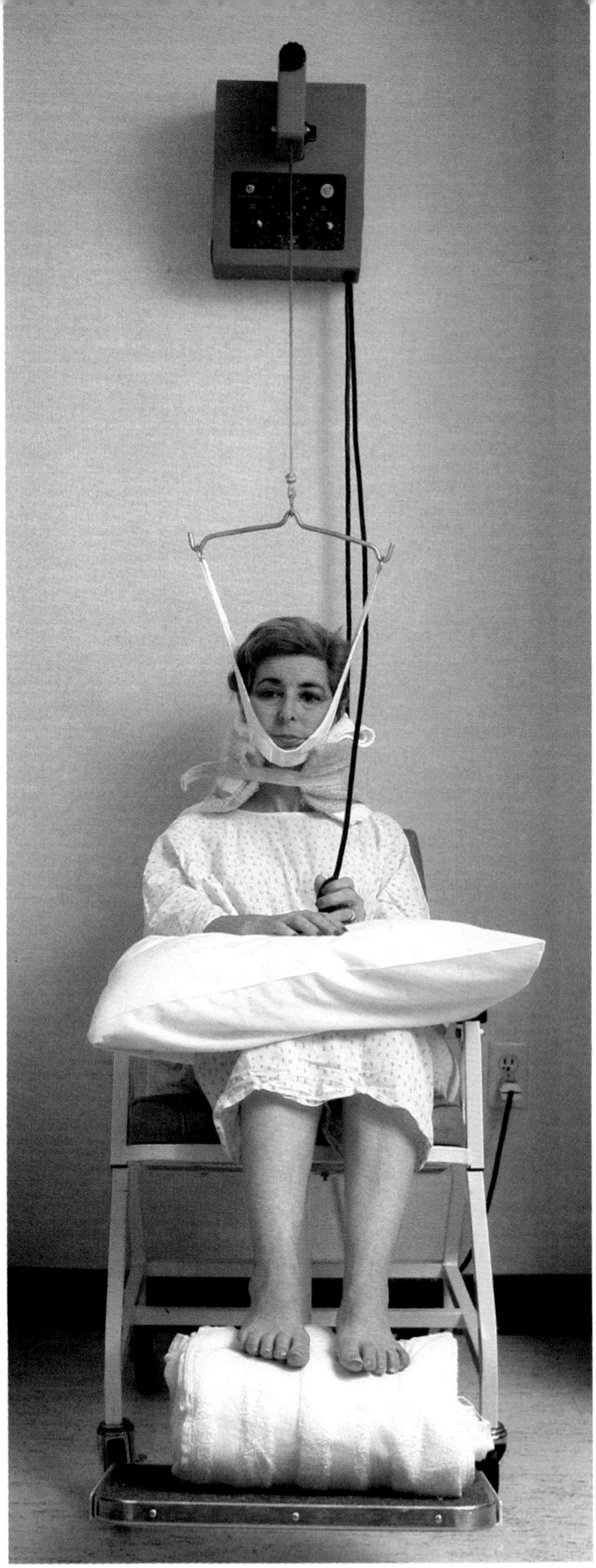

Her head suspended in a traction cradle, her neck supported by a cervical collar, a patient squeezes a hand control to activate the winch on the wall; the device will pull her head upward and stretch out tight neck muscles that contribute to head pain.

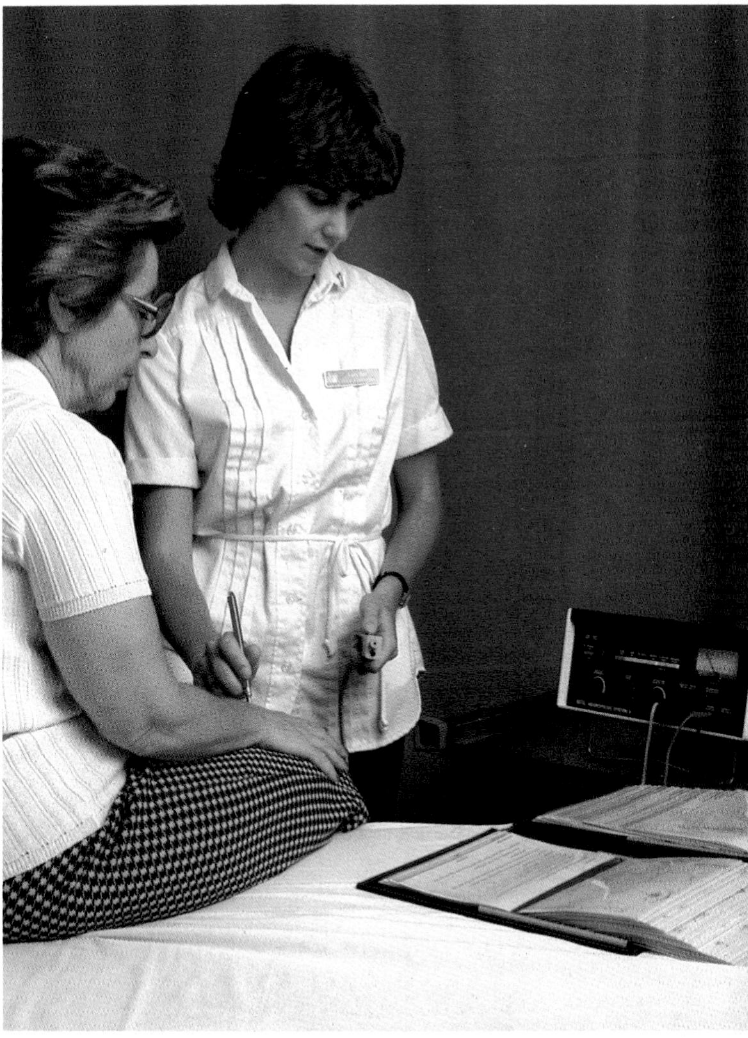

Eyes fixed on the dials of a meter that monitors the current, therapist Laura Dale touches the tip of an electrically charged wand to a patient's wrist. The current from the wand stimulates nerve signals in the forearm that, according to one plausible explanation of the procedure's action, override pain signals sent to the brain by nerves in the head.

Classes in relaxation

The most common therapies practiced at headache clinics are those that teach patients how to relax. In one kind, called progressive relaxation *(right),* patients do physical exercises that teach them how muscles feel when tense or relaxed.

In biofeedback therapy *(below),* an instrument monitors an internal function, such as muscle tension, and emits sounds to signal high or low tension. By listening to the machine's feedback and noting the physical sensations associated with it, the patient can, with practice, learn to control muscle tension and thereby manage one cause of headache.

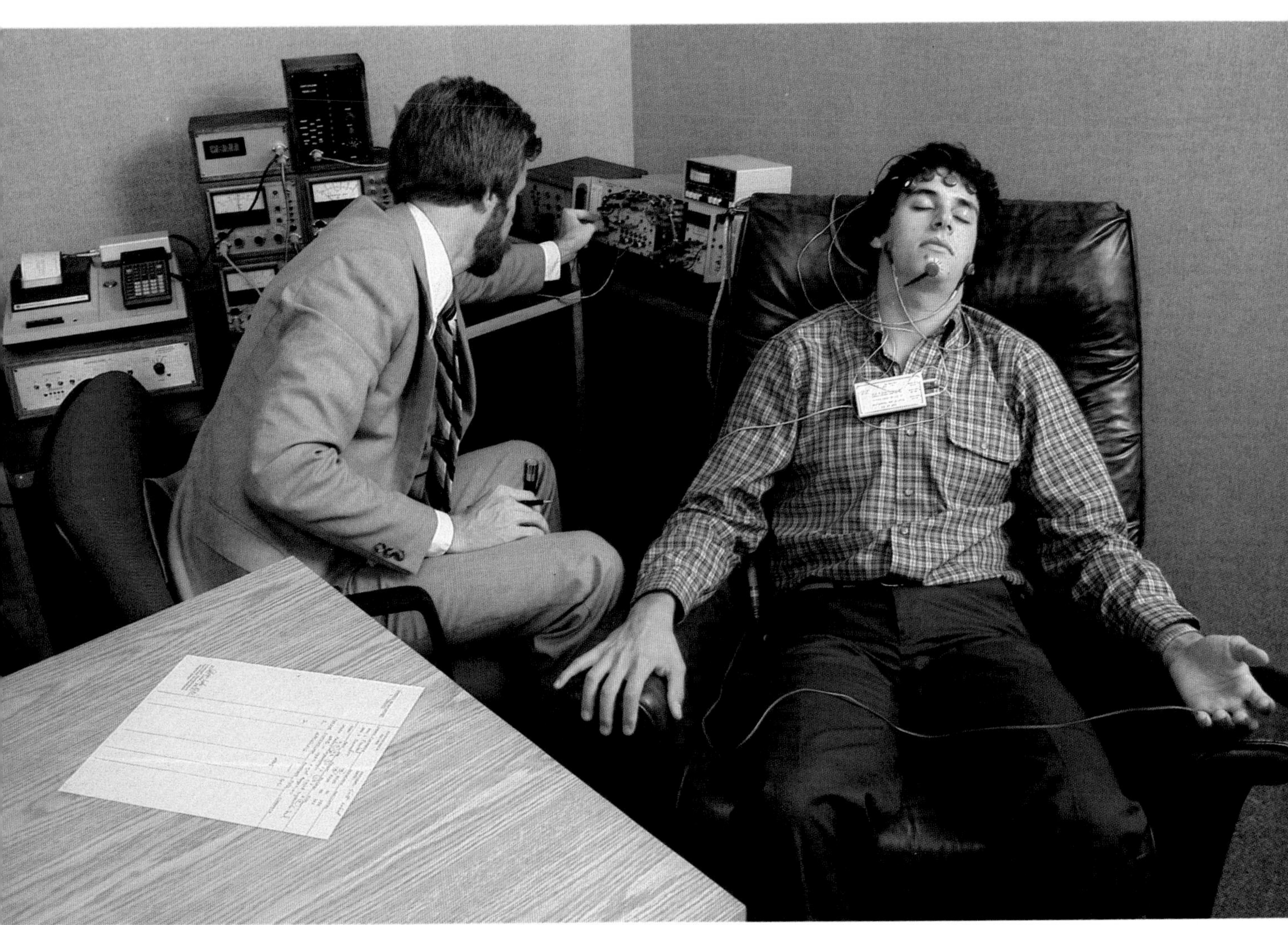

In a biofeedback session, psychologist Alvin E. Lake adjusts a device that measures muscle tension through sensors on the skin and emits a tone—the higher the tone, the greater the tension. The subject focuses on relaxing his muscles, lowering the tone.

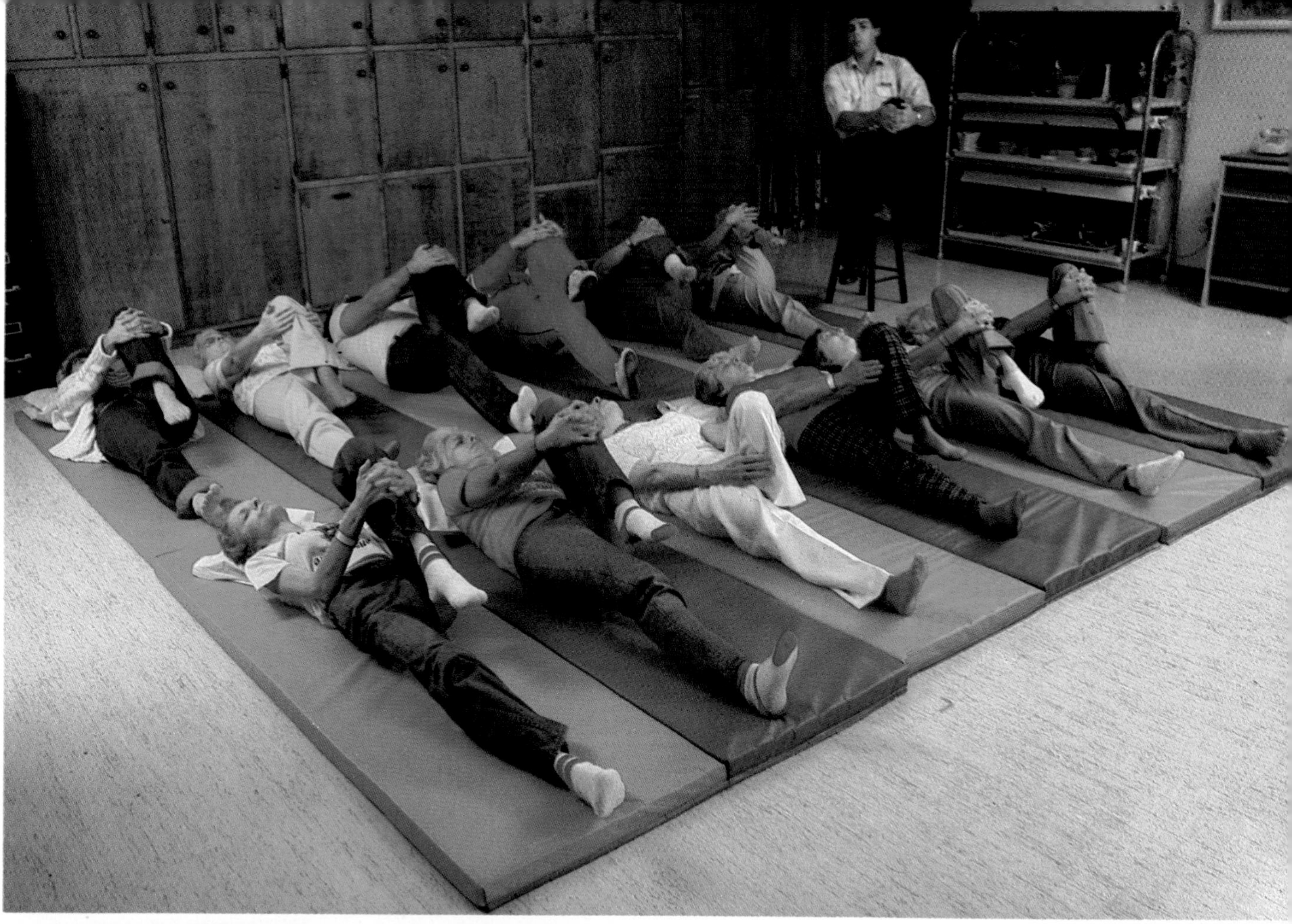

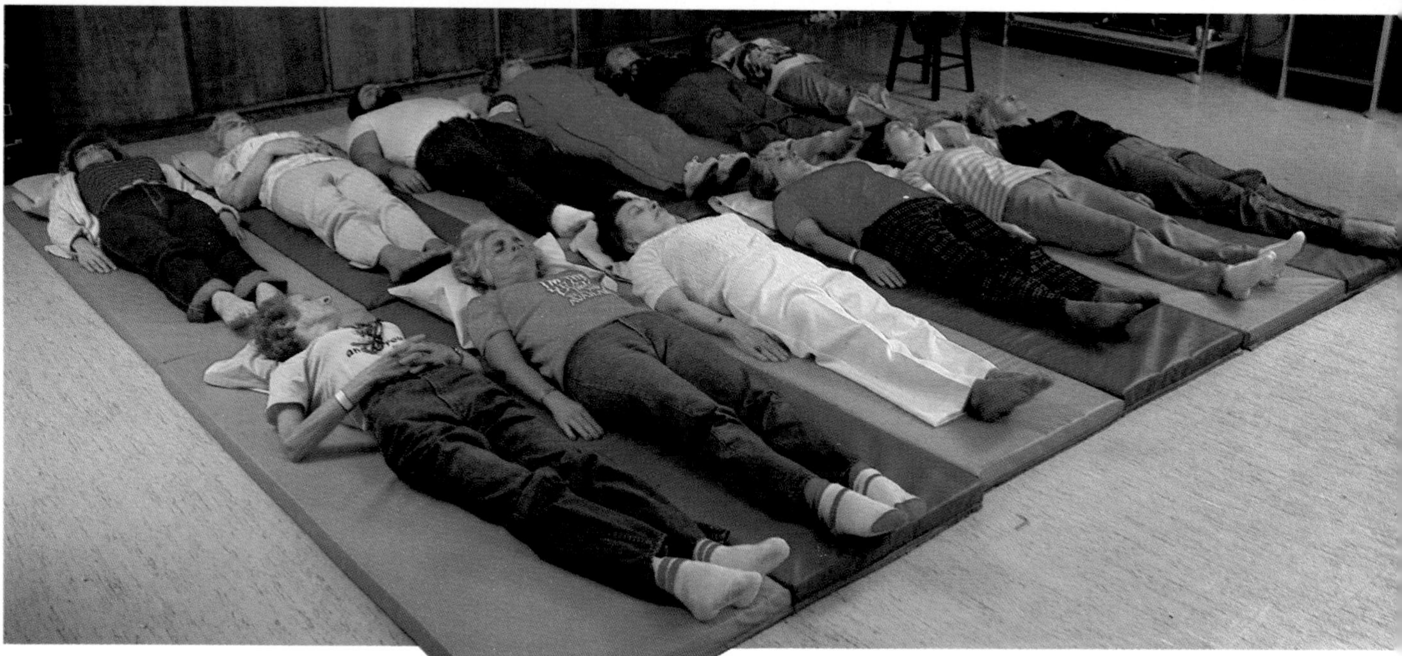

Recreational therapist Patrick Dolan leads headache patients in progressive relaxation. He instructs them first to draw their knees to their chest (top), tensing muscles in their legs and lower back, and then to relax totally (above).

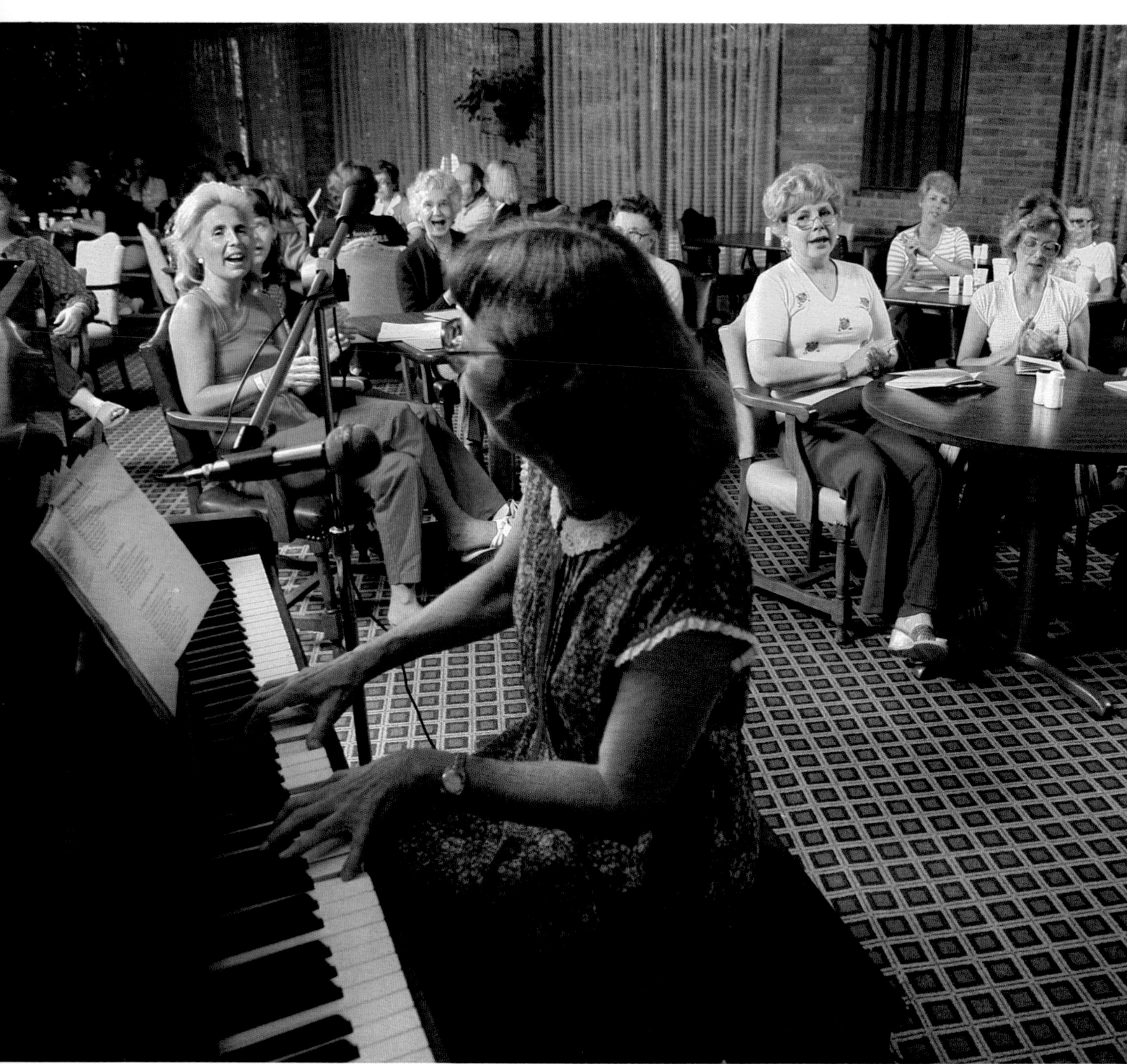

Headache patients assembled in a hospital dining room sing and clap along with piano music played by recreational therapist Alice Tite. Such activities help make normally tense people relax and laugh in spite of themselves.

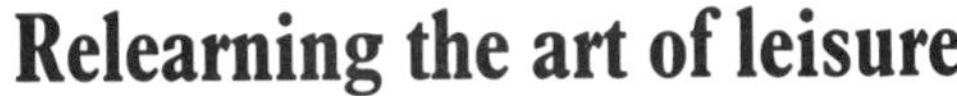

Relearning the art of leisure

Many clinic patients complain that they have lost the art of having fun. To this, headache specialists respond with activities ranging from bowling and bingo to crafts and songfests.

These pursuits have goals beyond recreation: "We try to get patients to focus on something outside their pain, since you can't focus on pain and an activity at the same time," explained Alice Tite, director of recreational therapy. After an hour of crafts or another project, she commented, many chronic sufferers tell her with amazement, "This is the first time I haven't been conscious of my headache."

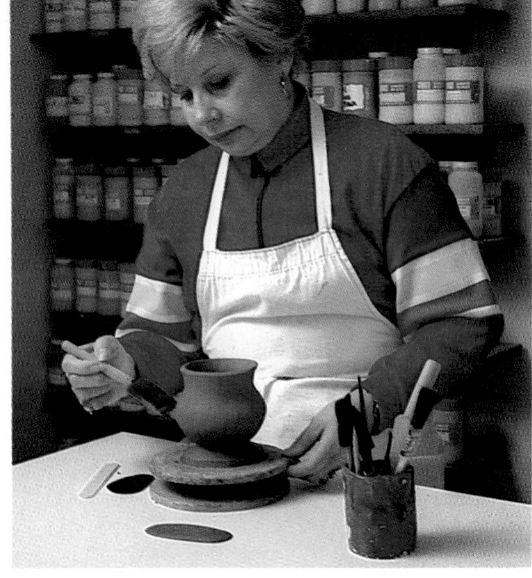

Headaches aside for now, a patient works on pottery.

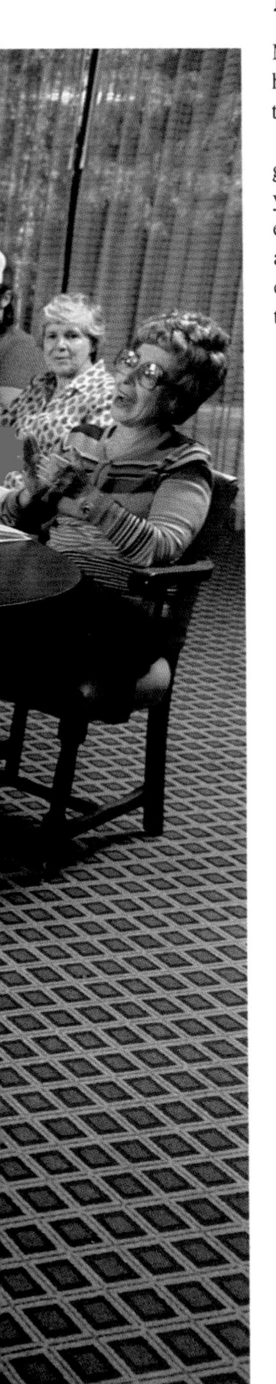

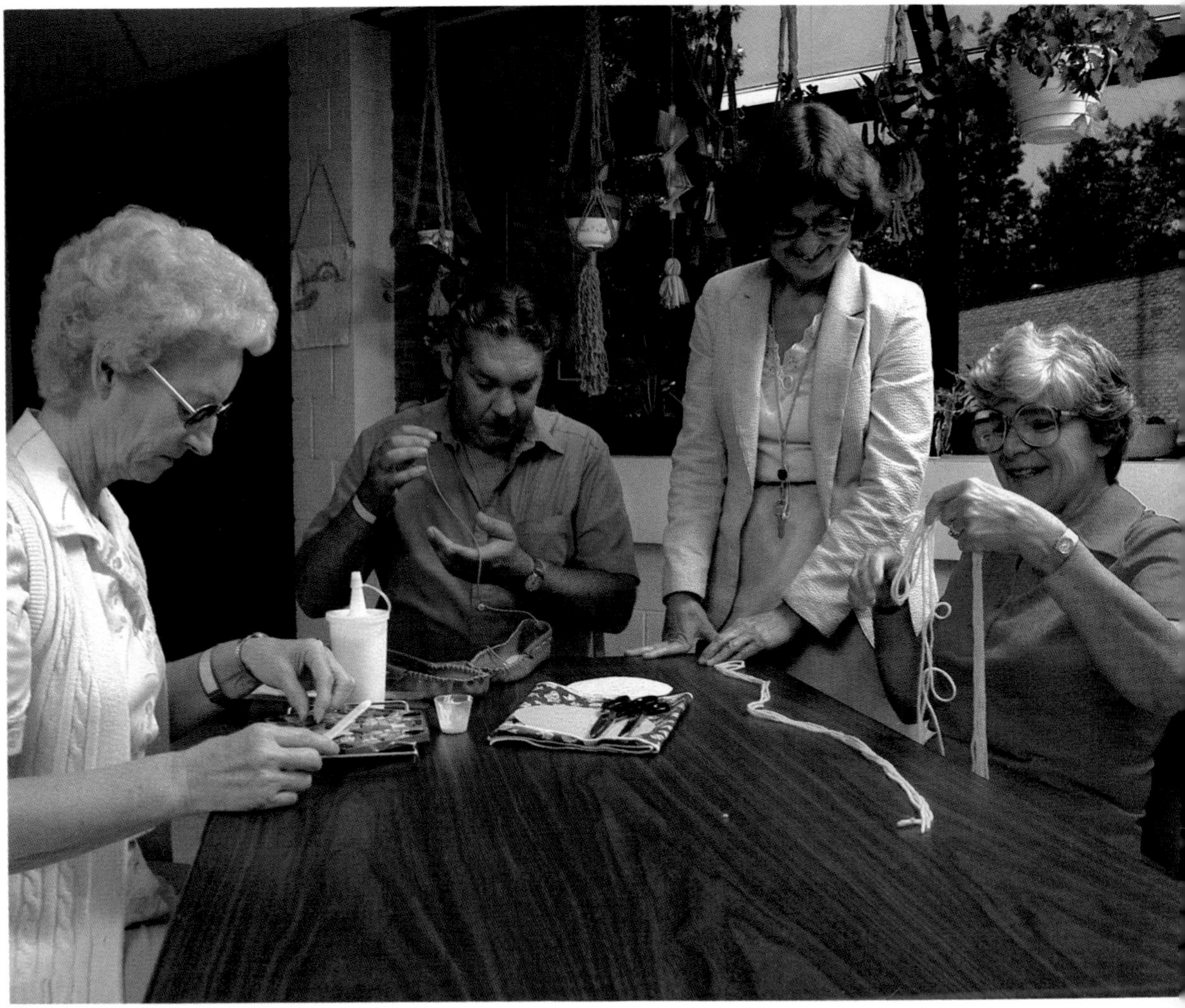

In a sunny therapy room, a woman makes a trivet of inlaid tile (left), a man laces leather moccasins and a third patient braids yarn into a spice-hanger—projects intended mainly to force them to concentrate on something besides pain.

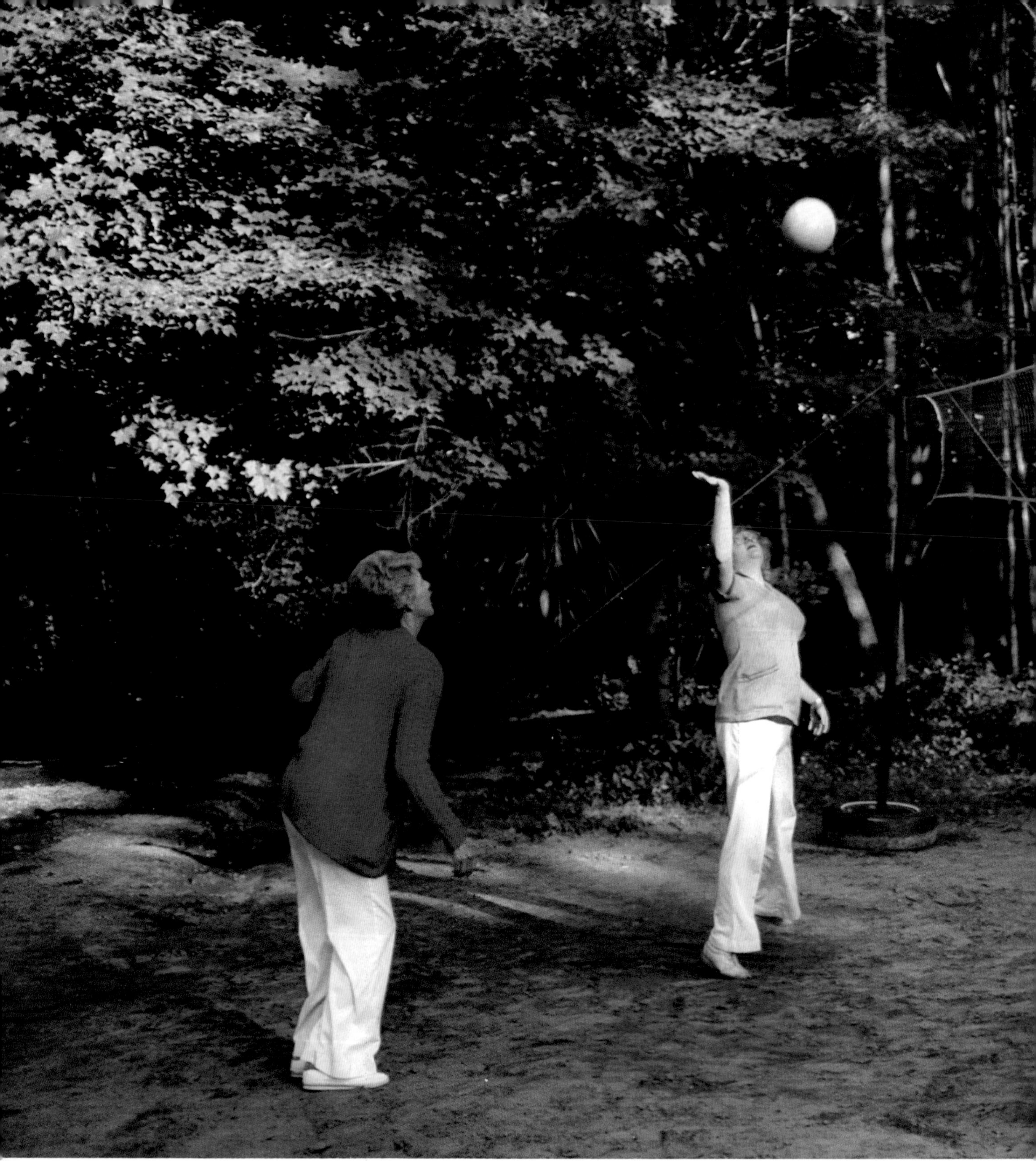

Patients join therapist Patrick Dolan (center) in an evening volleyball game. Such exercise helps prevent headaches because it releases nervous energy and muscle tension—and, said Dr. Saper, because it is fun. "We aren't running a 'headache camp' as some have affectionately called it," he said, "but still, medical care doesn't always necessarily have to be a serious business."

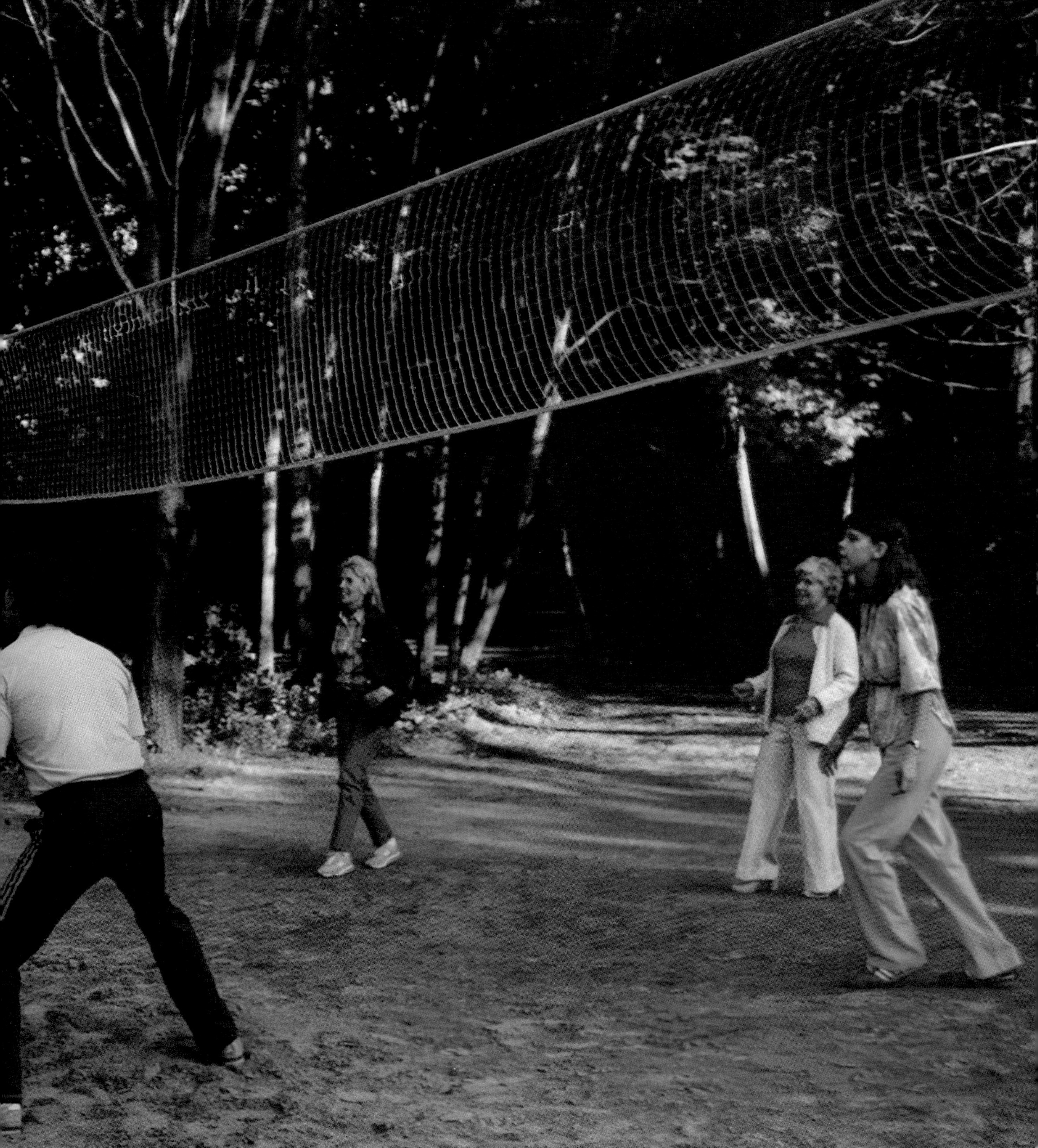

The remedies that work best

For most headaches, aspirin truly is, as its ubiquitous advertisements say, the drug doctors recommend most. But certain kinds of headaches demand different medicines. For some, a doctor may choose between a drug that attacks pain directly—a painkiller such as codeine—or one that addresses a possible source of the pain. The migraine drug methysergide, for example, inhibits the action of a nerve chemical, serotonin, thought to be involved in migraine attacks. For a muscle-tension headache, a doctor may recommend a painkiller, or a muscle relaxant and tranquilizer such as diazepam, or an antidepressant such as amitriptyline.

The table below, prepared with the assistance of Christopher S. Conner, Director of the Rocky Mountain Drug Consultation Center, shows the most frequently prescribed drugs effective for headache. They are listed by their generic chemical names, with asterisks designating those that contain more than one ingredient. The insignia Rx indicates that the drug requires a prescription.

When using these drugs, heed the following cautions. Pregnant women should consult a doctor before taking any drug. Drugs that cause drowsiness should not be mixed with alcohol or other depressants, nor should anyone taking such a drug drive or operate heavy machinery. See a physician if serious side effects appear: Sore throat, weakness, fever, unusual bruising or bleeding, or prolonged infection may indicate reduced blood counts; yellowing of the skin or of the whites of the eyes may suggest liver damage.

DRUG	Intended effect	Minor side effects	Serious side effects	Special cautions
ACETAMINOPHEN **DATRIL** **PHENAPHEN** **TYLENOL**	Relieves most common headaches as well as mild migraine	Dizziness; diarrhea; upset stomach	Liver damage or hepatitis; reduced white-blood-cell and platelet counts	Consult doctor before taking if you have liver disease. Overdose can cause liver damage, mainly in adults.
AMITRIPTYLINE (Rx) **ELAVIL** **ENDEP**	Prevents migraine	Drowsiness; dry mouth; dizziness; fatigue; headache	Blurred vision; chronic and severe constipation; difficulty urinating; irregular heartbeat; reduced white-blood-cell count; fainting; liver damage; convulsions	Consult doctor before taking if you have asthma, heart disease, high blood pressure, epilepsy, glaucoma, liver disease, or if you are recovering from a heart attack.
ASPIRIN	Relieves most common headaches as well as mild migraine	Upset stomach; ringing in the ears	Creation or activation of ulcers; allergic reactions, such as tightness in chest or wheezing; slowed blood clotting	Consult doctor before taking if you have peptic ulcer, liver disease, bleeding disorders, a history of allergies or asthma, or if you are taking drugs to prevent blood clots. Do not take tablets that smell like vinegar—odor indicates presence of acetic acid, a by-product of aspirin decomposition that can irritate the mouth or stomach. Stop taking a week before any surgery.
BUTALBITAL (Rx) **ANAPHEN*** **FIORINAL*** **FIORINAL with CODEINE***	Relieves mild migraine and muscle-tension headache when used in products that contain other pain relievers	Drowsiness; clumsiness; dizziness	Difficulty breathing; mental changes, such as confusion or excitement; liver damage; reduced white-blood-cell and platelet counts; slow heartbeat	Consult doctor before taking if you have lung or liver disease, or porphyria (a disorder of metabolism). Dependence may result with extended use.
CAFFEINE **CAFERGOT* (Rx)** **WIGRAINE* (Rx)**	Relieves migraine when used in products that contain ergotamine	Nausea; restlessness; insomnia	Rapid heartbeat; tremors	Consult doctor before taking if you have heart disease or high blood pressure.

* Combination drug. Refer also to other active ingredients on label.

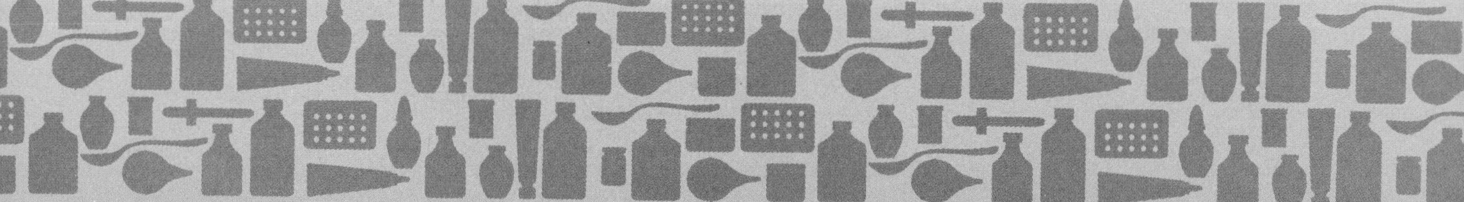

DRUG	Intended effect	Minor side effects	Serious side effects	Special cautions
CALCIUM CARBASPIRIN **CALURIN**	All effects similar to ASPIRIN			
CARBAMAZEPINE (Rx) **TEGRETOL**	Relieves pain of trigeminal neuralgia	Drowsiness; dizziness; nausea; vomiting; dry mouth; blurred vision	Reduced red- and white-blood-cell and platelet counts; severe skin rash; liver damage; kidney damage; confusion	Consult doctor before taking if you have liver or kidney disease, blood disorders, or are taking a drug to prevent blood clots.
CARISOPRODOL (Rx) **SOMA COMPOUND*** **SOMA COMPOUND with CODEINE***	Relieves muscle-tension headache when used in products that contain other pain relievers	Drowsiness; nausea; nervousness; headache	Severe dizziness or fainting; allergic reactions, such as skin rash, difficulty breathing, itching; mental or emotional change, such as depression or confusion; extreme weakness; temporary loss of limb control or vision	Consult doctor before taking if you have porphyria (a disorder of metabolism), or if you are allergic to meprobamate (a tranquilizer) or carbromal (a sedative).
CHOLINE MAGNESIUM TRISALICYLATE (Rx) **TRILISATE**	Relieves common, mild migraine and muscle-tension headache	Upset stomach; ringing in the ears	Severe nausea or vomiting; creation or activation of ulcers; hearing loss	Consult doctor before taking if you have a peptic ulcer. Notify doctor of persistent ringing in ears, headache or dizziness—signs of overdose. Risk of ulcers is increased if taken with alcohol or other drugs used for inflammation. Inform doctor of bloody or black, tarry stools—signs of stomach bleeding.
CHOLINE SALICYLATE **ARTHROPAN LIQUID**	All effects similar to CHOLINE MAGNESIUM TRISALICYLATE			
CLONIDINE (Rx) **CATAPRES**	Prevents migraine	Dry mouth and eyes; drowsiness; constipation; nausea; dizziness; light-headedness	Depression; nightmares; impotence; coldness of extremities; fluid retention and weight gain	Consult doctor before taking if you have kidney or heart disease, or if you have had a recent heart attack. Consult doctor before discontinuing this drug—severe increase in blood pressure can occur if this medicine is stopped abruptly. This drug can reduce the effects of levodopa, a drug used for Parkinson's disease.
CODEINE (Rx) **EMPIRIN with CODEINE*** **FIORINAL with CODEINE*** **TYLENOL with CODEINE***	Relieves migraine and muscle-tension headache	Constipation; appetite loss; upset stomach; drowsiness; dizziness; skin rash	Difficulty breathing; slow heartbeat; fainting	Consult doctor before taking if you have liver, lung or heart disease. Dependence may result with extended use.
CYPROHEPTADINE (Rx) **PERIACTIN**	Prevents migraine and cluster headache	Drowsiness; dizziness; dry mouth; constipation; difficulty urinating	Allergic reactions, such as skin rash or hives; delirium; confusion; hallucinations	Consult doctor before taking if you have glaucoma, high blood pressure, thyroid disease or urinary obstruction.

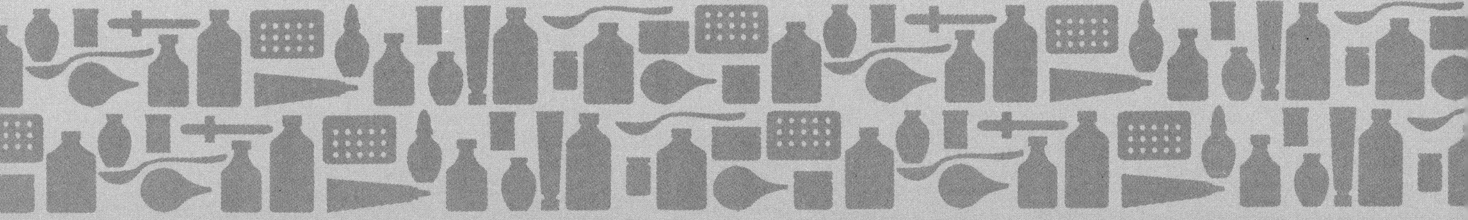

DRUG	Intended effect	Minor side effects	Serious side effects	Special cautions
DIAZEPAM (Rx) **VALIUM**	Relieves muscle-tension headache and mild migraine when used with other pain relievers	Drowsiness; slurred speech; weakness; clumsiness	Depression; excited or agitated behavior; confusion; liver damage; reduced white-blood-cell count; difficulty breathing	Dependence can result with extended use, even at recommended doses. Consult doctor before taking if you suffer from lung or liver disease. Consult doctor before discontinuing after extended use—withdrawal symptoms can occur. The effects of this drug are exaggerated when taken in combination with the ulcer drug cimetidine.
DIHYDROERGOTAMINE (Rx) **D.H.E. 45**	Relieves migraine and cluster headache	Tingling or coldness in hands or feet; nausea; dizziness; diarrhea; muscle pains	Chest pain; severely reduced blood flow to intestines, hands or feet	Consult doctor before taking if you have blood vessel disease, high blood pressure, heart disease, peptic ulcer, liver or kidney disease. Inform doctor of severe abdominal pain or persistent coldness or numbness of hands or feet—signs of reduced blood flow. Do not exceed 6 mg. in one day or 10 mg. in one week.
ERGOTAMINE (Rx) **BELLERGAL*** **CAFERGOT*** **ERGOMAR** **ERGOSTAT** **GYNERGEN** **WIGRAINE***	All effects similar to DIHYDROERGOTAMINE; Bellergal prevents migraine			
ETHOHEPTAZINE (Rx) **EQUAGESIC*** **ZACTIRIN***	Relieves muscle-tension headache and mild migraine	Nausea; vomiting; dizziness; drowsiness	None	Take with food or milk to lessen stomach upset.
HYDROMORPHONE (Rx) **DILAUDID**	Relieves migraine and severe muscle-tension headache	Constipation; dizziness; drowsiness; nausea; vomiting; appetite loss	Difficulty breathing; slow heartbeat; fainting	Consult doctor before taking if you have lung, liver or heart disease. Dependence may result with extended use.
IBUPROFEN (Rx) **MOTRIN**	Relieves tension headache	Diarrhea; nausea; dizziness; constipation; dry mouth	Ringing in the ears; severe fluid retention; creation or activation of stomach ulcer; impaired vision; severe skin rash; reduced platelet and white-blood-cell counts; kidney damage	Consult doctor before taking if you have ulcers or have had unusual reactions to aspirin or other drugs used to treat inflammation. Take with milk or food to lessen stomach upset. Inform doctor of bloody or black, tarry stools—signs of bleeding from the stomach. Inform doctor of swelling of the legs or feet—signs of excess fluid retention. Inform doctor of pain during urination or of blood in the urine.
IMIPRAMINE (Rx) **TOFRANIL**	All effects similar to AMITRIPTYLINE			
INDOMETHACIN (Rx) **INDOCIN**	Prevents cluster headache	Headache; nausea; vomiting; dizziness; ringing in the ears	Stomach ulcers and bleeding; damage to the cornea and retina with prolonged use; fluid retention; liver damage; reduced blood-cell counts	Consult doctor before taking if you have liver disease, ulcers or other stomach problems, or if you are taking drugs to prevent blood clots. Take with food or milk to decrease stomach upset. Notify doctor of blurred vision during prolonged use—a sign of eye damage. Inform doctor of bloody or black, tarry stools—signs of stomach bleeding. Risk of ulcers is increased if drug is taken with alcohol, or with aspirin or other drugs used for inflammation.

* Combination drug. Refer also to other active ingredients on label.

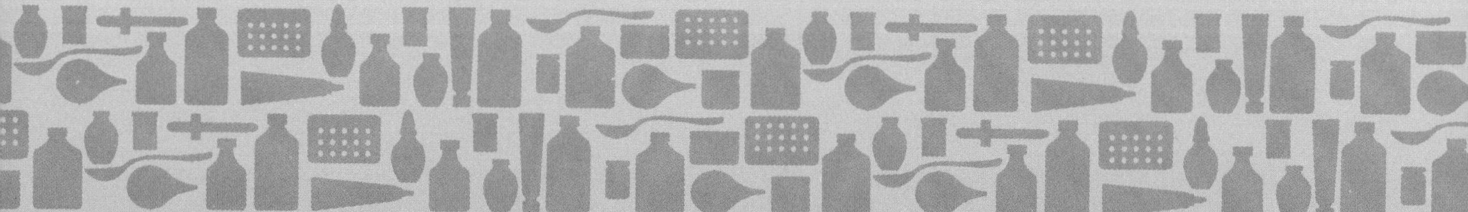

DRUG	Intended effect	Minor side effects	Serious side effects	Special cautions
ISOCARBOXAZID (Rx) **MARPLAN**	Prevents migraine	Dry mouth; dizziness; constipation; drowsiness; tiredness; weakness	Fainting; tremors; rapid heartbeat; liver damage; persistent diarrhea; swelling of legs or feet	This drug interacts with many other medicines—consult doctor before taking in combination with any other drug. Consult doctor before taking if you suffer from any of the following: diabetes, high blood pressure or heart, kidney, thyroid or liver disease. Avoid foods or beverages containing tyramine, such as cheeses, yogurt, raisins, sour cream, bananas, beer and wine—severe increases in blood pressure can result. Avoid other medicines and foods or beverages containing tyramine for at least two weeks after discontinuing this medication—severe blood pressure elevation can result. Avoid large amounts of caffeine-containing beverages, such as coffee, tea and colas—high blood pressure can result. Inform doctor of severe chest pain, headaches, nausea, vomiting or fever—signs of increased blood pressure. Prior to any type of surgery—including dental surgery—inform doctor you are taking this medicine.
ISOMETHEPTENE (Rx) **MIDRIN***	Relieves migraine and cluster headache	Dizziness; insomnia; nausea; vomiting; drowsiness	Disturbed heartbeat; weakness	Consult doctor before taking if you have glaucoma, high blood pressure or kidney, liver or heart disease.
LITHIUM (Rx) **ESKALITH** **LITHANE** **LITHONATE**	Prevents cluster headache	Increased thirst; diarrhea; dry mouth	Nausea; vomiting; drowsiness; confusion; weakness; tremors; slurred speech; seizures; thyroid dysfunction	Consult doctor before taking if you suffer from any of the following disorders: heart disease, epilepsy, Parkinson's disease or kidney disease. Drink plenty of water while taking this drug (consume at least two quarts daily). Avoid strenuous exercise in hot weather. Take with food or milk to decrease the likelihood of stomach upset. Inform doctor of dry or puffy skin or of unusual tiredness or weight gain—signs of thyroid gland dysfunction. The effects of this drug can be decreased by large amounts of salt or by stomach remedies containing sodium bicarbonate. The side effects of this drug can be increased by diuretics—drugs that promote fluid loss and lower blood pressure.
MEPERIDINE (Rx) **DEMEROL** **MEPERGAN FORTIS***	Relieves migraine and muscle-tension headache	Constipation; dizziness; drowsiness; nausea; vomiting; appetite loss	Difficulty breathing; slow heartbeat; fainting	Consult doctor before taking if you suffer from any of the following: lung, liver or heart disease. Avoid use with monoamine oxidase (MAO) inhibitors, used to treat depression—severe reactions can occur, such as sharp increases in blood pressure. Dependence may result with extended use.
MEPROBAMATE (Rx) **EQUAGESIC***	Relieves muscle-tension headache and mild migraine when used in products that contain other pain relievers	Drowsiness; dizziness; nausea; slurred speech	Confusion; reduced white-blood-cell and platelet counts; excitement; difficulty breathing; heart irregularities, including slow or irregular heartbeat	Consult doctor before taking if you have liver disease. Dependence may result with extended use. Consult doctor before discontinuing this drug after extended use—withdrawal symptoms can occur, including agitation and seizures.

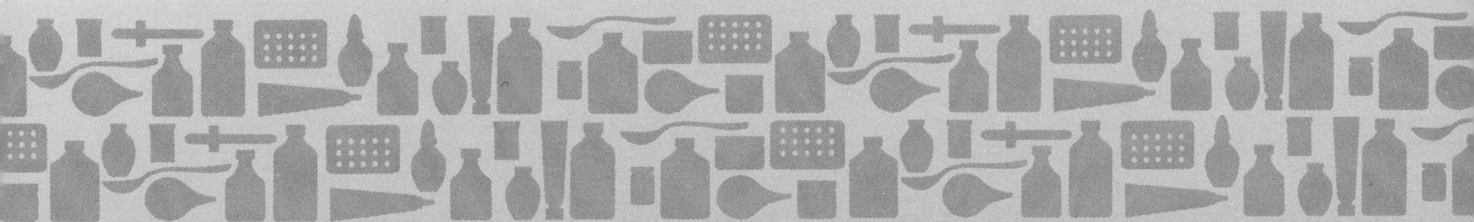

DRUG	Intended effect	Minor side effects	Serious side effects	Special cautions
METHYSERGIDE (Rx) **SANSERT**	Prevents migraine and cluster headache	Nausea; vomiting; weight gain; abdominal cramps; tingling or coldness of hands or feet	Abnormal tissue growth, primarily in the abdominal and pelvic areas; severely reduced blood flow to intestines, hands or feet; hallucinations; depression; chest pain	Consult doctor before taking if you suffer from any of the following disorders: blood vessel disease, high blood pressure, heart disease, peptic ulcer, liver or kidney disease, lung disease or arthritis. Inform doctor promptly if you experience severe abdominal pain or persistent coldness or numbness of hands or feet—signs of reduced blood flow. Inform doctor promptly if you experience chest pain, pain on urination, difficulty breathing, or kidney pain—signs of abnormal tissue growth.
METOCLOPRAMIDE (Rx) **REGLAN**	Prevents migraine	Drowsiness; constipation; dry mouth; nausea	Skin rash; muscle spasms; tremors or twitching; abnormal or uncontrolled body movements	Consult doctor before taking if you have epilepsy or Parkinson's disease.
ORPHENADRINE (Rx) **NORGESIC*** **NORGESIC FORTE***	Relieves muscle-tension headache and mild migraine when used in products that contain other pain relievers	Dry mouth; drowsiness; dizziness; nausea	Allergic reactions, such as skin rash or itching; fainting; confusion; rapid heartbeat	Consult doctor before taking if you have glaucoma, heart disease, ulcers, or urinary or intestinal obstruction.
OXYCODONE (Rx) **PERCOCET-5*** **PERCODAN*** **TYLOX***	Relieves migraine and severe muscle-tension headache	Drowsiness; constipation; dizziness; upset stomach	Shortness of breath; slow heartbeat	Consult doctor before taking if you suffer from any of the following disorders: liver, heart or lung disease. Dependence may result with extended use.
PENTAZOCINE (Rx) **TALWIN**	Relieves migraine and severe muscle-tension headache	Drowsiness; nausea; dizziness; constipation	Hallucinations; confusion; difficulty breathing	Consult doctor before taking if you suffer from any of the following disorders: epilepsy or liver, kidney, heart, prostate or lung disease, or if you have had a recent head injury. Dependence can result with extended use.
PENTOBARBITAL (Rx) **CAFERGOT P-B***	Relieves migraine when used in combination products that contain ergotamine	Drowsiness; clumsiness; dizziness	Difficulty breathing; liver damage; reduced white-blood-cell and platelet counts; slow heartbeat; mental or emotional changes, including confusion and excitement	Consult doctor before taking if you have porphyria (a disorder of metabolism) or lung or liver disease. Dependence may result with extended use. Do not discontinue abruptly after extended use—withdrawal symptoms, such as agitation and seizures, may occur.
PHENELZINE (Rx) **NARDIL**	All effects similar to ISOCARBOXAZID			
PHENOBARBITAL (Rx) **BELLERGAL***	All effects similar to PENTOBARBITAL			
PHENYLTOLOXAMINE **PERCOGESIC*** **PERCOGESIC with CODEINE* (Rx)**	Relieves muscle-tension headache and mild migraine when used in products that contain other pain relievers	Drowsiness; dizziness; dry mouth; blurred vision; difficulty urinating	Rapid heartbeat; confusion; delirium	Consult doctor before taking if you have glaucoma, heart disease, high blood pressure, or urinary or intestinal obstruction.

* Combination drug. Refer also to other active ingredients on label.

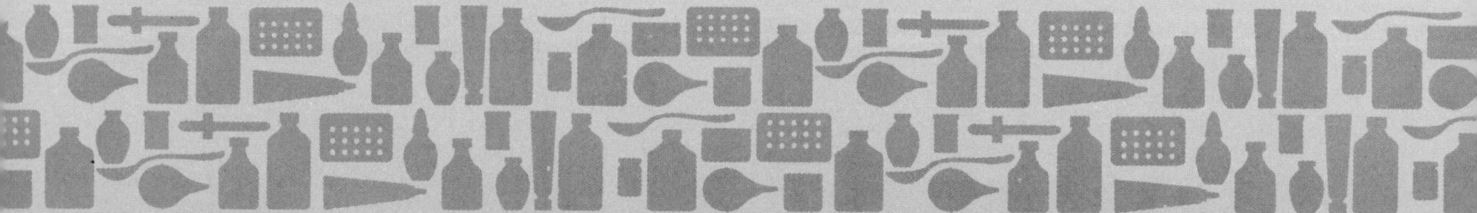

DRUG	Intended effect	Minor side effects	Serious side effects	Special cautions
PREDNISONE (Rx) **DELTASONE** **ORASONE** **PARACORT**	Prevents cluster headache; relieves migraine	Nausea; indigestion; menstrual irregularities; weight gain; insomnia; nervousness; muscle cramps	Mental or emotional disturbances; potassium loss; bone disease; peptic ulcer; increased glucose levels in blood—diabetes; inflammation of the pancreas—pancreatitis; increased pressure inside the eye—glaucoma; high blood pressure; impaired immune response	Consult doctor before taking if you are taking digoxin or digitoxin, drugs that control heartbeat—the combination may increase risk of irregular heartbeat. Consult doctor before taking if you suffer from any of the following disorders: heart disease, diabetes mellitus, fungus infections, peptic ulcer or tuberculosis. Take with food or milk to lessen stomach upset. Inform doctor of bloody or black, tarry stools—signs of stomach bleeding. Inform doctor of persistent muscle cramps or unusual tiredness—signs of potassium loss. Do not discontinue abruptly after prolonged use—withdrawal reactions can occur, such as fever, weakness and dangerous decreases in blood pressure. Do not submit to any vaccinations or skin tests without consulting your doctor. Risk of ulcers is increased when this drug is taken with alcohol, or with aspirin or other drugs used for inflammation. May interfere with drugs used to prevent blood clots or to treat diabetes.
PROPOXYPHENE (Rx) **DARVOCET-N*** **DARVON** **DARVON COMPOUND-65*** **DARVON-N**	Relieves mild migraine and muscle-tension headache	Drowsiness; dizziness; nausea; constipation	Confusion; difficulty breathing; liver damage	Consult doctor before taking if you have liver disease. Dependence may result with extended use.
PROPRANOLOL (Rx) **INDERAL**	Prevents migraine and cluster headache	Dizziness; nausea; diarrhea; tiredness; cold hands and feet; dry mouth	Decreased blood pressure; mental confusion; difficulty breathing; reduced heart rate; reduced platelet and white-blood-cell counts; severe depression; increased risk of bronchial asthma; possible congestive heart failure	Consult doctor before taking if you have allergies or asthma, diabetes, emphysema or liver disease. Inform doctor of persistent dizziness or lightheadedness—signs of low blood pressure. May produce excessive increases in blood pressure when taken with monoamine oxidase (MAO) inhibitors, used to treat depression. Do not discontinue this drug abruptly—risk of heart complications increases.
SALSALATE (Rx) **ARCYLATE** **DISALCID**	All effects similar to ASPIRIN			
SODIUM SALICYLATE **URACEL**	All effects similar to CHOLINE MAGNESIUM TRISALICYLATE			
TRIAMCINOLONE (Rx) **ARISTOCORT** **KENACORT**	All effects similar to PREDNISONE			
ZOMEPIRAC (Rx) **ZOMAX**	Relieves muscle-tension headache	Headache; upset stomach (nausea); dizziness; diarrhea; drowsiness	None	None

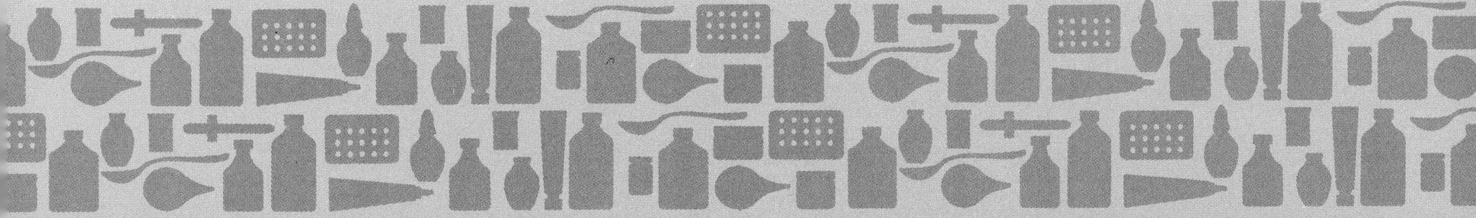

An encyclopedia of symptoms

Headaches are of so many types and arise from so many different causes that telling one from another can be crucial to treatment. Some remedies for the common tension headache, for instance, are likely to make the other common type—vascular—feel worse. Even more important, headaches are sometimes only a by-product of serious illness or injury. In such cases, recognizing distinctions among types of headaches can be vital.

The headache types and the diseases or injuries for which headaches may be a symptom are described below, listed alphabetically by conditions that can be felt or seen. The disorder associated with each symptom—or each group of symptoms—is named in small capital letters. These descriptions are simplified; if you have any doubt about any symptom you encounter, consult a doctor.

ABDOMINAL PAIN. Most stomach-aches are short-lived and are related to minor dietary indiscretions. Head pain is associated with abdominal pain only in certain conditions.

- **Abdominal pain that is accompanied by throbbing pain on one side of the head** may be a sign of either CLASSIC or COMMON MIGRAINE (see HEAD PAIN). The abdominal pain is frequently associated with nausea and vomiting, and with an extreme sensitivity to light and sound.
- **Abdominal pain that is not accompanied by throbbing head pain** but that strikes a victim of either CLASSIC or COMMON MIGRAINE may suggest MIGRAINE EQUIVALENTS—symptoms of MIGRAINE encountered without the head pain. The abdominal pain may be accompanied by nausea, vomiting or diarrhea. Some people experience dizziness or an increased heart rate.
- **Abdominal pain that comes and goes and is associated with frequent or continuous head pain** may be a sign of DEPRESSION. Other symptoms include sleeplessness, fatigue and constipation. Consult a physician if any of these problems recur frequently.

APPETITE LOSS. A temporary loss of appetite is seldom a matter for much concern, but it can be a symptom of more serious medical conditions, including CANCER, and it sometimes accompanies certain headaches.

If loss of appetite is accompanied by throbbing pain on one side of the head, the cause may be either CLASSIC or COMMON MIGRAINE (see HEAD PAIN). Other symptoms include nausea, vomiting and abdominal pain. Appetite usually returns to normal within a day after the head pain passes. Consult a physician.

If appetite loss is associated with frequent or continuous head pain, the cause may be DEPRESSION. Other symptoms may include sleeplessness, fatigue and constipation. Consult a physician if such symptoms are persistent.

BEHAVIOR CHANGES. Behavior changes, either subtle or dramatic, can include confusion, decreased alertness, clumsiness, memory loss and dramatic mood swings. Some temporary behavior changes associated with headaches accompany migraine attacks, but others may signal the presence of serious conditions requiring prompt medical attention.

- **Behavior changes that are accompanied by head pain** not associated with migraine may be symptoms of dangerous injury to the brain or skull.

If behavior changes and head pain occur suddenly and are associated with a feeling of weakness or with paralysis, the cause may be either a TRANSIENT ISCHEMIC ATTACK (TIA), a temporary reduction in blood flow to the brain; or a STROKE, a complete blockage of blood flow to part of the brain. Get medical attention immediately.

If behavior changes and severe head pain occur suddenly and are associated with drowsiness, nausea or vomiting, the cause may be SUBARACHNOID HEMORRHAGE, bleeding around the brain, or INTRACRANIAL HEMORRHAGE, bleeding within the brain. Get medical attention immediately.

If behavior changes and head pain occur after a head injury and are associated with dizziness or convulsions, the cause may be either a SUBDURAL or an EPIDURAL HEMATOMA, varieties of blood clots on the brain. Get medical attention immediately.

If behavior changes and head pain occur after a head injury, the cause may be CONCUSSION, a sudden temporary loss of consciousness following a blow to the head; or a SKULL FRACTURE, broken bones surrounding the brain. Other symptoms include nausea, vomiting, drowsiness and dizziness. Get in touch with a physician immediately.

- **Behavior changes in a person having persistent or recurrent head pain** may indicate a BRAIN TUMOR, an abnormal growth in the brain. Consult a physician promptly.
- **Behavior changes** can sometimes accompany or precede an attack of MIGRAINE (see HEAD PAIN).

If behavior changes come on suddenly, last for less than 30 minutes, and are followed by throbbing pain on one side of the head, the cause may be CLASSIC MIGRAINE. Other symptoms of this disorder include temporary vision or language disturbances, and numbness and tingling of the hands. Consult a physician if the changes persist.

If behavior changes develop gradually for a day or so and are then followed by throbbing pain on one side of the head, the cause may be COMMON MIGRAINE. There can also be weight gain, swelling or irritability. Consult a physician.

CONVULSIONS. Convulsions can range from a brief period of staring into space to a severe shaking episode with uncontrolled muscle movements and loss of consciousness. They are caused by electrical surges in the brain and can be brought on by withdrawal from alcohol; by EPILEPSY, a condition of generally unknown origin that produces recurrent seizures; by BRAIN TUMORS, abnormal growths in the brain; or by BRAIN INFECTIONS. Head pain, confusion and drowsiness are often present after recovery from a convulsion. Consult a physician promptly.

DIZZINESS. Unless it occurs after an injury, occasional dizziness accompanying headache is seldom a sign of anything serious. The feeling generally passes quickly; sit down and bend forward at the waist until it does.

• **Dizziness and steady aching head pain after an injury** may indicate that harm has been done to the neck, skull or brain; such a pain should not ignored.

If dizziness and head pain follow a neck injury and are associated with a stiff neck, nausea or blurred vision, the cause may be a CERVICAL STRAIN, a stretching or tearing of the muscles of the neck. Such "whiplash" injuries are often caused by rear-end automobile collisions. Consult a physician promptly.

If dizziness and head pain occur after a head injury, the cause may be CONCUSSION, a sudden temporary loss of consciousness following a blow to the head; or a SKULL FRACTURE, broken bones surrounding the brain. Other symptoms of these conditions include nausea, vomiting, drowsiness and behavior changes. Consult a physician immediately.

If dizziness and head pain occur after a head injury and are associated with drowsiness, behavior changes or convulsions, the cause may be a SUBDURAL or an EPIDURAL HEMATOMA, varieties of blood clots on the brain. Get medical attention immediately.

• **Dizziness and head pain unconnected with injury** have a variety of causes.

If dizziness and severe head pain occur in association with drowsiness, nausea or vomiting, the cause may be SUBARACHNOID HEMORRHAGE, bleeding around the brain; or INTRACRANIAL HEMORRHAGE, bleeding within the brain. This is an emergency: Get medical attention immediately.

If dizziness and throbbing head pain occur with nausea and vomiting, the cause may be CLASSIC or COMMON MIGRAINE (see HEAD PAIN). Consult a physician.

If dizziness and throbbing head pain are associated with sweating and a tightness or burning in the chest or face, the cause may be CHINESE-RESTAURANT SYNDROME, a reaction to monosodium glutamate (MSG), a seasoning used in Oriental cooking and in some canned, powdered and frozen foods. Symptoms usually begin 15 to 30 minutes after eating foods containing MSG and usually pass within an hour. The only treatment is avoidance of MSG—check labels on prepared-food packages and insist on MSG-free dishes in Oriental restaurants.

If dizziness and throbbing head pain are associated with upset stomach, thirst, fatigue and recent consumption of alcoholic beverages, the cause may be HANGOVER. Rest, relax, take aspirin and drink beverages containing caffeine.

• **Dizziness that is accompanied by steady, aching head pain or tightness in the head** may be due to TENSION HEADACHE (see HEAD PAIN). Dizziness usually is mild and is sometimes described as a "swimming" feeling. Lie down, relax and take aspirin.

DROWSINESS. If drowsiness is accompanied by head pain, a serious problem may exist. Get medical treatment promptly.

• **Drowsiness and head pain that are associated with behavior changes, dizziness or convulsions** may indicate EPIDURAL or SUBDURAL HEMATOMA, types of blood clots on the brain; or the presence of a BRAIN TUMOR, an abnormal growth in the brain. Consult a physician immediately.

EAR PAIN. Ear pain may be caused by wax in the ear or by an ear infection, but when it also is accompanied by headaches it may suggest a disorder that is not in the ear itself. Sometimes it indicates a dental problem or trouble with the sinuses or jaw joint. For any persistent pain in the ear, consult a physician.

• **Ear pain that is accompanied by pain or tenderness localized at the front of the head or face,** and that is associated with fever or nasal discharge, may be evidence of SINUSITIS, an infection of the sinuses. Apply warm, wet compresses to the face and take aspirin if the symptoms are mild. Consult a physician if pain is severe or if fever persists.

• **Ear pain that occurs suddenly and strikes right in front of the ear,** at the outer edge of the cheek, may be a sign of TEMPOROMANDIBULAR JOINT SYNDROME (TMJ), a misalignment of the jaw joint. The cause usually is improper alignment of the teeth or bite. If pain is persistent, consult a dentist specializing in TMJ.

EYE PAIN. Pain in the eyes most often is caused by an irritating object or substance that gets into the eye, but it may also be connected with a headache.

Pain that is deep in the eye or behind it may indicate EYESTRAIN, a headache-causing eye-muscle imbalance that eyeglasses normally can correct. Or it may signal GLAUCOMA, a disease marked by increased pressure in the eye. Consult a physician.

If pain around or behind one eye occurs with redness and watering, and with a clogged nostril and flushed skin on the same side of the face as the eye pain, it may indicate the very painful CLUSTER HEADACHE (see HEAD PAIN). Attacks occur suddenly, often at night, and produce a severe stabbing or burning pain that lasts about 30 minutes. Consult a physician.

FACIAL PAIN. Several face pains, which may be agonizing and difficult to treat, are associated with headaches.

- **Facial pain that is confined to one side of the face**—usually in the cheek, chin, gum or forehead—and that is of a burning or stabbing variety may indicate TRIGEMINAL NEURALGIA, unusual sensitivity in a facial nerve. The condition sometimes is called TIC DOULOUREUX. Such pain usually occurs suddenly, continues for a few seconds or several minutes and frequently is triggered by a touch to the face or gum. When it strikes, the pain is often severe. Facial muscle spasms occasionally accompany this pain. Consult a physician.
- **Facial pain that occurs suddenly in the upper face or around the eye** and that is accompanied by a red or tearful eye, or by a clogged nostril and flushed skin on the same side as the pain, may indicate CLUSTER HEADACHE. The pain, often described as a burning, boring or stabbing feeling, usually starts near or behind the eye, or in the temple or forehead. Attacks often begin at night, recur at the same time each day for several weeks and last for about 30 minutes. Consult a physician.
- **Facial pain in the forehead, nose or ears that occurs suddenly after the eating or drinking of cold food** may indicate ICE CREAM HEADACHE, caused by sensitivity of nerves in the back of the mouth and throat to cold. Pain is usually intense but brief, and it may affect the mouth and throat as well. To avoid this condition, eat cold foods only in small portions and allow them to warm slightly at the front of the mouth.
- **Facial pain, swelling and tenderness over the forehead, nose or cheek** that is accompanied by fever and nasal discharge may indicate SINUSITIS, an infection of the sinuses. Apply warm, wet compresses to the face and take aspirin if symptoms are mild. Consult a physician if pain is severe or if fever persists.

FATIGUE. This condition is often accompanied by head pain. It can indicate such disorders as INFLUENZA or INFECTIOUS MONONUCLEOSIS, two viral infections; or a chronic illness such as ANEMIA, too few red blood cells or lack of iron in the blood; or CANCER. Consult a physician if fatigue is accompanied by persistent fever or pale skin, or if it has no ready explanation.

- **Persistent fatigue can be a sign of** DEPRESSION, a chronic state of poor mental health, sometimes caused by chemical imbalances in the brain. Other symptoms include frequent or continuous head pain, difficulty sleeping, abdominal pain, constipation, loss of appetite and a gloomy outlook on life. Consult a physician if any of these symptoms are persistent or if they interfere with daily life.
- **Fatigue that follows the consumption of alcoholic beverages and is accompanied by throbbing head pain,** an upset stomach, malaise or thirst may suggest HANGOVER. Rest, relax, take aspirin and drink beverages that contain caffeine.

FEVER. For mild fever and head pain, rest, drink plenty of liquids and take aspirin.

- **If fever and head pain are accompanied by stiff neck, difficulty breathing or a cough that produces thick mucus,** PNEUMONIA might be the problem. Consult a physician.
- **Fever that occurs in an old person and is accompanied by sharp head pain, scalp tenderness or burning** may be a symptom of TEMPORAL ARTERITIS, an inflammation of blood vessels in the scalp. Consult a physician.

HEAD PAIN. Probably the best way to identify headache cause is by precise location of the pain or of accompanying aches (see EAR PAIN, EYE PAIN, FACIAL PAIN, JAW PAIN, NECK PAIN, SINUS PAIN). For example, an otherwise mysterious headache is likely to be a result of sinus infection if there is also pain in an ear. However, many common head pains are not so easily located, and the cause of the pain must be recognized by its characteristic sensations and by the other symptoms that occur with it.

- **Steady, dull, aching head pain, either generalized or localized,** normally suggests TENSION HEADACHE, produced by prolonged contraction of the neck, scalp or face muscles. This is the most common cause of head pain. Pain may be felt in the forehead, at the back of the head or neck, at the temples, on one or both sides of the head, or all the way around the head at the level of the hatband. The pain often is described as a squeezing pressure or tightness. For occasional symptoms, rest, relax and take aspirin. Heat, gentle massage and stretching exercises may also help.
- **Sharp, severe pain that is centered around one red, tearful eye and that is associated with a clogged nostril and flushed skin on that side of the face** may suggest CLUSTER HEADACHE. This condition usually afflicts adult males, occasionally awakening them from sleep. Consult a physician.

• **Dull pain in the face, nose, mouth or throat that occurs after consuming cold food or drink** may suggest ICE CREAM HEADACHE, caused by sensitivity of nerves in the mouth and throat to cold. Pain may travel to the top of the head or to the ears. Consume any cold food or drink in small portions, and allow it to warm slightly at the front of the mouth.

• **Throbbing pain localized at one side of the head** may indicate one of the two forms of MIGRAINE.

If throbbing one-sided head pain is accompanied by nausea and vomiting and sensitivity to light and noise, the cause may be COMMON MIGRAINE, in which blood vessels in the scalp dilate. (In a minority of cases, the pain affects both sides of the head.) Consult a physician so that treatment can be started.

If throbbing, one-sided head pain is preceded by a 15- to 30-minute period of unusual visual disturbances, language disturbances or other unsettling sensations such as tingling or numbness of the hands, the cause may be CLASSIC MIGRAINE, a condition in which blood vessels first narrow, then dilate to cause pain. Additional associated symptoms are the same as those that accompany COMMON MIGRAINE—nausea and vomiting and sensitivity to light and sound. Consult a physician so that a treatment program can be started.

• **Throbbing pain over the temples and a tightness around the forehead** that occurs shortly after eating certain foods may suggest CHINESE-RESTAURANT SYNDROME, a reaction to monosodium glutamate (MSG). This seasoning is found in Oriental foods and also in many canned, powdered or frozen foods. Associated symptoms are dizziness or a tight feeling across the chest. Avoid foods containing MSG.

• **Throbbing head pain that is either localized or generalized and that follows the consumption of alcohol** may suggest HANGOVER. Other symptoms include upset stomach, thirst, fatigue and general malaise. Rest, relax, drink beverages containing caffeine and take aspirin.

• **Throbbing head pain that occurs after eating preserved meats** suggests HOT DOG HEADACHE, pain resulting from a sensitivity to nitrate or nitrite preservatives. These chemicals are present in preserved meats such as ham, bacon, bologna and salami as well as hot dogs.

JAW PAIN. Jaw pain accompanied by headache normally results from misaligned teeth or jaws. Yet because of stress, many people unconsciously keep their jaw muscles in a constant state of partial or complete contraction; this occasionally produces the pain of TENSION HEADACHE. To avoid such pain, relax jaw muscles by letting your jaw hang loosely.

• **Jaw pain upon awakening** may indicate BRUXISM, or grinding of the teeth during sleep. This grinding action can leave the jaw muscles tense and contracted, bringing on a tension headache. Consult a physician.

• **Jaw pain that occurs suddenly, often while chewing or yawning, and that is associated with a clicking or locking of the jaw joint** may indicate TEMPOROMANDIBULAR JOINT SYNDROME (TMJ), misalignment of the jaw joint. This condition is painful in itself, but it also can produce TENSION HEADACHE. Consult a dentist specializing in TMJ if such jaw pain is a frequent problem.

LANGUAGE DISTURBANCE. Slurred words, difficulty in expression or inability to understand what others are saying may be a symptom of dangerous harm to skull or brain, especially when these problems are accompanied by head pains.

If language disturbance occurs suddenly and is accompanied by either head pain, weakness or paralysis of one side of the body, the cause may be a STROKE, a complete blockage of blood flow to part of the brain. Get medical attention immediately.

If language disturbance and head pains occur suddenly, but without weakness or paralysis, a serious medical condition such as a BRAIN TUMOR, an abnormal growth in the brain, may exist. Consult a physician promptly.

If language disturbance occurs suddenly, lasts for 15 to 30 minutes and is then replaced by throbbing head pain, the cause may be CLASSIC MIGRAINE. Other symptoms include visual disturbances, nausea, vomiting, or tingling or numbness in the hands. Consult a physician.

If language disturbance and severe head pain are associated with drowsiness, dizziness, nausea or vomiting, the cause may be SUBARACHNOID HEMORRHAGE, bleeding around the brain, or INTRACRANIAL HEMORRHAGE, bleeding within the brain. Get medical attention immediately.

NAUSEA. When nausea and vomiting accompany head pains, they may indicate nothing more than influenza or an upset stomach, but they sometimes are symptoms of serious illness or dangerous harm to the head.

• **Nausea and vomiting that are accompanied by throbbing pain on one side of the head** may suggest either CLASSIC or COMMON MIGRAINE. Other symptoms of these disorders can include abdominal pain or excessive sensitivity to light and sound. Consult a physician.

• **Nausea and vomiting associated with severe generalized head pain and a stiff neck** may be evidence of MENINGITIS, an infection of the lining of the brain and spinal cord; or they may indicate SUBARACHNOID HEMORRHAGE, bleeding around the brain. Get medical attention immediately.

• **Nausea and vomiting associated with generalized head pain, behavior changes or drowsiness** may be symptoms of either EPIDURAL or SUBDURAL HEMATOMA, types of blood clots on the brain, or a BRAIN TUMOR, an abnormal growth in the brain. Get medical attention immediately.

If nausea, vomiting and head pain occur after a head injury, the cause may be CONCUSSION, a sudden temporary loss of consciousness following a blow to the head, or a SKULL FRACTURE, broken bones surrounding the brain. Other symptoms include behavior changes, drowsiness and dizziness. Consult a doctor at once.

NECK PAIN. Neck pain and stiffness frequently accompany or bring on TENSION HEADACHE (see HEAD PAIN). Such pain and stiffness often can be easily explained—they are caused by sleeping in an unusual position, for instance, or hunching over a desk for hours. In older people, neck stiffness can be a sign of OSTEOARTHRITIS, a degenerative disorder of the joints in the neck. For mild symptoms, rest, relax and take aspirin. Heat, massage and gentle stretching exercises can also help.

If severe neck pain and stiffness are associated with sudden, severe and unremitting head pain, the cause may be a SUBARACHNOID HEMORRHAGE, bleeding around the brain. Other symptoms can include vomiting, drowsiness, behavior changes, sweating or fever. Get medical attention immediately.

If severe neck stiffness is accompanied by head pain, fever, lethargy, nausea, vomiting or rash, the cause may be MENINGITIS, an infection of the lining of the brain and spinal cord. Get medical attention immediately.

If neck pain and stiffness occur after a neck injury such as that sustained in a rear-end automobile collision, the cause may be a CERVICAL STRAIN, also known as WHIPLASH—a stretching or tearing of the muscles that support the neck. A dull constant ache or tightness of the upper back, the neck or the entire head may accompany this type of injury. Other symptoms include dizziness, nausea or blurred vision. Consult a physician promptly.

RINGING IN THE EARS. Unusual hearing disturbances—ringing, roaring, buzzing, whistling, or hissing—sometimes accompany various kinds of head pain. The sounds, if mild and temporary, are nothing to worry about, vanishing with the disappearance of the head pain, but they can be signs of serious disease if they are severe or persistent, if they recur frequently in only one ear or if they appear seemingly without cause. Consult a physician.

If ringing in the ears is associated with dizziness, hearing loss or head pain, the cause may be ACOUSTIC NEUROMA, a tumor on the nerve to the ear. Consult a physician promptly.

• **Ringing in the ears can be a symptom of drug toxicity.**

If ringing in the ears is of recent onset, and if you regularly take large doses of aspirin, of the malaria medicine quinine or of the heart medicine quinidine, the ringing may indicate sensitivity to these drugs. Head pain may also be present. Consult a physician.

SEXUAL DISTURBANCES. Headaches before, during or after intercourse are common. Some of these headaches are of psychological origin, some have physical causes. In rare instances they can be a symptom of physical problems, for sexual activity places a heavy burden on the circulatory system.

If steady, aching, tight head pain develops gradually during sexual activity, it may indicate TENSION HEADACHE. To prevent recurrent episodes, try to relax completely before sexual activity; loosen tight neck and shoulder muscles with a gentle massage.

If a pounding or throbbing pain occurs suddenly just before or along with orgasm, it may indicate BENIGN ORGASMIC CEPHALGIA, a condition brought about by sudden dilation of blood vessels in the brain, caused by increased blood pressure and heart rate. Consult a physician immediately if pain persists or worsens.

If severe head pain occurs suddenly during sexual activity, and if the pain is persistent and unremitting and is accompanied by neck pain, vomiting or behavior changes, the cause may be a SUBARACHNOID HEMORRHAGE, bleeding around the brain. Get medical attention immediately.

• **Persistent or continuous head pain that frequently interferes with sexual relations** may be an indication of DEPRESSION. Consult a physician.

SINUS PAIN. Contrary to common belief, the sinuses are not a leading cause of pain in the head. Occasionally these pockets within the bones of the skull and face do become infected and painful, but most people who complain of sinus headache have nothing wrong with their sinuses and are really suffering from TENSION HEADACHE or MIGRAINE.

• **If sinus pain occurs after a common cold, influenza or nasal allergy**—suggesting SINUSITIS, an infected sinus—look for other symptoms indicating infection. They include fever and nasal discharge as well as tenderness and swelling over the nose, cheeks or forehead. Apply warm wet compresses to the face and take aspirin if symptoms are mild. Consult a physician if pain is severe or if fever persists.

• **Pain in the face, forehead, mouth, nose or throat that occurs when you swallow cold food or liquids** may indicate ICE CREAM HEADACHE, caused by excessive sensitivity to cold in the nerves in the back of the mouth and throat. Pain may travel from the face to the top of the head, throughout the head, or to the ears. To avoid it, eat cold foods in small portions, and allow them to warm slightly at the front of the mouth.

SLEEP DISTURBANCES. The worries that bring on many common headaches may also cause difficulty sleeping at night. However, some combinations of sleeplessness and head pain arise from less usual causes.

• **If you are frequently plagued by troubled sleep,** or if you wake up very early every morning, it may be a sign of DEPRESSION. Consult a physician.

• **Head pain that wakes you from a sound sleep** may suggest MIGRAINE, which is marked by throbbing pain on one side of the head, or CLUSTER HEADACHE, which is signaled by pain near the eye, redness and watering of the eye, nasal congestion and a flushed face. Consult a physician.

STUFFED-UP NOSE. Only rarely is nasal congestion associated with head pain.

• **Nasal congestion associated with pain, tenderness, or swelling over the forehead, cheeks or nose,** as well as with fever and a thick or blood-tinged nasal mucus, may be a sign of SINUSITIS, an infection of the sinuses. Take aspirin and apply warm wet compresses to the forehead and nose. Consult a physician if pain is severe or if fever persists.

• **Nasal congestion or runny nose that occurs suddenly on one side** and is associated with sudden, severe pain around one eye, with flushing of one side of the face and with a red and watering eye may indicate a CLUSTER HEADACHE. Consult a physician.

VISUAL CHANGES. Blurred, double or dimmed vision is a serious symptom, possibly indicating BRAIN INJURY, the potentially blinding pressure of GLAUCOMA, or the inflammation of TEMPORAL ARTERITIS. When vision changes are associated with head pain, however, they usually are caused by MIGRAINE.

If visual changes occur suddenly, last for only 15 to 30 minutes, and are followed by throbbing pain on one side of the head, the cause may be CLASSIC MIGRAINE. The changes most often include blind spots, zigzag lines, flashing lights or hallucinations of distorted figures or shapes. These migraine "auras" are generally experienced for 15 to 30 minutes before the pain of migraine arrives, but some people have the auras without suffering a headache afterward. Consult a physician.

VOMITING. *See NAUSEA.*

WEAKNESS. Generalized malaise very commonly accompanies the headaches of the common cold or influenza and is no cause for alarm, but persistent weakness or paralysis can indicate a variety of more serious illnesses.

• **Weakness or paralysis that occurs suddenly, with or without head pain, may indicate** a STROKE, a blockage of blood flow to part of the brain. Get medical attention immediately.

• **Weakness or paralysis that occurs suddenly, is accompanied by visual disturbances,** lasts 15 to 30 minutes and is followed by throbbing head pain on one side may indicate CLASSIC MIGRAINE.

Bibliography

BOOKS

Adams, Raymond D., and Maurice Victor, *Principles of Neurology*. McGraw-Hill, 1977.

Alexopoulos, Constantine John, *Introductory Mycology*. John Wiley & Sons, 1962.

AMA Drug Evaluations. American Medical Association, 1980.

Appenzeller, Otto, ed., *Pathogenesis and Treatment of Headache*. Spectrum, 1976.

Beeson, Paul B., et al., eds., *Cecil Textbook of Medicine*. W. B. Saunders, 1979.

Benson, Herbert, *The Relaxation Response*. Avon Books, 1975.

Berde, B., and H. O. Schild, eds., *Ergot Alkaloids and Related Compounds*. Springer-Verlag, 1978.

Berkow, Robert, ed., *The Merck Manual*. Merck Sharp & Dohme Research Laboratories, 1977.

Berland, Theodore, and Robert George Addison, *Living with Your Bad Back*. St. Martin's Press, 1972.

Bernstein, Douglas A., and Thomas D. Borkovec, *Progressive Relaxation Training: A Manual for the Helping Professions*. Research Press, 1973.

Bianchini, Francesco, and Francesco Corbetta, *Health Plants of the World: Atlas of Medicinal Plants*. Newsweek Books, 1977.

Bond, Michael R., *Pain: Its Nature, Analysis and Treatment*. Churchill Livingstone, 1979.

Bonica, John J., *The Management of Pain*. Lea & Febiger, 1953.

Bove, Frank James, *The Story of Ergot*. S. Karger, 1970.

Brena, Steven F., ed., *Chronic Pain: America's Hidden Epidemic*. Atheneum/SMI, 1978.

Bresler, David E., *Free Yourself from Pain*. Simon and Schuster, 1979.

Brown, Barbara B., *Stress and the Art of Biofeedback*. Bantam Books, 1977.

Bullock, Theodore Holmes, et al., *Introduction to Nervous Systems*. W. H. Freeman, 1977.

Curtis, Helena, *Biology*. Worth, 1979.

Dalessio, Donald J., ed., *Wolff's Headache and Other Head Pain*. Oxford University Press, 1980.

Davis, Audrey, and Toby Appel, *Bloodletting Instruments in the National Museum of History and Technology*. Smithsonian Institution Press, 1979.

de Sahagun, Bernardino, *Florentine Codex: General History of the Things of New Spain*. The School of American Research and the University of Utah, 1950-1970.

Diamond, Seymour, and William Barry Furlong, *More Than Two Aspirin: Hope for Your Headache Problem*. Avon Books, 1976.

Diamond, Seymour, and Donald J. Dalessio, *The Practicing Physician's Approach to Headache*. Williams & Wilkins, 1978.

Duke, Marc, *Acupuncture*. Pyramid Communications, 1972.

Freese, Arthur S., *Headaches: The Kinds and the Cures*. London: George Allen & Unwin Ltd., 1976.

Friedman, Arnold P. and Shervert H. Frazier, Jr., *The Headache Book*. Dodd, Mead, 1973.

Fuller, John G., *The Day of St. Anthony's Fire*. Macmillan, 1968.

Gelb, Harold, and Paula M. Siegel, *Killing Pain Without Prescription*. Harper & Row, 1980.

Gerald, Michael C., *Pharmacology: An Introduction to Drugs*. Prentice-Hall, 1974.

Gilman, Alfred G., et al., *Goodman and Gilman's: The Pharmacological Basis of Therapeutics*. Macmillan, 1980.

Gray, Henry, *Anatomy, Descriptive and Surgical*. Bounty Books, 1977.

Green, Elmer and Alyce, *Beyond Biofeedback*. Delacorte, 1977.

Guyton, Arthur C., *Textbook of Medical Physiology*. W. B. Saunders, 1981.

Hass, Frederick J., and Edward F. Dolan, Jr., *What You Can Do About Your Headaches*. Henry Regnery, 1973.

Hanington, Edda, *The Headache Book*. Technomic, 1980.

Huard, Pierre, and Ming Wong, *Chinese Medicine*. McGraw-Hill, 1968.

Inglis, Brian, *The Book of the Back*. Hearst Books, 1978.

Irwin, Yukiko, *Shiatzu: Japanese Finger Pressure for Energy, Sexual Vitality and Relief from Tension and Pain*. Lippincott, 1976.

Isselbacher, Kurt J., et al., eds., *Harrison's Principles of Internal Medicine*. McGraw-Hill, 1980.

Jacobson, Edmund, *You Must Relax*. McGraw-Hill, 1976.

Kamiya, Joe, *Biofeedback and Self-Control*. Aldine Atherton, 1971.

Karlins, Marvin, and Lewis M. Andrews, *Biofeedback: Turning on the Power of Your Mind*. Warner, 1972.

Kaufman, John E., ed., *IES Lighting Handbook*. Illuminating Engineering Society of North America, 1981.

Kingsbury, John M., *Poisonous Plants of the United States and Canada*. Prentice-Hall, 1964.

Kudrow, Lee, *Cluster Headache: Mechanisms and Management*. Oxford University Press, 1980.

Lagerwerff, Ellen B., and Karen A. Perlroth, *Mensendieck: Your Posture and Your Pains*. Anchor, 1973.

Lance, James W.:
Headache: Understanding, Alleviation. Charles Scribner's Sons, 1975.
Mechanism and Management of Headache. Butterworth, 1978.

Lankford, T. Randall, *Integrated Science for Health Students*. Reston, 1979.

Lennox, William Gordon, *Science and Seizures: New Light on Epilepsy and Migraine*. Harper & Brothers, 1946.

Levy, Charles Kingsley, *Biology: Human Perspectives*. Goodyear, 1979.

Leyel, C. F., ed., *Culpeper's English Physician & Complete Herbal*. Wilshire, 1972.

Linde, Shirley, *How to Beat a Bad Back*. Rawson, Wade, 1980.

Long, James W., *The Essential Guide to Prescription Drugs: What You Need to Know for Safe Drug Use*. Harper & Row, 1977.

Lyons, Albert S., and R. Joseph Petrucelli II, *Medicine: An Illustrated History*. Abrams, 1978.

MacKinney, Loren, *Medical Illustrations in Medieval Manuscripts*. University of California Press, 1965.

Madders, Jane, *Stress and Relaxation*. Arco, 1979.

Mann, Felix, *Acupuncture: The Ancient Chinese Art of Healing*. Vintage Books, 1972.

Masunaga, Shizuto, *Zen Shiatsu: How to Harmonize Yin and Yang for Better Health*. Japan Publications, 1977.

McQuade, Walter, and Ann Aikman, *Stress: What It Is, What It Can do to Your Health, How to Fight Back*. Bantam Books, 1975.

Melzack, Ronald, *The Puzzle of Pain*. Basic Books, 1973.

Miller, Sigmund S., ed., *Symptoms: The Complete Home Medical Encyclopedia*. Avon Books, 1978.

Mines, Samuel, *The Conquest of Pain*. Grosset & Dunlap, 1974.

Noback, Charles R., and Robert J. Demarest, *The Nervous System: Introduction and Review*. McGraw-Hill, 1972.

Ostfeld, Adrian M., *The Common Headache Syndromes: Biochemistry, Pathophysiology, Therapy*. Charles C. Thomas, 1962.

Parish, Peter, *The Doctors and Patients Handbook of Medicines and Drugs*. Knopf, 1980.

Physicians' Desk Reference. Litton Industries, 1981.

Raskin, Neil H., and Otto Appenzeller, *Headache, Volume XIX*. W. B. Saunders, 1980.

Ricciuti, Edward R., *The Devil's Garden: Facts and Folklore of Perilous Plants*. Walker, 1978.

Roe, Daphne A., *Alcohol and the Diet*. AVI, 1979.

Rose, F. Clifford, and M. Gawel, *Migraine: The Facts*. Oxford University Press, 1979.

Ryan, Robert E., Sr., and Robert E. Ryan, Jr., *Headache and Head Pain: Diagnosis and Treatment*. C. V. Mosby, 1978.

Saper, Joel R., and Kenneth R. Magee, *Freedom from Headaches: A Personal Guide for Understanding and Treating Headache, Face, and Neck Pain*. Simon and Schuster, 1978.

Schindler, Paul E., Jr., *Aspirin Therapy*. Walker, 1978.

Singer, Charles, *From Magic to Science: Essays on the Scientific Twilight*. Dover, 1958.

Soyka, Fred, *The Ion Effect: How Air Electricity Rules Your Life and Health*. Dutton, 1977.

Speer, Frederic A., *Migraine*. Nelson-Hall, 1977.

Starobinski, Jean, *A History of Medicine*. Hawthorn Books, 1964.

Stern, Robert M., and William J. Ray, *Biofeedback: Potential and Limits*. University of Nebraska Press, 1977.

Stollerman, Gene H., ed., *Advances in Internal Medicine*. Year Book Medical Publishers, Inc., 1979.

Sulman, Felix Gad, *Health, Weather and Climate*. S. Karger, 1976.

Thomson, William A. R., *A Change of Air: Climate and Health*. Charles Scribner's Sons, 1979.

United States Pharmacopeia Dispensing Information. United States Pharmacopeial Convention, 1981.

Vander, Arthur J., et al., *Human Physiology: The Mechanisms of Body Function*. McGraw-Hill, 1980.

Werner, Joan K., *Neuroscience: A Clinical Perspective*. W. B. Saunders, 1980.

PERIODICALS

Atkinson, Ruth A., and Otto Appenzeller, "Deer Woman." *Headache,* Vol. 17, No. 6, January 1978.

Behrens, Myles M., "Headaches and Head Pains Associated with Diseases of the Eye." *Research and Clinical Studies in Headache,* Vol. 4, 1976.

Damrau, Frederic, and Arthur H. Goldberg, "Adsorption of Whisky Congeners by Activated Charcoal: Chemical and Clinical Studies Related to Hangover." *Southwestern Medicine,* Vol. 52, No. 9, September 1971.

Damrau, Frederic, and Emma Laddy, "Hangovers and Whisky Congeners: Comparison of Whisky with Vodka." *Journal of the National Medical Association,* July 1960.

Diamond, Seymour, "Biofeedback and Headache." *Headache,* Vol. 19, No. 3, April 1979.

Ekbom, K., and T. Greitz, "Carotid Angiography in Cluster Headache." *Acta Radiologica Diagnosis,* 1970.

Every, R. G., "The Significance of Extreme Mandibular Movements." *The Lancet,* July 2, 1960.

Friedman, Arnold P.:
"Characteristics of Tension Headache: A Profile of 1,420 Cases." *Psychosomatics,* Vol. 20, No. 7, July 1979.
"The Headache in History, Literature, and Legend." *Bulletin of the New York Academy of Medicine,* Vol. 48, No. 4, May 1972.
"Muscle Contraction Headache." *American Family Physician,* November 1979.
"Nature of Headache." *Headache,* Vol. 19, No. 3, April 1979.

Gelb, Harold, "TMJ Syndrome: The Tell-Tale Click." *Behavioral Medicine,* March 1978.

Graham, John R., "Migraine Headache: Diagnosis and Management." *Headache,* Vol. 19, No. 3, April 1979.

Kellaway, Peter, "The Part Played by Electric Fish in the Early History of Bioelectricity and Electrotherapy." *Bulletin of the History of Medicine,* Vol. 20, No. 2, July 1946.

Kudrow, Lee, "Cluster Headache: Diagnosis and Management." *Headache,* Vol. 19, No. 3, April 1979.

Kuehl, Frederick A., Jr., and Robert W. Egan, "Prostaglandins, Arachidonic Acid, and Inflammation." *Science,* Vol. 210, November 28, 1980.

Martin, M. J., et al., "Muscle-Contraction Headache: A Psychiatric Review." *Research and Clinical Studies in Headache,* Vol. 1, 1967.

Martin, Maurice J.:
"Psychogenic Factors in Headache." *Medical Clinics of North America,* Vol. 62, No. 3, May 1978.
"Tension Headache, A Psychiatric Study." *Headache,* Vol. 6, May 1966.

"Migraine, Headache, and Related Conditions—Panel 7." *Archives of Neurology,* Vol. 36, November 16, 1979.

"A New Approach to Pain." *Emergency Medicine,* March 1974.

Okihiro, Michael M., et al., "Relaxation Skills Training—An Alternative in the Treatment of Headache." *Hawaii Medical Journal,* Vol. 39, No. 5, May 1980.

Pike, P. M. H., "Transcutaneous Electrical Stimulation: Its Use in the Management of Postoperative Pain." *Anaesthesia,* Vol. 33, 1978.

Ramwell, Peter W., "Biologic Importance of Arachidonic Acid." *Archives of Internal Medicine,* Vol. 141, February 23, 1981.

Rapoport, Alan, and Fred Sheftell, "Headaches." *Runner's World,* Vol. 15, No. 7, July 1980.

"A Script for Deep Muscle Relaxation." *Diseases of the Nervous System,* Vol. 38, 1977.

Smith, Stephen D., "Head Pain and Stress from Jaw-Joint Problems: Diagnosis and Treatment in Temporomandibular Orthopedics." *Osteopathic Medicine,* February 1980.

Snyder, Solomon H., "Opiate Receptors and Internal Opiates." *Scientific American,* March 1971.

Stone, P. T., "Light and the Eyes at Work." *The Ophthalmic Optician,* Vol. 20, No. 1, January 5, 1980.

Werner, David, "Healing in the Sierra Madre." *Natural History,* November 1970.

OTHER PUBLICATIONS

Runck, Bette, "Biofeedback—Issues in Treatment Assessment." U.S. Department of Health and Human Services, National Institutes of Mental Health, 1980.

Zimmermann, M., "Peripheral and Central Nervous Mechanisms of Nociception, Pain, and Pain Therapy: Facts and Hypotheses." From *Advances in Pain Research & Therapy,* Raven Press, 1979.

Acknowledgments

The index for this book was prepared by Barbara L. Klein. For their help in the preparation of this volume, the editors wish to thank the following: Dr. Otto Appenzeller, University of New Mexico School of Medicine, Albuquerque; Dr. Ruth Atkinson, University of New Mexico School of Medicine, Albuquerque; François Avril, Bibliothèque Nationale, Paris; Dr. Jeffery L. Barker, National Institute of Neurological and Communicative Disorders and Stroke, Bethesda, Md.; Michael R. Barnat, Michigan Headache and Neurological Institute, Ann Arbor; Dr. Steven Baskin, The New England Center for Headache, Cos Cob, Conn.; Bayer AG, Leverkusen; Loring Chapman, University of California School of Medicine, Davis; Dr. Donald J. Dalessio, Scripps Clinic and Research Foundation, La Jolla, Calif.; Janine Delerue, *France Soir,* Paris; Dr. Seymour Diamond, Diamond Headache Clinic, Chicago, Ill.; Dr. Karl Ekbom, Söder Hospital, Stockholm; Jane Elshami, National Capital Poison Center, Washington, D.C.; Dr. Albert Fanchamps, Sandoz Ltd., Basel; Gilberta N. Fouquet, Sandoz, Inc., East Hanover, N.J.; Dr. Arnold P. Friedman, Neurological Associates of Tucson, Tucson, Ariz.; Dr. Harold Gelb, University of Medicine and Dentistry of New Jersey, New York, N.Y.; Dr. Elmer Green, Menninger Foundation, Topeka, Kans.; Howard Haynes, Illuminating Engineering Society of North America, New York, N.Y.; Dr. Neill S. Hirst, Michigan Headache and Neurological Institute, Ann Arbor; Kent Kraft, University of Georgia, Athens; Dr. Lee Kudrow, California Medical Clinic for Headache, Encino; Alvin E. Lake, Michigan Headache and Neurological Institute, Ann Arbor; Grace Lewandowski, Michigan Headache and Neurological Institute, Ann Arbor; David Mech, North Central Forest Experiment Station, St. Paul, Minn.; E. Merck, Darmstadt; William Mino, Riker Laboratories, Inc., Northridge, Calif.; Derek R. Mullis, The Migraine Trust, London; Ronald P. Olmstead, Chelsea Community Hospital, Chelsea, Mich.; Dr. Gaston L. S. Pawan, Middlesex Hospital, London; Dr. Edward Perl, University of North Carolina School of Medicine, Chapel Hill; Dr. F. Clifford Rose, Princess Margaret Migraine Clinic, London; Lucille St. Hoyme, National Museum of Natural History, Washington, D.C.; Dr. Joel R. Saper, Michigan Headache and Neurological Institute, Ann Arbor; Federigo Sicuteri, University of Florence, Italy; Dr. Egilius Spierings, University Hospital, Rotterdam; Dr. Brendan C. Stack, National Capital Center for Craniofacial Pain, Vienna, Va.; Dr. William Sweet, Boston; Alice R. Tite, Chelsea Community Hospital, Chelsea, Mich.; Dr. Robert Toltzis, National Heart, Lung, and Blood Institute, Bethesda, Md.; Margie J. Van Meter, Michigan Headache and Neurological Institute, Ann Arbor; David Werner, Hesperian Foundation, Palo Alto, Calif.; Iwao Yoshizaki, Japan Publications, Inc., Tokyo.

Picture credits

The sources for the illustrations that appear in this book are listed below. Credits for the illustrations from left to right are separated by semicolons, from top to bottom by dashes.

Cover: Enrico Ferorelli. 7: Library of Congress. 9: Walter Hilmers Jr. from HJ Commercial Art. 11: David Werner (2); Nathan Benn from Woodfin Camp & Associates. 14: Lee Kudrow, M.D., California Medical Clinic for Headache. 17: G. Hausman from The Image Bank; Walter Hilmers Jr. from HJ Commercial Art. 18: Dan McCoy from Rainbow. 20: Lenare, London; Library of Congress—The Mansell Collection, London. 22: National Library of Medicine. 23: Photo Bulloz, courtesy Musée du Petit-Palais, Paris. 24: National Museum of Natural History, Washington, D.C., catalog no. 178473, and Provenience Huarochiri, Peru; Hamburgisches Museum für Völkerkunde, Hamburg. 25: Giraudon, courtesy Musée Condé, Chantilly; Jean-Loup Charmet, courtesy Musée de l'Histoire de la Médecine, Paris. 26: Yale University Library. 27: Guido Sansoni, courtesy Biblioteca Medicea Laurenziana, Florence. 28: Copied by Marcello Vivarelli, courtesy Biblioteca Casanatense, Rome—Yale University Library. 29: Austrian National Library, Vienna; Guido Sansoni, courtesy Biblioteca Medicea Laurenziana, Florence. 30, 31: Photo Bulloz, courtesy Musée des Beaux-Arts, Saint-Omer, France. 33: Ernst Haas. 35: Drawing by Trudy Nicholson. 36: Yale S. Palchick, D.D.S., F.A.G.D. 38, 39: John Dominis for *Life;* Udo Hirsch from Bruce Coleman Ltd., London—© Leonard Lee Rue III from Photo Researchers, Inc. 42, 43: Frederic F. Bigio from B-C Graphics. 44: Walter Hilmers Jr. from HJ Commercial Art. 47: Lane Stewart for *Sports Illustrated.* 50-59: Fil Hunter. 61: Richard Jeffery. 63: Adapted from a chart by G. L. S. Pawan, M.D., that appeared in *Nutrition and Food Science,* January 1976, Forbes Publications Ltd., London. 64-67: Fil Hunter. 69: Erik Leigh Simmons from The Image Bank. 71: Frederic F. Bigio from B-C Graphics. 75: © 1979 Peter Angelo Simon. 77: Jean-Loup Charmet, Paris. 81-83: Hildegard von Bingen, *Scivias,* Otto Müller Verlag, Salzburg. 84: Leslie Crespin. 86: © 1980 Dan McCoy from Rainbow. 88: Frederic F. Bigio from B-C Graphics. 92: *Acta Radiologica,* Stockholm, courtesy of Dr. Karl Ekbom and Professor Torgny Greitz. 94: Philadelphia Museum of Art: Wilstach Fund. 95: Courtesy of the New York Public Library, Astor, Lenox and Tilden Foundations. 96: *France-Soir,* Paris. 97: James Whitmore for *Life.* 98-101: Sandoz Ltd., Basel. 102, 103: Fil Hunter. 105: Jeffery L. Barker and Joseph H. Neale. 108: John Senzer. 110: Jean-Loup Charmet, Paris—Ciba-Geigy, Basel. 111: Excedrin/Reproduced with permission of the copyright owner, Bristol-Myers Company © 1979; E. Merck; Darmstadt. 112: Courtesy of the Archives, Hahnemann Medical College & Hospital of Philadelphia. 113: Top, Photographic Department, Wellcome Research Laboratories, Beckenham, Kent. 115, 118: © 1974 Lennart Nilsson from *Behold Man,* Little, Brown and Co. 119: Drawing by Trudy Nicholson. 120: Jeffery L. Barker and Donald Schmechel. 121: Drawing by Trudy Nicholson. 122: Micrograph produced by John Heuser, M.D., Washington University, St. Louis. 123: Drawing by Trudy Nicholson. 124: © 1974 Lennart Nilsson from *Behold Man,* Little, Brown and Co. 125: Drawing by Trudy Nicholson. 127: Dan McCoy from Rainbow. 134: Hartley Film Foundation, Inc. 136: Don Richards, The Menninger Foundation. 137: Library of Congress—Medtronic, Inc., Neuro Division. 138: Nathan Benn from Woodfin Camp & Associates. 139: Photo by Mark Sexton, Peabody Museum of Salem; © 1977 Brian Brake from Photo Researchers, Inc. 140, 141: Japan Publications, Inc. 142-157: John Senzer.

Index

Page numbers in italics indicate an illustration of the subject mentioned.